Oxford University Press

Oxford   New York
Athens   Auckland   Bangkok   Bombay
Calcutta   Cape Town   Dar es Salaam   Delhi
Florence   Hong Kong   Istanbul   Krachi
Kuala Lumpur   Madras   Madrid   Melbourne
Mexico City   Nairobi   Paris   Singapore
Taipei   Tokyo   Toronto

and associated companies in
Berlin   Ibadan

Library of Congress Cataloging-in-Publication Data
The public health consequences of disasters /
edited by Eric K. Noji.
p.   cm.   Includes bibliographical references and index.
ISBN 0-19-509570-7
1. Disaster medicine.   2. Public health.
I. Noji, Eric K.
[DNLM: 1. Environmental Health.
2. Disasters.   3. Epidemiologic Methods.
4. Disease Outbreaks.   5. Disaster Planning—methods.
WA   30   P977   1977]   RA645.5.P83   1977   362.1—dc20
DNLM/DLC   for Library of Congress   96-25497

9 8 7 6 5 4 3 2 1

Printed in the United States of America
on acid-free paper

Foreword

In the last half of the twentieth century there has been heightened recognition of the value of epidemiologic methods in defining and managing problems related to public health. For example, epidemiologic studies of both acute and chronic diseases have provided health professionals with critical data to use for prevention and control. Furthermore, decision-makers have increasingly acknowledged the importance of setting up surveillance systems to collect relevant health data that can be used as a scientific basis for action on public health problems.

During the last few decades, most epidemiologic studies have centered on the more common diseases and health conditions, which means that the treatments for these conditions have improved the most. On the other hand, the consequences to human health of unexpected natural and technological disasters have been relatively neglected. Reasons for such lack of attention include (1) the rarity, unpredictability, and suddenness of disaster occurrence; (2) the mind-set that nature's behavior and its aftermath cannot be controlled; (3) the emphasis during a crisis on providing curative medicine rather than on analyzing causes; (4) the difficulty in getting useful data on the health consequences of disasters during and soon after such catastrophes; and (5) the belief of many that public health methods of analyzing the causes and determinants of disease contribute little to the understanding of the consequences to human health of such disasters.

Although many, if not all, of these reasons may explain the relatively few health studies related to disasters in the past, these reasons may not pertain in the future. A body of information related to the adverse health effects of disasters is now accumulating, but it requires scientific analysis so we can apply the lessons learned during one disaster to the management of the next. This book provides the results of scientific analyses, and recommendations about how to apply lessons learned, and more. With years of on-site experience, the authors—mostly from the Centers for Disease Control and Prevention—give the reader ample technical descriptions of each kind of disaster, pertinent summaries of previous disasters, and copious data on what has been learned from past epidemiologic investigations of the public health consequences of disasters. In addition, always emphasizing the use of proven surveillance and epidemiologic methods, the contributors challenge the health professions with questions that must still be answered by future studies in the field during or shortly after a disaster.

Carefully planned epidemiologic studies address in advance the problems of selecting control subjects, determining adequate statistical power, recognizing possible biases, and the like. However, in the midst of real disasters and under immense pressure to prevent and control as much disease or death as possible, an epidemiologic field team may view these concerns as academic, out of reach, or even irrelevant. Consequently, as discussed in this book, ''quick and dirty'' investigations may have to be done at the expense of some of the robust and rigorous standards of a more leisurely epidemiologic study.

Yet collecting and analyzing relevant data by scientifically accepted methods is paramount and must be taken into consideration despite the need to respond under severe time pressure.

The Public Health Consequences of Disasters will serve as the essential desk reference not only for health professionals responsible for preparing for and responding to disasters, but for decision makers answerable to the public they serve.

Guilford, Vermont   *Michael B. Gregg*

Acknowledgments

First and foremost, I would like to thank my wife, Pam, who has endured virtual widowhood during the year of the editing process. Without her unyielding support, this book would not have been possible.

Acknowledgments to Michael B. Gregg, Jean French, Suzanne Binder, Lee M. Sanderson, and Elliott Churchill for their work on the CDC monograph *The Public Health Consequences of Disasters 1989*—a work that served as the basis and inspiration for this book.

I would also like to thank Stephen B. Thacker, Henry Falk, and Thomas Sinks of the National Center for Environmental Health for their support of this project and for their fostering of the growth of disaster epidemiology at this institution for the past several years.

Many thanks to Helen McClintock, Elizabeth Fortenberry, Dorothy Sussman, Kevin Moran, and Mariane Schaum of Publications Activities, National Center for Environmental Health, who helped in both the early stages of this endeavor and in the monumental task of editing the final manuscript.

Much appreciation to Elizabeth Cochran, Martha Hunter, Jane House, and Jessie Thompson of the Graphics Group, National Center for Environmental Health, for their help in preparing many of the figures for this book.

Finally, thanks and much appreciation to Jeffrey House of Oxford University Press, for his patience, constant support, and encouragement. He has shared our excitement and commitment to the idea behind this work.

E. K. N.

Table of Contents

II   Geophysical Events

III   Weather-Related Problems

IV   Human-Generated Problems

Contributors

Eric K. Noji, M.D., M.P.H.
Chief, Disaster Assessment & Epidemiology
  Section
National Center for Environmental Health
Centers for Disease Control & Prevention

Peter J. Baxter, M.D.
Consultant Occupational Physician
University of Cambridge Clinical School
Addenbrooke's Hospital
Cambridge, England

R. Elliott Churchill, M.A.
Special Projects Coordinator
Epidemiology Program Office
Centers for Disease Control & Prevention

Ruth A. Etzel, Ph.D., M.D.
Chief, Air Pollution & Respiratory Health
  Branch
National Center for Environmental Health
Centers for Disease Control & Prevention

Brian W. Flynn, Ed.D.
Chief, Emergency Services and Disaster
  Relief Branch
Center for Mental Health Services
Substance Abuse and Mental Health
  Services Administration

Jean G. French, Ph.D.
Adjunct Professor of Epidemiology
Department of Epidemiology
University of North Carolina School of
  Public Health

Ellen T. Gerrity, Ph.D.
Acting Chief
Violence and Traumatic Stress Research
  Branch
National Institute of Mental Health

Edwin M. Kilbourne, M.D.
Assistant Director
Epidemiology Program Office
Centers for Disease Control & Prevention

Scott R. Lillibridge, M.D.
Associate Director for International and
  Intergovernmental Affairs
National Center for Environmental Health
Centers for Disease Control & Prevention

Josephine Malilay, Ph.D.
Epidemiologist
Disaster Assessment & Epidemiology
  Section
National Center for Environmental Health
Centers for Disease Control & Prevention

Michael Sage, M.S.
Deputy Chief, Radiation Studies Branch
National Center for Environmental Health
Centers for Disease Control & Prevention

Lee M. Sanderson, Ph.D.
Senior Epidemiologist, Division of Health
  Assessment and Consultation
Agency for Toxic Substances & Disease
  Registry

Michael J. Toole, M.D., DTM&H
Head, International Health Unit
Macfarlane Burnet Centre for Medical
  Research
Melbourne, Australia

Scott F. Wetterhall, M.D., M.P.H.
Assistant Director for Science
Division of Surveillance & Epidemiology
Epidemiology Program Office
Centers for Disease Control & Prevention

Robert C. Whitcomb, Jr., M.S.
Physical Scientist
Environmental Dosimetry Section
Radiation Studies Branch
National Center for Environmental Health
Centers for Disease Control & Prevention

Ray Yip, M.D.
Chief, Maternal and Child Health Branch
Division of Nutrition
National Center for Chronic Disease
  Prevention & Health Promotion
Centers for Disease Control & Prevention

Introducti

My true love is out there somewhere and they can go fuck themselves.

www.someecards.com

With both disasters and the number of their victims increasing, disasters constitute a major public health problem. According to the International Federation of Red Cross and Red Crescent Societies in 1993, the number of people affected by disasters (killed, injured, or displaced) rose from 100 million in 1980 to 311 million in 1991. Sudden-impact natural disasters such as earthquakes may result in large numbers of injured persons, many of whom are handicapped for life. Health facilities can be destroyed, and national health care development efforts may be set back for years. Denser settlement patterns, established as a result of urban migration and population growth, mean that more people are exposed. The increasingly sophisticated and technical physical infrastructure of human culture is similarly more vulnerable to destruction than were the systems of habitation and culture built in past generations. The result is that today the damage from natural and technological disasters tends to be more and more extensive if proper precautions are not taken.

Because of the massive adverse impact of natural disasters on human settlements, the United Nations General Assembly has declared the 1990s the International Decade for Natural Disaster Reduction (IDNDR) and has called for a global scientific, technical, and political effort to reduce the impact of catastrophic acts of nature. The UN resolution is both an invitation and a challenge to the public health community to give special priority in the next few years to programs and projects that will help minimize the impact of natural disasters. The "Decade" represents a real opportunity to pull together the wealth of technical expertise and experience we have gained worldwide to institute effective and proven public health measures that will prevent much of the death, injury, and economic disruption caused by disasters.

The importance of disasters as a public health problem is now widely recognized. Many research centers have been established, among them collaborative centers under the sponsorship of the World Health Organization. Courses and workshops organized by the World Health Organization, by the Pan American Health Organization, and by academic institutions include basic disaster epidemiology and information systems for disasters.

The Centers for Disease Control and Prevention (CDC), based in Atlanta, Georgia, has major responsibilities to prepare for and respond to public health emergencies such as disasters, as well as to conduct investigations into the health effects and medical consequences of disasters. For the past quarter century, the CDC has had a rich and diversified history of responding to natural and technological disasters, both domestically and internationally. During the Nigerian Civil War in the late 1960s, 20 CDC Epidemic Intelligence Service (EIS) officers helped maintain public health programs for millions of displaced civilians who were deprived of their basic needs by that war. The EIS officers also assisted in the development of techniques for rapidly assessing people's nutritional status and for conducting surveys to identify populations in need of medical assistance. CDC has also attempted to adapt traditional epidemiologic techniques and public health programs to the realities of disaster situations, refugee camps, and scattered, famine-affected communities. A major aim of disaster research conducted by the CDC is to assess risk for death and injury and to develop strategies for preventing or mitigating the impact of future disasters. As a result, a considerable body of knowledge and experience has been accumulated by the CDC. This knowledge and that of other investigators has been compiled in this book for dissemination and for providing guidance on certain technical subjects for those involved in future disaster-relief programs. The goal is to make the public health response to disasters more efficient and effective, but that goal can be attained only if the approach is based on sensible, organized, well-conceived, and scientific principles. This approach can make prevention more effective, relief more relevant, and management more efficient at the local, national, and international levels. Ultimately, this will help save more lives.

Since the CDC Disaster Monograph was first published in 1989, a score or so of important disaster studies have added substantially to the body of knowledge on the public health consequences of disasters and have actually changed disaster relief practices (e.g., the Armenia earthquake, Hurricanes Hugo and Andrew, the Loma Prieta earthquake, the ''Great Midwest Flood of 1993,'' and the Kurdistan, Somalia, Bosnia, and Zaire refugee emergencies). Some historical review has been included in this book to orient the reader and provide a better perspective on the subject. We have attempted to address major issues covered in the earlier monograph as well as to summarize the most pertinent, recent, and useful advances in disaster epidemiology, information management, and hazards research.

More and more the global community is witnessing complex emergencies resulting from the breakdown of traditional state structures, armed conflict, and the upsurge of ethnicity and micronationalism (e.g., Bosnia, Somalia, Rwanda, Chechnya). The number of refugees affected by a combination of natural and man-made disasters has increased in the mid-1990s to an estimated 17 million, and the number of persons displaced through other causes, though difficult to estimate, is probably just as large. Not surprisingly, the causes of these emergencies as well as the assistance to the afflicted are influenced by intense levels of complex political, social, and economic considerations. Because of the profound public health impact of such situations, we have added a special chapter on complex emergencies, including population displacements and refugee situations.

In many chapters there is some overlap of material because of the nature of the topics. This repetition serves as a reminder that some disasters significantly affect our population in diverse yet similar and predictable ways. As UN Secretary General Boutros Boutros Ghali stated:

> There is no hard-and-fast division—in terms of their effects on civilian populations—between conflicts and wars, and natural disasters. Droughts, floods, earthquakes and cyclones are just as destructive for communities and settlements as wars and civil confrontation. Just as preventive diplomacy can foresee and prevent the outbreak of war, so the effects of natural disasters can be foreseen and contained.

The contents of this book are divided into several major sections: General Issues, Geophysical Events, Weather-Related Problems, and Human-Generated Problems. The first section, a kind of primer, describes

- the overall public health effects of disasters common to most catastrophic events
- practical applications of epidemiologic methods to disasters, including the role of the epidemiologist in disasters
- concepts and role of surveillance and epidemiology
- environmental health (e.g., water supply, solid and liquid waste disposal, basic shelter-related public health concerns)
- important considerations relating to communications efforts between health officials and the news media in times of disaster
- communicable disease control following natural disasters
- the emotional and mental health impact of disasters

The other chapters, which cover discrete types of natural and human-generated disasters, emphasize such areas as the history and nature of the disasters, as well as causative factors for the natural disaster that may influence morbidity and mortality. Each chapter then addresses the public health implications of such events, including (1) prevention and control measures, (2) critical knowledge gaps, (3) methodologic problems of epidemiologic studies, and (4) research recommendations in areas in which the public health practitioner needs more useful information. Most of the chapters follow this outline, but in some instances the format is slightly different because of the nature of the subject material. In all chapters, however, the underlying approach and the considerations taken by the authors emphasize the level of epidemiologic knowledge of each subject. Since epidemiology is the basic science of public health, and since public health directs its attention toward prevention and control of unnecessary morbidity and premature mortality, our intention has been to review what is known from an epidemiologic viewpoint and to emphasize that additional epidemiologic information is needed for a fuller comprehension of the particular problem. Woven into the content of most chapters are discussions of exposure-, disease-, or health-event surveillance, because no meaningful epidemiologic analyses or appropriate public health action can follow without reliable, objective data. It will be apparent to the reader that, with a few exceptions, epidemiologic methods have not been frequently or thoroughly applied to natural and human-generated disasters and that much more information and many more analyses are needed. Within each chapter, controversial areas are acknowledged and special considerations that may affect management are noted. A common theme in this book is that the effects of disasters on public health can be avoided or minimized through application of effective prevention strategies.

We hope that this book will aid public health professionals in the assessment and management of natural and technological disasters. By necessity, this book is unable to cover all aspects of emergency preparedness and response. The recommendations provided here will not be effective unless they are supported by adequate preparedness planning, coordination, communications, logistics, personnel management, and relief-worker training. Although there are several acceptable approaches to dealing with disasters, we have attempted to delineate an approach based on the latest accepted knowledge, technology, and methods found in the literature, taking into account the extensive emergency experience of the contributing authors, most of whom work at the Centers for Disease Control and Prevention in Atlanta, Georgia. From their work and that of other investigators over the past several years, we have gained greater insight and made advances that should further the important overall goal of minimizing the impact of natural and human-made catastrophes on human communities. I am indebted for each author's enthusiastic support of this work.

Atlanta, Ga
March 1996

E.K.N.

Recommended Readings

Centers for Disease Control. Health status of Kampuchean refugees—Sakaeo, Thailand. *MMWR* 1979;28:545–546.

Centers for Disease Control. Public health consequences of acute displacement of Iraqi citizens—March to May, 1991. *MMWR* 1991;40:443–446.

Foege W, Conrad RL. *IKOT IBRITAM Nutritional Project (Nigeria): Report to the International Committee of the Red Cross*, March, 1969.

French JG, Falk H, Caldwell GC. Examples of CDC's role in the health assessment of environmental disasters. *The Environmental Professional* 1982;4:11–14.

Glass RI, Nieburg P, Cates W, Davis C, *et al.* Rapid assessment of health status and preventive-medicine needs of newly arrived Kampuchean refugees, Sakaeo, Thailand. *Lancet* 1980; 868–872.

Gregg MB, editor. *The public health consequences of disasters*. Atlanta, Georgia: Centers for Disease Control, 1989.

International Federation of Red Cross and Red Crescent Societies. *World disasters report*. Dordrecht, the Netherlands: Martinus Nijhoff Publishers, 1993, 1–124.

Koplan JP, Falk H, Green G. Public health lessons from the Bhopal chemical disaster. *J Am Med Assoc* 1990;264:2795–2796.

Noji EK. Natural disasters. *Crit Care Clin* 1991;7:271–292.

Noji EK. Public health challenges in technological disaster situations. *Archives of Public Health* 1992;50:99–104.

Noji EK. The Centers for Disease Control: Disaster preparedness and response activities. *Disasters: The International Journal of Disaster Studies and Practice* 1992;16:175–177.

Noji EK. Progress in disaster management. *Lancet* 1994:343:1239–1240.

Parrish RG, Falk H, Melius JM. Industrial disasters: classification, investigation and prevention. *Recent Advances in Occupational Health* 1987;3:155–168.

Toole MJ, Waldman RJ. Nowhere a promised land: The plight of the world's refugees *Encyclop Br. Med Health* 1991; Annual:124–141.

Toole MJ, Galson S, Brady W. Are war and public health compatible? *Lancet* 1993;341:935–938.

Western K. *The epidemiology of natural and man-made disasters: The present state of the art* [dissertation]. London: University of London, 1972.

I

GENERAL ISSUES

1

The Nature of Disaster: General Characteristics and Public Health Effects

ERIC K. NOJI

Thou shalt be visited by the Lord of Hosts with Thunder, and with Earthquakes and Great Noise, with Storm and Tempest, and the Flame of Devouring Fire.

—Isaiah 29:6

Natural disasters such as earthquakes, tropical cyclones, floods, and volcanic eruptions have claimed approximately 3 million lives worldwide during the past 20 years, have adversely affected the lives of at least 800 million more people, and have caused more than $50 billion in property damage (1, 2) (Tables 1-1 and 1-2). Worldwide, a major disaster occurs almost daily, and natural disasters that require international assistance for affected populations occur weekly (3).

Unfortunately, the threats posed by disasters will likely be even worse in the future. Increasing population densities in floodplains, along vulnerable coastal areas, and near dangerous faults in the earth's crust; the development and transportation of thousands of toxic and hazardous materials; and rapid industrialization in developing countries all point to the probability of future catastrophic disasters with the potential for millions of casualties (4, 5) (Fig. 1-1). Indeed, our planet will experience many natural hazards during the next decade:

- 1 million thunderstorms
- 100, 000 floods
- tens of thousands of landslides, damaging earthquakes, wildfires, and tornadoes
- several hundred to several thousand tropical cyclones, and hurricanes, tsunamis, drought episodes, and volcanic eruptions

3

Table 1-1 Selected Natural Disasters of the Twentieth Century*

Year	Event	Location	Approximate Death Toll
1900	Hurricane	USA	6,000
1902	Volcanic eruption	Martinique	29,000
1902	Volcanic eruption	Guatemala	6,000
1906	Typhoon	Hong Kong	10,000
1906	Earthquake	Taiwan	6,000
1906	Earthquake/Fire	USA	1,500
1908	Earthquake	Italy	75,000
1911	Volcanic eruption	Philippines	1,300
1915	Earthquake	Italy	30,000
1916	Landslide	Italy, Austria	10,000
1919	Volcanic eruption	Indonesia	5,200
1920	Earthquake/Landslide	China	200,000
1923	Earthquake/Fire	Japan	143,000
1928	Hurricane/Flood	USA	2,000
1930	Volcanic eruption	Indonesia	1,400
1932	Earthquake	China	70,000
1933	Tsunami	Japan	3,000
1935	Earthquake	India	60,000
1938	Hurricane	USA	600
1939	Earthquake/Tsunami	Chile	30,000
1945	Floods/Landslides	Japan	1,200
1946	Tsunami	Japan	1,400
1948	Earthquake	USSR	100,000
1949	Floods	China	57,000
1949	Earthquake/Landslide	USSR	20,000
1951	Volcanic eruption	Papua, New Guinea	2,900
1953	Floods	North Sea coast	1,800
1954	Landslide	Austria	200
1954	Floods	China	40,000
1959	Typhoon	Japan	4,600
1960	Earthquake	Morocco	12,000
1961	Typhoon	Hong Kong	400
1962	Landslide	Peru	5,000
1962	Earthquake	Iran	12,000
1963	Tropical cyclone	Bangladesh	22,000
1963	Volcanic eruption	Indonesia	1,200
1963	Landslide	Italy	2,000
1965	Tropical cyclone	Bangladesh	17,000
1965	Tropical cyclone	Bangladesh	30,000

4

Table 1-1 (*Continued*)

Year	Event	Location	Approximate Death Toll
1965	Tropical cyclone	Bangladesh	10,000
1968	Earthquake	Iran	30,000
1970	Earthquake/Landslide	Peru	70,000
1970	Tropical cyclone	Bangladesh	500,000
1971	Tropical cyclone	India	30,000
1972	Earthquake	Nicaragua	6,000
1976	Earthquake	China	250,000
1976	Earthquake	Guatemala	24,000
1976	Earthquake	Italy	900
1977	Tropical cyclone	India	20,000
1978	Earthquake	Iran	25,000
1980	Earthquake	Italy	1,300
1982	Volcanic eruption	Mexico	1,700
1985	Tropical cyclone	Bangladesh	10,000
1985	Earthquake	Mexico	10,000
1985	Volcanic eruption	Columbia	22,000
1988	Hurricane Gilbert	Caribbean	343
1988	Earthquake	Armenia SSR	25,000
1989	Hurricane Hugo	Caribbean	56
1990	Earthquake	Iran	40,000
1990	Earthquake	Philippines	2,000
1991	Tropical cyclone	Philippines	6,000
1991	Volcanic eruption	Philippines	800
1992	Earthquake	Turkey	500
1992	Hurricane Andrew	United States	42
1992	Tsunami	Indonesia	2,000
1993	Earthquake	India	10,000
1995	Earthquake	Japan	5,400

*Disasters selected to represent global vulnerability to rapid-onset disasters.

Sources: Office of US Foreign Disaster Assistance. Disaster history: significant data on major disasters worldwide, 1900–present. Washington, D.C.: Agency for International Development, 1995. *(2)* National Geographic Society. Nature on the rampage: our violent earth. Washington, D.C.: National Geographic Society, 1987.

Every state and territory in the United States has communities that are at risk from one or more natural hazards: earthquakes, volcanic eruptions, severe storms (hurricanes and tornadoes), floods, landslides, wildfires, tsunamis, and drought *(6)*.

The disasters unfolding in the 1990s—in Somalia, the former Yugoslavia, Cambodia, Afghanistan, Rwanda, and in many republics of the former Soviet Union (e.g., Chechnya)—bear witness to the fact that today there are few simple cases of cause and

Table 1-2 The Ten Worst Natural Disasters Worldwide 1945–1990

Year	Location	Type of Disaster	Number of Deaths
1948	USSR	Earthquake	100,000
1949	China	Flood	57,000
1954	China	Flood	40,000
1965	Bangladesh	Cyclone	30,000
1968	Iran	Earthquake	30,000
1970	Peru	Earthquake	70,000
1970	Bangladesh	Cyclone	500,000
1971	India	Cyclone	30,000
1976	China	Earthquake	250,000
1990	Iran	Earthquake	40,000

Sources: Office of US Foreign Disaster Assistance. Disaster history: significant data on major disasters worldwide, 1900–present. Washington, D.C.: Agency for International Development, 1995. *(2)* National Geographic Society. Nature on the rampage: our violent earth. Washington, D.C.: National Geographic Society, 1987.

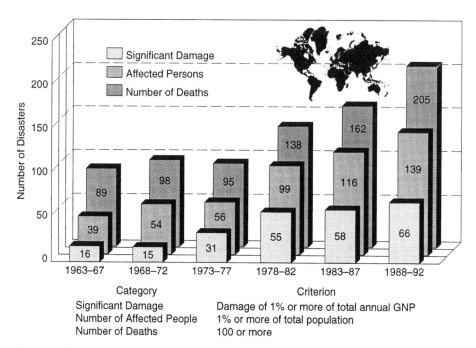

Figure 1-1. Major disasters around the world, 1963–1992. Significant disasters based on: damage, affected persons, deaths.

effect. The disasters of today involve economic dislocation; the collapse of political structures; violence ranging from banditry, through civil conflict, to all-out international war; famine; and mass population displacements. Chronic warfare rages in approximately 130 locations throughout the world. A range of factors, from conflict to rapid industrialization, means that disasters are also becoming more complex, to the point that entire countries or societies have become ''disaster sites'' *(7, 8)*.

Much of the destruction caused by natural disasters can be avoided. For almost every natural disaster in the 1990s, ''an ounce of prevention'' or preparedness would have made a real difference. In many cases building codes were ignored, communities were located in dangerous areas, warnings were not issued or followed, or plans were forgotten. We now know much about the cause and nature of disasters and about populations at risk, and that knowledge allows us to anticipate some of the effects a disaster may have on the health of an affected community *(9)*. Understanding the way that people are killed and injured in disasters is a prerequisite for preventing or reducing deaths and injuries during future disasters.

Definition of Disaster

There are many definitions of disasters. From the standpoint of health care providers, a disaster should be defined on the basis of its consequences on health and health services. A pragmatic definition follows:

> A disaster is the result of a vast ecological breakdown in the relation between humans and their environment, a serious and sudden event (or slow, as in a drought) on such a scale that the stricken community needs extraordinary efforts to cope with it, often with outside help or international aid *(10, 11)*.

From a public health perspective, disasters are defined by what they do to people; otherwise, disasters are simply interesting geological or meteorological phenomena. What might constitute a disaster for one community might not necessarily be considered a disaster in a different community.

Disasters can be further divided into two broad categories—those caused by natural forces and those that are caused by people or generated by humans *(12)* (Table 1-3). Natural disasters arise from the forces of nature, such as earthquakes, volcanic eruptions, hurricanes, floods, fire, tornadoes, and extremes of temperature. Disasters or emergency situations caused by people (human-generated) are those in which the principal direct causes are identifiable human actions, deliberate or otherwise. Disasters generated by humans can be divided further into three broad categories: (1) complex emergencies; (2) technological disasters; and (3) disasters such as transportation disasters, material shortages resulting from energy embargoes, and dam breaks that are not caused by natural hazards but that occur in human settlements. Complex emergencies usually

Table 1-3 Classification of Disasters

I. Natural disasters

    A. Sudden impact or acute onset (e.g., geological and climatic hazards such as earthquakes, tsunamis, tornadoes, floods, tropical storms, hurricanes, cyclones, typhoons, volcanic eruptions, landslides, avalanches, wildfires). This category also includes epidemics of water-, food-, or vector-borne diseases and person-to-person transmission of diseases.

    B. Slow or chronic-onset (e.g., drought, famine, environmental degradation, chronic exposure to toxic substances, desertification, deforestation, pest infestation [e.g., locusts])

II. Disasters generated by people (human-generated)

    A. Industrial/technological (e.g., system failures/accidents, chemical/radiation, spillages, pollution, explosions, fires, terrorism)

    B. Transportation (vehicular)

    C. Deforestation

    D. Material shortages

    E. Complex emergencies (e.g., wars and civil strife, armed aggression, insurgency, and other actions resulting in displaced persons and refugees)

involve situations in which civilian populations suffer casualties and loss of property, basic services, and a means of livelihood as a result of war, civil strife, or other political conflict. In many cases, people are forced to flee their homes temporarily or permanently; others become refugees in other countries. Technological disasters are those in which large numbers of people, property, infrastructure, or economic activity are directly and adversely affected by major industrial accidents, severe pollution incidents, unplanned nuclear releases, major fires, or explosions from hazardous substances such as fuel, chemicals, explosives, or nuclear materials. The distinction between natural disasters and those caused by people may be blurred, for a natural disaster or phenomenon may trigger secondary disasters—such as fires after an earthquake, hazardous air-pollution conditions resulting from a temperature inversion, or release of toxic materials into the environment in the aftermath of floods—that are associated with the vulnerability of the human environment. Such combination, or synergistic, disasters have become known as "NA-TECHS." An example of a NA-TECH disaster occurred in the former Soviet Union when windstorms spread radioactive materials across the country, increasing by 30% to 50% the land area contaminated in an earlier nuclear disaster.

    Natural disasters and those generated by people can be divided into acute- or sudden-impact events, such as earthquakes and tropical cyclones, and those events of slow or chronic genesis (the so-called "creeping" disasters), such as droughts leading to famine and gradually developing environmental catastrophes that result from chronic exposure of the community to harmful chemicals or to radiation in local industry or toxic disposal sites (Table 1-3).

Table 1-4 Crude Disaster Mortality by Type of Disaster, 1960–1969, 1970–1979, and 1980–1989:

Disaster Type	Deaths		
	1960–69	1970–79	1980–89
Floods	28,700	46,800	38,598
Cyclones	107,500	343,600	14,482
Earthquakes	52,500	389,700	53,740
Hurricane			1,263
Other disasters			1,011,777
Total			1,119,860

Source: Office of US Foreign Disaster Assistance. *Disaster history: significant data on major disasters worldwide, 1900–present.* Washington, D.C.: Agency for International Development, 1995. *(2)*

Global Magnitude of Disaster Impact

From 1980 through 1990, floods were the most frequent type of natural disaster statistically, accounting for more than one-third of all disasters occurring in that decade *(2)*. Windstorms (e.g., hurricanes and tornadoes) were the next most frequent disaster (one quarter of the total number), whereas earthquakes caused the greatest numbers of deaths and monetary loss *(13)* (Tables 1-4 and 1-5). From 1965 to 1992, more than 90% of

Table 1-5 Ten Major Types of Disasters Ranked by the Number of Lives Lost Worldwide during the Period 1947–1980

Type of Disaster	Number of Deaths
Tropical cyclones, hurricanes, typhoons	499,000
Earthquakes	450,000
Floods (other than those associated with hurricanes)	194,000
Thunderstorms and tornadoes	29,000
Snowstorms	10,000
Volcanoes	9,000
Heatwaves	7,000
Avalanches	5,000
Landslides	5,000
Tidal waves (tsunamis)	5,000

Source: Shah BV. Is the environment becoming more hazardous? Global survey 1947–1980. *Disasters* 1983;7:202–209. *(18)*

Table 1-6 Top Ten Countries by Number of Disasters (1966–1990)

Industrialized Countries		Developing Countries	
Countries	Number	Countries	Number
Hong Kong	220	Philippines	272
Australia	154	India	216
USA	114	China	157
New Zealand	89	Indonesia	139
Japan	80	Bangladesh	100
Soviet Union	67	Peru	73
Italy	51	Iran	64
Canada	38	Mexico	62
France	37	Vietnam	41
Greece	37	Turkey	41
Total	887	Total	1165

Source: Disaster ranking over 25 years from CRED disaster events database. *CRED Bulletin.* Brussels: Centre for Research on the Epidemiology of Disasters (CRED), 1993.

Table 1-7 Top Twenty Countries by Number of Deaths and Number of People Affected (1966–1990)

Countries	Total No. of Deaths (in thousands)	Countries	Total No. of Affected (in millions)
Ethiopia	611.8	India	1551.8
Bangladesh	365.5	China	298.6
China	292.8	Bangladesh	214.0
Pakistan	214.2	Brazil	51.3
Mozambique	212.2	Ethiopia	49.7
Sudan	152.4	Philippines	36.1
Iran	106.5	Vietnam	28.8
Peru	91.4	Mozambique	25.3
India	87.0	Sudan	15.1
Philippines	26.8	Pakistan	14.6
Soviet Union	26.0	Sri Lanka	14.5
Colombia	24.6	Peru	12.5
Guatemala	24.2	Argentina	11.2
Indonesia	24.1	Thailand	8.5
Somalia	22.2	Indonesia	8.2
Turkey	20.3	Niger	7.8
Nigeria	13.6	Senegal	7.3
Mexico	12.1	Mauritania	7.0
Honduras	11.2	Burkina Faso	6.9
Nicaragua	10.4	Korea	6.6
Total	2349.3	Total	2375.8

Source: Office of US Foreign Disaster Assistance. *Disaster history: significant data on major disasters worldwide, 1900–present.* Washington, D.C.: Agency for International Development, 1995. *(2)*

Table 1-8 Natural Disasters in the United States by Type of Disaster, 1945–1989

Type	Number of Disasters	Number of Deaths	Deaths per Disaster
Storms	58	3,968	68
Tornadoes	39	3,033	78
Hurricanes	15	3,075	205
Other weather	24	3,745	156
Geological	6	551	92
All Other	3	164	55
Total	145	14,536	100

Source: Glickman TS, Silverman ED. *Acts of God and acts of man. Discussion Paper CRM 92-02.* Washington D.C.: Center for Risk Management, Resources for the Future, 1992: 1–65. *(15)*

all natural-disaster victims lived in Asia and Africa *(14)*. The following is a rough ratio for major natural-disaster occurrences per year: Asia, 15; Latin America and Africa, 10; North America, Europe, and Australia, 1. Whether disasters in a region are measured by economic loss or by numbers of deaths and injuries, data show that Asia is the most natural-disaster-prone part of the world; Latin America and Africa are the second most prone; and North America, Europe, and Australia are the least prone *(14)* (Tables 1-6 and 1-7). In the United States, for example, 145 natural disasters caused 14, 536 deaths in the years between 1945 and 1989 *(15)* (Tables 1-8 and 1-9).

Factors Contributing to Disaster Occurrence and Severity

Natural hazards such as earthquakes, hurricanes, floods, droughts, and volcanic eruptions usually spring to mind when the word "disaster" is mentioned. Yet these events are in fact only natural agents that transform a vulnerable human condition into a disaster. The hazards themselves are not disasters but rather are factors in causing a

Table 1-9 Natural Disasters in the United States by Time Period 1945–1959, 1960–1974, and 1975–1989

	Number of Events	Number of Deaths	Deaths per Event	Deaths per Year
1945–1959	47	4,452	95	297
1960–1974	49	4,634	95	309
1975–1989	49	5,450	111	363
Total	145	14,536	100	323

Source: Glickman TS, Silverman ED. *Acts of God and acts of man. Discussion Paper CRM 92-02.* Washington D.C.: Center for Risk Management, Resources for the Future, 1992:1–65. *(15)*

disaster. Particularly in developing countries, these major factors contribute to disaster occurrence and severity:

- human vulnerability resulting from poverty and social inequality
- environmental degradation resulting from poor land use
- rapid population growth, especially among the poor

Anderson estimated that 95% of the deaths that are the result of natural disasters occur among 66% of the world's population that lives in the poorest countries *(16)*. For example, more than 3,000 deaths per disaster occur in low-income countries compared with the average of 500 deaths per disaster that occur in high-income countries. The poor are probably most at risk because they (1) are least able to afford housing that can withstand seismic activity; (2) often live along coasts where hurricanes, storm surges, or earthquake-generated tidal waves strike or live in floodplains subject to inundation; (3) are forced by economic circumstances to live in substandard housing built on unstable slopes that are susceptible to landslides or are built next to hazardous industrial sites; and (4) are not educated as to the appropriate lifesaving behaviors or actions that they can take when a disaster occurs *(17)*.

The underlying natural causes of disaster have not changed, but the human impact of disasters has increased as the world's population has grown *(18)*. In 1920, about 100 million people lived in cities in the developing world. By 1980, this number had increased by a factor of ten to about a billion people. At current trends, by the year 2000, the number of urban dwellers in developing countries will have almost doubled again—to 1.9 billion, a number equal to the total of all people who lived on earth in 1920. By the year 2000, 20 cities in the world will have populations greater than 10 million people; a significant number of these cities are located in areas that are at extremely high risk for natural disasters *(16)*. These cities include Mexico City, São Paolo, Calcutta, Greater Bombay, Shanghai, Rio de Janeiro, Delhi, Buenos Aires, Cairo, Jakarta, Baghdad, Tehran, Karachi, Istanbul, Dacca, Manila, Beijing, and Bangkok. In addition, industrial and technological development near these cities has introduced new types of hazards that have created catastrophes like those in 1984 in Bhopal and in 1986 at Chernobyl.

Clearly, industrialized countries are buffered from disasters by their ability to (1) forecast severe storms, (2) enforce strict codes for aseismic and fireproof construction, (3) use communication networks to broadcast disaster warnings and alerts, (4) provide emergency medical services, and (5) engage in contingency planning to prepare the population and public institutions for possible disasters. The low mortality associated with recent disasters in the United States, such as Hurricanes Hugo (1989) and Andrew (1992) and earthquakes in San Francisco (1989) and Los Angeles (1994), attest to the success of such measures *(19)*. In many developing countries, such measures either are not available or have not been implemented, and the populations remain increasingly vulnerable to the adverse health consequences from natural disasters. Effective measures and technology for natural-disaster reduction exist now, and one of the goals of the International Decade for Natural Disaster Reduction is to make them available to all countries.

Phases of a Disaster (The Disaster Cycle)

Sudden-impact disasters can be viewed as a continuous time sequence of five different phases: interdisaster, predisaster, impact, emergency, and rehabilitation *(20)*. For each phase, new knowledge exists about how to design appropriate prevention measures for different types of natural disasters *(21)*. These phases may last from just a few seconds to months or years, with one phase merging into the next *(22)*.

The Nondisaster or Interdisaster Phase

Long before a disaster strikes, officials should have in place disaster-prevention and -preparedness measures and should conduct disaster training and education programs for the community *(23)*. Several activities essential for appropriate emergency management should be undertaken, including mapping the specific locations of potential disasters and pinpointing potential associated risks; conducting a vulnerability analysis; taking inventory of existing resources for coping with a potential disaster in order to facilitate the rapid mobilization of all available resources during the emergency; planning the implementation of appropriate preventive, preparedness, and mitigation measures; and conducting education and training of health personnel and the community.

The Predisaster or Warning Phase

Before a disaster strikes, officials should issue timely warnings, take protective actions, and possibly evacuate the population. The effectiveness of protective actions will depend largely on the level of preparedness of the population, particularly at the community level. During this phase, several essential emergency-management activities should be undertaken, including issuing early warnings on the basis of predictions of the impending disaster and implementing protective measures (on the basis of the community's preparedness and contingency plans).

The Impact Phase

When disaster strikes, destruction, injuries, and death occur. The disaster may last a few seconds, as is the case with earthquakes, or for days or weeks, as is the case with floods or drought. The impact of a disaster on human health varies widely according to different factors, such as the nature of the disaster itself (e.g., the suddenness of onset and degree of warning given), population density, predisaster health and nutritional status, climate, and the organization of health services.

The Emergency Phase (also called the Relief or Isolation Phase)

The emergency phase starts immediately after impact and is the time for providing relief and assistance to the victims. This phase requires actions that are necessary to save lives, including search-and-rescue operations; first aid; emergency medical assistance; restoration of emergency communications and transportation networks; public health surveillance; and in some cases, evacuation from areas still vulnerable to the hazard (e.g., evacuating people from damaged buildings at risk from earthquake aftershocks or from low-lying areas that are at risk for further riverine flooding) *(24)*. In the immediate postimpact period, the local community is isolated (isolation period), and many of the most pressing rescue tasks are accomplished by the survivors themselves, by using locally available resources. The existence of district- and community-preparedness plans greatly increases the self-reliance and effectiveness of assistance, contributing to the reduction of disaster-related mortality and morbidity.

The Reconstruction or Rehabilitation Phase

As the emergency or relief phase ends, restoration of predisaster conditions begins. The reconstruction phase, which should lead to the restoration of predisaster conditions, includes reestablishing normal health services and assessing, repairing, and reconstructing damaged facilities and buildings. This phase is also the time for thinking about the lessons learned from the recent disaster that could assist in improving current emergency-preparedness plans. This phase actually represents the beginning of a new interdisaster phase. The time span for reconstruction or recovery is often difficult to define. It may start fairly early, even during the emergency period, and may last for many years.

General Public Health Effects of Disasters

Disasters affect a community in numerous ways. Roads, telephone lines, and other transportation and communication links are often destroyed. Public utilities (e.g., water supply and sewage-disposal services) and energy supplies (e.g., gas and electricity) may be disrupted. Substantial numbers of victims may be rendered homeless. Portions of the community's industrial or economic base may be destroyed or damaged *(25)*. Casualties may require medical care, and damage to food sources and utilities may create significant public health threats *(26)*.

Disasters may be considered a public health problem for many reasons:

- They may cause an unexpected number of deaths, injuries, or illnesses in the affected community, exceeding the therapeutic capacities of the local health services and requiring external assistance.

- Disasters may destroy local health infrastructures such as hospitals, which will therefore not be able to respond to the emergency. Disasters might also disrupt the provision of routine health services and preventive activities, leading to long-term health consequences in terms of increased morbidity and mortality.
- Some disasters may have adverse effects on the environment and the population, increasing the potential risk for communicable diseases and environmental hazards that will increase morbidity, premature death, and diminished quality of life in the future (27).
- Disasters may affect the psychological and social behavior of the stricken community (28). Generalized panic, paralyzing trauma, or antisocial behavior rarely occurs after major disasters, and survivors rapidly recover from their initial shock. However, anxiety, neuroses, and depression may occur after either sudden- or slow-onset emergencies.
- Some disasters may cause a shortage of food with severe nutritional consequences, such as starvation or specific micronutrient deficiencies—vitamin A deficiency, for example (see Chapter 15, ''Famine'').
- Disasters may cause large, spontaneous or organized population movements, often to areas where health services cannot cope with the new situation, thus leading to an increase in morbidity and mortality (see Chapter 20, ''Complex Emergencies''). Displacing large populations may also increase the risk for outbreaks of communicable diseases both in the displaced and host communities, where large populations of displaced persons may be crowded together and share unsanitary conditions or contaminated water. A review of the disaster epidemiology literature that describes numerous disasters indicates that such epidemics are uncommon after natural disasters (see Chapter 5, ''Communicable Diseases and Disease Control'').

Specific medical and health problems tend to occur at different times after a disaster's impact (29). Thus, severe injuries requiring immediate trauma care occur mainly at the time and place of impact, whereas the risks for increased disease transmission take longer to develop, with the greatest danger occurring in those areas where crowding and poor sanitation exist (30). Effective medical and public health response depends on anticipating these different medical and health problems as they arise and delivering the appropriate interventions at the precise times and places where they are needed most (31).

After a disaster, the pattern of health care needs will change—rapidly in sudden-impact natural disasters, more gradually in famine or refugee situations—from casualty and acute patient care management toward provision of primary health services (e.g., maternal and pediatric health care, services to people with chronic diseases). Priorities will also shift after the emergency phase from health care to such environmental health concerns as supplying water, disposing of excreta and solid waste, ensuring food safety, providing shelter, attending to personal hygiene needs and vector control, treating injuries that occur as a result of cleanup activities, and conducting public health surveillance *(32)*. Mental health interventions and rehabilitation planning are frequently required as well.

The long-term impact of disasters expresses itself in various ways. For example, a community's economic infrastructure may be so badly damaged by a disaster that the community's ability to provide health services could be impaired for years to come (e.g., in some countries, disasters have depleted the entire annual budget for infrastructure development, including that for health care) *(33)*. Under such conditions, one catastrophic disaster can make sustainable development virtually impossible *(34)*. In flooding disasters, saltwater contamination of subsistence and marginal land may result in the loss of not just one, but the next several years' worth of harvests. For nutritionally and economically fragile populations, the loss of one or more harvest seasons may result in a rise in mortality as a secondary effect of the disaster. Consequently, more people may die from the long-term impact than died from the disaster's initial impact.

On a more individual level, disaster-induced death and disability of the primary wage earner of a family can mean a lifetime's loss of revenue and possible destitution for the surviving members of the family for many years. These effects are most pronounced in developing countries, where government-sponsored social security is either nonexistent or less developed than in industrialized countries. Similarly, the deaths of a herdsman's breeding stock or the loss of capital or tools of trade due to water damage, cyclones, or earthquakes can effectively destroy the means of livelihood for families.

Clearly, considerable research needs to be done in order to evaluate accurately the complete health impact of a disaster on the health of populations *(28, 35)*. More accurate epidemiologic knowledge than currently exists about the causes of death and the types of injuries and illnesses caused by disasters is essential to determine appropriate relief supplies, equipment, and personnel needed to respond effectively. Results of surveys have shown that each kind of disaster has its own common epidemiologic profile and pathological characteristics, and these similarities and differences are crucial in planning, in designing and implementing prevention activities, and in executing disaster medical-aid programs *(36, 37)* (Table 1-10). Therefore, since each type of disaster is characterized by different morbidity and mortality patterns and thus has different health care requirements *(3, 38)*, emergency responders must become experts in handling the type of disaster most prevalent in their own communities. For example, hospitals along the Gulf Coast of the United States should plan for hurricanes, whereas those in California should plan for earthquakes *(38–40)*.

Disasters are accompanied by a variety of health problems related to the effects of the disaster on the environment. Although occasional exceptions have been reported, outbreaks of communicable diseases have generally been absent after modern disasters (see Chapter 5, "Communicable Diseases and Disease Control After Disasters"). In our society, growing numbers of older people depend on medical equipment and daily medications for treating cardiovascular, respiratory, or metabolic conditions. A major management problem during the immediate disaster response is interruption of medical

Table 1-10 Short-term Effects of Major Natural Disasters

Effect	Earthquakes	High Winds (without flooding)	Tsunamis/Flash Flood	Floods
Deaths	Many	Few	Many	Few
Severe injuries requiring extensive care	Overwhelming	Moderate	Few	Few
Increased risk for communicable diseases	Potential (but small) risk after all major disasters (probability rises as overcrowding increases and sanitation deteriorates)			
Food scarcity	Rare (may occur because of factors other than food shortage)	Rare	Common	Common
Major population movements	Rare (may occur in heavily damaged urban areas)	Rare	Common	Common

Source: Table adapted from *Emergency health management after natural disaster.* Office of Emergency Preparedness and Disaster Relief Coordination: Scientific Publication No. 407. Washington, D.C., Pan American Health Organization, 1981. *(36)*

care to such chronically ill residents. The physical stress of a disaster also appears to aggravate chronic conditions, and increases in cardiovascular morbidity and mortality have been reported after numerous disasters, notably earthquakes.

Myths and Realities of Disasters

The Pan American Health Organization has identified many myths and erroneous beliefs that are widely associated with the public health impact of disasters; all disaster planners and managers should be familiar with them *(41)*. These include the following:

Myth #1:   Foreign medical volunteers with any kind of medical background are needed.

Reality: The local population almost always covers immediate lifesaving needs. Only medical personnel with skills that are not available in the affected country may be needed.

Myth #2:   Any kind of international assistance is needed, and it is needed now!

Reality: A hasty response that is not based on an impartial evaluation only contributes to the chaos. It is better to wait until genuine needs have been assessed. As a matter of fact, most needs are met by the victims themselves and their local government and agencies, not by foreign intervenors.

Myth #3:   Epidemics and plagues are inevitable after every disaster.
Reality: Epidemics do not spontaneously occur after a disaster, and dead bodies
             will not lead to catastrophic outbreaks of exotic diseases. The key to
             preventing disease is to improve sanitary conditions and educate the
             public.

Myth #4:   Disasters bring out the worst in human behavior (e.g., looting, rioting).
Reality: Although isolated cases of antisocial behavior exist, most people re-
             spond spontaneously and generously.

Myth #5:   The affected population is too shocked and helpless to take responsi-
             bility for its own survival.
Reality: On the contrary, many people find new strength during an emergency,
             as evidenced by the thousands of volunteers who spontaneously united
             to sift through the rubble in search of victims after the 1985 Mexico
             City earthquake.

Myth #6:   Disasters are random killers.
Reality: Disasters strike hardest at the most vulnerable group—the poor, and
             especially women, children, and the elderly.

Myth #7:   Locating disaster victims in temporary settlements is the best alternative.
Reality: It should be the last alternative. Many agencies use funds normally spent
             for tents to purchase building materials, tools, and other construction-
             related support in the affected country.

Myth #8:   Food aid is always required for natural disasters.
Reality: Natural disasters only rarely cause loss of crops. Therefore, victims do
             not require massive food aid.

Myth #9:   Clothing is always needed by the victims of a disaster.
Reality: Used clothing is almost never needed; it is almost always culturally
             inappropriate, and though accepted by disaster victims, it is almost never
             worn.

Myth #10:   Things are back to normal within a few weeks.
Reality: The effects of a disaster last a long time. Disaster-affected countries
             deplete much of their financial and material resources in the immediate
             postimpact phase. Successful relief programs gear their operations to
             the fact that international interest wanes as needs and shortages become
             more pressing.

Summary

Sound epidemiologic knowledge of the morbidity and mortality caused by disasters is
essential when determining what relief supplies, equipment, and personnel are needed

to respond effectively in emergency situations. All disasters are unique because each affected region of the world has different social, economic, and baseline health conditions. Some similarities exist, however, among the health effects of different types of disasters; recognition of these effects can ensure that the limited health and medical resources of the affected community are well managed.

References

1. Advisory Committee on the International Decade for Natural Hazard Reduction. Confronting natural disasters: an International Decade for Natural Hazard Reduction. Washington, D.C.: National Academy Press, 1987.
2. Office of US Foreign Disaster Assistance. *Disaster history: significant data on major disasters worldwide, 1900–present*. Washington, D.C.: Agency for International Development, 1995.
3. Binder S, Sanderson LM. The role of the epidemiologist in natural disasters. *Ann Emerg Med* 1987;16:1081–84.
4. Hagman G. *Prevention better than cure*. Stockholm: Swedish Red Cross, 1984.
5. Wijkman A, Timberlake L. *Natural disasters: acts of God or acts of man*. New York: Earthscan, 1984.
6. Hays WW. Perspectives on the International Decade for Natural Disaster Reduction. *Earthquake Spectra* 1990;6:125–145.
7. Waeckerle JF, Lillibridge SR, Burkle FM, Noji EK. Disaster medicine: challenges for today. *Ann Emerg Med* 1994;23:715–718
8. International Federation of Red Cross and Red Crescent Societies. *World disasters report*. Dordrecht, the Netherlands: Martinus Nijhoff Publishers, 1993.
9. Sanderson LM. Toxicologic disasters: natural and technologic. In: Sullivan JB, Krieger GR, editors. *Hazardous materials toxicology: clinical principles of environmental health*. Baltimore, MD: Williams & Wilkins, 1992:326–331.
10. Gunn SWA. *Multilingual dictionary of disaster medicine and international relief*. Dordrecht, The Netherlands: Kluwer Academic Publishers, 1990.
11. Lechat MF. Disasters: a public health problem. *Workshop on health aspects of disaster preparedness. 1984 Oct 15–20; Trieste*. Brussels: Centre for Research on the Epidemiology of Disasters, 1984.
12. Rutherford WH, de Boer J. The definition and classification of disasters. *Injury* 1983;15:10–12.
13. Berz G. Research and statistics on natural disasters in insurance and reinsurance companies. *The Geneva Papers on Risk and Insurance* 1984;9:135–157.
14. IDNDR Promotion Office. *Natural disasters in the world: statistical trends on natural disasters*. Tokyo: National Land Agency, 1994.
15. Glickman TS, Silverman ED. *Acts of God and acts of man. Discussion Paper CRM 92–02*. Washington D.C.: Center for Risk Management, Resources for the Future, 1992.
16. Anderson MB. Which costs more: prevention or recovery? In: Kreimer A, Munasinghe M, editors. *Managing natural disasters and the environment*. Washington, D.C.: World Bank, 1991.
17. Guha-Sapir D, Lechat MF. Reducing the impact of natural disasters: why aren't we better prepared? *Health Policy and Planning* 1986;1:118–126.

18. Shah BV. Is the environment becoming more hazardous: a global survey, 1947–1980. *Disasters* 1983;7:202–209.
19. Lechat MF. Updates: the epidemiology of health effects of disasters. *Epidemiol Rev* 1990; 12:192–197.
20. Lechat MF. Disasters and public health. *Bull World Health Organ* 1979;57:11–17.
21. Noji EK, Sivertson KT. Injury prevention in natural disasters: a theoretical framework. *Disasters* 1987;11:290–296.
22. Cuny FC. Introduction to disaster management. Lesson 5: technologies of disaster management. *Prehospital and Disaster Medicine* 1993;6:372–374.
23. United Nations Disaster Relief Organization (UNDRO). *Disaster prevention and mitigation: preparedness aspects*, vol 11. New York: UNDRO, 1984.
24. Burkle FM, Sanner PH, Wolcott BW, editors. *Disaster medicine*. New York: Medical Examination Publishing Co., 1984.
25. UNDP/UNDRO Disaster Management Training Programme. *An overview of disaster management*, 2nd ed. New York: UNDP/UNDRO, 1992.
26. Baskett P, Weller R. *Medicine for disasters*. London: Wright, 1988.
27. de Ville de Goyet C, Lechat MF. Health aspects of natural disasters. *Trop Doct* 1976;6:152–157.
28. Logue JN, Melick ME, Hansen H. Research issues and directions in the epidemiology of health effects of disasters. *Epidemiol Rev* 1981;3:140–162.
29. World Health Organization: Emergency care in natural disasters. Views of an international seminar. *WHO Chronicles* 1980;34:96–100.
30. Sidell VW, Onel E, Geiger JH, Leaning J, Foege WH. Public health responses to natural and man-made disasters. In: Last J, Wallace R, editors. *Maxcy-Rosenau-Last. Public health and preventive medicine*, 13th ed. Norwalk, CT: Appleton and Lange; 1992:1173–1185.
31. UNA-USA Policy Studies Panel on International Disaster Relief: Acts of nature, acts of man. *The global response to natural disasters*. New York: UNA-USA, 1977.
32. Pan American Health Organization (PAHO). *Health services organization in the event of disaster*. Washington, D.C.: PAHO, 1983.
33. Cuny FC. *Disasters and development*. Oxford: Oxford University Press, 1983.
34. US National Committee for the Decade for Natural Disaster Reduction: *Facing the challenge. The US national report to the IDNDR World Conference on Natural Disaster Reduction*. Washington, D.C.: National Academy Press, 1994.
35. Seaman J. *Epidemiology of natural disasters: contributions to epidemiology and biostatistics*. Basel, Switzerland: Karger, 1984.
36. Pan American Health Organization (PAHO): *Emergency health management after natural disaster*. Scientific Publication No. 407. Washington, D.C.: PAHO Office of Emergency Preparedness and Disaster Relief Coordination, 1981.
37. Noji EK. Natural disasters. *Crit Care Clin* 1991;7:271–292.
38. Guha-Sapir D, Lechat MF. Information systems and needs assessment in natural disasters: an approach for better disaster relief management. *Disasters* 1986;10:232–237.
39. Contzen H. Preparations in hospital for the treatment of mass casualties. *Journal of the World Association for Emergency and Disaster Medicine* 1985;1:118–119.
40. Katz LB, Pascarelli EF. Planning and developing a community hospital disaster program. *Emergency Medical Services* 1978;Sept./Oct.:70.
41. de Ville de Goyet C. *The role of WHO in disaster management: relief, rehabilitation, and reconstruction*. Geneva: World Health Organization, 1991.

2

The Use of Epidemiologic Methods in Disasters

ERIC K. NOJI

Epidemiology, as classically defined, is the quantitative study of the distribution and determinants of health-related events in human populations *(1)*. It is less concerned with events affecting a single individual than it is with the patterns of events in populations. The fundamental axiom of epidemiology is that adverse health outcomes do not occur randomly within a population but rather occur in somewhat predictable patterns. Such patterns may be manifested as clusters of disease, injuries, or other health outcomes in time, space, or certain groups of people.

Similarly, epidemiologic methods can be used to measure and describe the adverse health effects of natural and human-caused disasters and the factors that contribute to those effects; the overall objective of such epidemiologic investigations is to assess the needs of disaster-affected populations, match available resources to needs, prevent further adverse health effects, evaluate program effectiveness, and permit better contingency planning *(2, 3)*. By identifying risk factors for specific outcomes such as death and injury, epidemiologists can help develop effective strategies to prevent future disaster-related morbidity and mortality. Epidemiologic data can, for example, be used in designing appropriate warning and evacuation systems, in developing guidelines for preparedness training, and in increasing public awareness through targeted education *(4)*. In addition, epidemiologists play an important role in providing informed advice about the probable future health effects of a disaster, in establishing priorities for action by public health authorities, and in emphasizing the need for valid and timely data collection and analysis as the basis of immediate decision-making *(5)*.

Epidemiologic studies of disasters can include the following: surveillance; evaluations of the public health impact of a disaster; evaluations of the natural history of the disaster's acute health effects; analytic studies of risk factors for adverse health effects; clinical investigations of the efficacy and effectiveness of particular approaches to diagnosis and treatment; population-based studies of long-term health effects; studies of the psychosocial impact of a disaster; and evaluations of the effectiveness of various types of assistance and the long-term effects of disaster-relief aid on restoring public health to predisaster conditions (6, 7).

Historical Development of Disaster Epidemiology

Over the past 20 years, the epidemiology of disasters has emerged as an area of special interest. The uses of epidemiology in disaster situations have been reviewed in a number of reports, and periodic updates on the "state of the art" have appeared every few years (7–11).

In 1957, in one of the earliest reviews on the role of epidemiology during natural disasters, Saylor and Gordon considered disasters as epidemics and suggested using well-defined epidemiologic parameters such as time, place, and person to describe disasters (12). However, the practical application of epidemiology to disaster management really began with the massive international relief operations mounted during the civil war in Nigeria in the late 1960s. Epidemiologists from the Center for Disease Control (CDC) helped to develop techniques for the rapid assessment of nutritional status and to conduct surveys to identify the population in need. Epidemiologists developed survey tools (such as the quakstick) and survey methods with which to rapidly assess the nutritional status of large displaced populations so that relief could be targeted to those groups in greatest need (7). Subsequently, surveillance was critical in monitoring how the nutritional status of the population was affected by the quantity and type of foods delivered. Rapid epidemiologic assessment proved invaluable in evaluating food-distribution practices in the face of rapidly changing conditions of health and relief (13). Since then, nutritional surveillance has become a routine part of relief work in famine areas and in refugee populations and is essential in determining problems of food distribution (14, 15) (see Chapter 15, "Famine").

During the 1970s, the need for disaster epidemiology was apparent in many disaster-relief operations (16, 17). Disaster managers and planners with no public health expertise and no reliable information on the health of the population affected by disasters were forced to direct major relief efforts. In the absence of an adequate field assessment, their response was often dictated by the relief and medical assistance made available by donors or was based on stereotyped forms of assistance assumed to be appropriate by donor agencies. As a result, disaster scenes were often cluttered by unnecessary, outdated, or unlabeled drugs, vaccines for cholera and typhoid fever that were not needed or effectively used, medical and surgical teams without proper support, and relief programs that did not address immediate local needs *(18)*. Disasters also often prompt an altruistic urge among health professionals, not all of whom are qualified to work in disaster situations. For example, no fewer than 30, 000 physicians and nurses from the United States, Europe, Latin America, and Asia volunteered to work with Cambodian refugees in 1979–80. However, many of these people lacked the special skills and experience required, and the task of screening for the proper personnel was often difficult. These problems of coordinating a disaster response are compounded by the conditions generally created by a disaster, including difficult logistics, a lack of communication, transportation, and local supplies and support. Since these relief operations were often conducted under the watchful eye of the media, medical-relief efforts were often pejoratively called "the second disaster" *(11)*. Ironically, although many governments and volunteer agencies have developed extensive disaster-response capabilities, the underuse and lack of coordination of disaster assessment has contributed to a pervasive cycle of inappropriate, and often ineffective, disaster relief *(19)*.

Experts realized that the effects of disasters on the health of populations were, in theory, amenable to study by epidemiologic methods and that certain common patterns of morbidity and mortality following certain disasters could be identified *(7)*. In the early 1970s, the Centre for Research on the Epidemiology of Disasters was established at the Catholic University of Louvain in Belgium. For the first time, specialized emergency units were established by the World Health Organization and the Pan American Health Organization. Important epidemiologic studies conducted following the 1976 earthquake in Guatemala pinpointed important logistical deficiencies in the international disaster-relief system and identified important risk factors for death and injury from earthquakes; the findings of these studies suggested potentially effective prevention strategies *(20, 21)*. The 1980 eruption of Mount St. Helens in the United States served as a major milestone in shaping the way the federal government responds to disasters, particularly in its coordination of the responses of dozens of different federal and state agencies to a national emergency *(22)*.

Drought in the African Sahel, floods in Bangladesh, and earthquakes in Mexico City and Armenia may not have much in common, but in the investigation of all three, the epidemiologic approach has proved powerful *(23, 24)*. Results of epidemiologic research on disasters have formed the scientific basis for increasingly effective prevention and intervention strategies to decrease mortality in several disaster situations *(5)*. For example, epidemiologic studies of tornadoes have resulted in changes in local housing laws designed to reduce the danger of living in mobile homes and have led to government guidelines describing what people can do to reduce their risk of serious injury or death *(25)*. Many studies have been done on the causes of food shortages and the effects of these shortages on populations in the developing world; and techniques of surveillance and assessment developed during the crises in the West African Sahel, Ethiopia, Bangladesh, and Uganda have become a routine part of relief work in famine areas and among refugee populations. Results of epidemiologic investigations of a wide spectrum of adverse medical and health consequences of disasters have allowed us to target specific interventions to prevent specific disaster-related health effects (e.g., improved warning and evacuation before flash floods and tropical cyclones *[26]*, the identification of effective safety actions that building occupants should take during earthquakes *[27]*, the development of measures to avoid cleanup injuries following hurricanes *[28, 29]*, and effective measles vaccination efforts, which have reduced the frequency and magnitude of measles outbreaks in refugee camps in Africa and Asia *[30]*), to measure the effectiveness of disaster-prevention and -preparedness programs, and to help local communities develop better emergency-preparedness and -mitigation programs.

During the late 1980s and early 1990s, interest in the epidemiology of disasters clearly accelerated *(31)*. New professional societies and scientific forums for the presentation of original work in this field appeared. Several university research centers now concentrate on the health and medical effects of disasters, including collaborating centers under the sponsorship of the World Health Organization *(32)*. Some of these institutions also have developed curricula that include basic disaster epidemiology and information systems for disasters *(33)*. With natural, technological, and complex disasters becoming an increasing threat to the health of people in both industrialized and developing countries, schools of public health need to offer more training opportunities in the public health consequences of disasters *(34, 35)*.

As relief agencies have come to accept the role of epidemiology in disaster responses, their reliance on the crisis-management approach has lessened, and rates of disaster-related morbidity and mortality have fallen *(36)*. Various efforts have been made to develop rapid and valid epidemiologic assessment techniques *(37, 38)*. Guha-Sapir and Lechat, for example, have developed useful needs-assessment indicators for use following natural disasters (''quick and dirty'' surveys). These have highlighted simplicity, speed of use, and operational feasibility *(39, 40)*. An organized approach to data collection in disaster situations also helps disaster managers make crucial decisions and predict the variety of options that they will face during the different phases of a disaster *(41)*.

Application of Epidemiologic Methods to Disasters

In recent years, epidemiologic techniques have been demonstrated to be of value before, during, and after disasters.

Before a Disaster

The greatest potential for preventing the adverse effects of natural disasters exists during the preimpact phase *(42)*. There are clear parallels between the concept of preventive medicine and that of disaster mitigation, which is defined as actions taken to reduce the effects of a disaster before it occurs. Thus, during the preimpact phase, disaster epidemiology involves delineating at-risk populations (vulnerability analysis), assessing the level of emergency preparedness and the flexibility of the existing surveillance systems, educating defined populations at risk, and training health and safety personnel *(43)*.

As mentioned above, epidemiologic methods can be used in community hazards analyses and in vulnerability analyses *(44)*. Hazards analysis involves collecting and assessing data on the nature, causes, frequency, distribution, and effects of past events in order to make predictions about future events. Health personnel should use the results of a hazard analysis to plan for those disasters most likely to occur in their community. For example, hospitals along the Gulf Coast of the United States should plan for hurricanes, while those in California should plan for earthquakes. It is very important to have knowledge of those disasters most prevalent in one's community, because different disasters are characterized by very different morbidity and mortality patterns and thus health care requirements. For example, earthquakes cause many immediate deaths and severe injuries, whereas hurricanes cause much property damage but relatively few deaths and usually only minor injuries.

Vulnerability analysis is the analysis of a population's risk when a hazard of a given magnitude occurs. Determining community vulnerability is often difficult because of the lack of good baseline data. Information necessary to complete a vulnerability analysis includes the density and geographical distribution of the population, the location of lifeline systems and structures with high occupancy (such as hospitals, schools, and factories), and the proximity of people and these structures to the potential dangers identified in the hazard analysis (e.g., faults, floodplains, industrial plants, and airports). Unfortunately, such information may not exist or be readily available. Hazard and vulnerability studies both require a careful examination of past disasters.

The results of hazard and vulnerability analyses can be combined to model or simulate natural and technological disasters. This is accomplished by projecting how a given type of disaster of particular intensity will affect a human population that has been characterized by a particular vulnerability to that event. For example, in the case of earthquakes, researchers have been able to establish probabilistic relationships between the level of shaking, the type of construction, and the severity of medical and public health impacts to be anticipated *(45)*. Such predicted health impacts of different types of disasters can then be used as the basis for many disaster-planning, -mitigation, and -preparedness activities. For example, these predictions can be used in developing more realistic drills and simulations and in designing appropriate warning, evacuation, and sheltering protocols.

During a Disaster

The critical component of any disaster response is the early conduct of a proper damage assessment to identify urgent needs and to determine relief priorities for an affected population *(46)*. Disaster assessment provides relief managers objective information about the effects of the disaster on a population, generated on the basis of rapidly conducted field investigations. These assessments are used to match available resources to a population's emergency needs and will maximize the efficacy with which finite medical resources are allocated. The early completion of this task and the subsequent mobilization of resources to address urgent medical and environmental needs can significantly reduce the adverse public health consequences of a disaster.

The techniques used to collect information (primarily sample and systematic surveys and simple reporting systems) are methodologically straightforward, and if suitable personnel and transportation are available, they should provide reasonably accurate and rapid estimates of the relief needs of disaster-affected populations (see Chapter 3, "Surveillance and Epidemiology"). Information from such rapidly undertaken epidemiologic investigations may be invaluable for the medical management of victims.

Public health surveillance is defined as the ongoing, systematic collection, analysis, and interpretation of data on specific health events for use in the planning, implementation, and evaluation of public health programs (47). A now well-established application of epidemiology is the surveillance and control of communicable diseases and other health hazards after disasters (48–54). Surveillance provides accurate and timely information that can be used by emergency managers, health care providers, emergency workers, and the public at large (see Chapter 3, "Surveillance and Epidemiology").

The success of an epidemic investigation after a disaster can be measured directly by how rapidly data collected and analyzed can be used to identify appropriate prevention strategies and how effectively decision-makers implement these strategies to direct relief and reduce ongoing morbidity (55). A successful investigation thus requires active coordination between the epidemiologist, who gathers data and identifies issues or strategies, and the decision-maker, who must understand the data and strategies presented by the epidemiologist and implement the required policies. During the time immediately following a disaster when no information is available about the medical needs of the population, the epidemiologist also has an important role to play in providing informed advice about the probable health effects that may arise, in establishing priorities for action, and in emphasizing the need for accurate information as the basis for relief decisions. As the value of basing relief decisions on reliable epidemiologic information becomes more widely recognized, epidemiology will become one of the most important components of relief operations.

After a Disaster

Generally, epidemiologic studies of natural disasters, including studies of the preimpact and impact phases, are conducted during the postimpact phase. Valuable information gathered during the hours, days, months, and years following a disaster can lead to policies and practices that reduce the risk of loss of death (56). For example, Glass has emphasized the need for such postdisaster epidemiologic follow-up studies to identify risk factors for death and injury that can then serve as the basis for planning strategies to prevent or reduce impact-related morbidity and mortality in future disasters (57).

Specific interventions (e.g., aseismic housing codes; early warning, preparation, and evacuation procedures; and lifesaving actions) can then be suggested to mitigate the negative consequences of disasters for high-risk populations (e.g., the aged, people living alone, mobile-home dwellers, and people dependent on life-support systems).

Subsequent evaluation of the effectiveness of these prevention measures can then lead to the development of actions that are even more effective in preventing morbidity and mortality directly attributable to disasters. For example, calculations of death rates can be used to evaluate the effectiveness of prevention measures aimed at mitigating the effects of disasters, such as assessing the adequacy of warning and evacuation in an area hit by flash floods or determining the safety of different types of building construction in an area where a strong earthquake has occurred.

Epidemiologists have employed a great variety of data-collection methods and strategies to study the postdisaster health effects of major disasters involving acute events such as earthquakes and tropical cyclones. Primarily using descriptive epidemiology, they have collected large amounts of epidemiologic data through case studies of new and previous disasters (16, 20). Examples of some of the few analytic epidemiologic studies conducted include studies of risk factors for morbidity and mortality in Guatemala (21), Italy (58), Armenia (27), the Philippines (59), and Puerto Rico (60). Such analytic studies have usually been of a case-control design. For example, why did some people die while their neighbors, family members, or others survive? Isolated case studies of the relationship between death or injuries and the type of traditional housing structures have provided clear indications regarding simple measures to be implemented in order to reduce human losses. Such analyses following disasters have yielded new information that has altered traditional thinking about the prevention of disaster-related mortality. More analytic studies such as these are needed to test conventional warnings and public safety advisories.

Practical, applied, operational research can also be useful in planning medical and public health responses to future disasters as well as in providing information useful for individual patient care. Ideally, the results of such retrospective epidemiologic studies would be used in formulating predictive indices that would allow emergency managers to assess the public health impact of a subsequent disaster from a few essential elements (indicators) and thus develop an appropriate relief response. For example, attack rates for various types of illnesses or conditions in survivors could be calculated, and the indices derived from these calculations could be used in determining what kinds of supplies, equipment, and personnel are most urgently needed.

During the postimpact phase, information is also needed on the complicated process of long-term rehabilitation and health services reconstruction (61). After a disaster, epidemiologic methods can be used to evaluate the effectiveness of health-intervention programs (62). Such evaluations in which what actually happened is compared with what was intended should be an integral part of the entire relief operation. In assessing disaster management, the evaluator would be looking at the ''actual'' results versus the ''intended'' results on two levels—the overall outcome of disaster-management efforts and the impact of each discrete category of relief efforts (e.g., provision of food and shelter, delivery of medical care, management of communications) *(63)*. For example, studies of the role and effectiveness of outside medical and rescue volunteers following disasters should help settle the controversy regarding their usefulness and provide public health authorities and emergency managers with guidelines and criteria for constructively using such volunteers. Unfortunately, there are no quantifiable measures of volunteer effectiveness and no agreed-upon methodology for evaluating the assistance that is provided by external sources.

Thus, epidemiologic studies are essential to understanding the consequences of disasters for the health of the population concerned. They are a prerequisite for the effective management and organization of disaster-relief operations. By evaluating the effectiveness of relief plans, epidemiologists can identify problems and suggest ways of improving those plans. Furthermore, by identifying risk factors for adverse public health outcomes, epidemiologic studies provide public health officials and others the data necessary to develop strategies to mitigate the harmful effects of disasters *(43)*.

Challenges and Problems Facing Epidemiologists Following a Disaster

Epidemiologists face numerous complex problems in disaster situations. These include problems related to the political environment and problems caused by rapidly changing social conditions and demographics. To solve these problems, epidemiologists must be innovative and able to adapt to new situations *(4)*. Reasonably objective data must be collected rapidly under highly adverse environmental conditions during the immediate emergency period. Critical information on the immediate effects of disasters on people (e.g., locations of where people are trapped, details about the victim-extrication process used, and the quality of on-site medical care); the extent of damage to buildings, personal property, and community ''lifelines'' (e.g., public utilities such as water and electricity); economic activities; and natural resources must be gathered within the first few hours to days because evidence is rapidly lost during rescue, cleanup, and recovery. Such data, which has been described by experienced disaster researchers as ''perishable,'' is usually irretrievably lost unless collected early.

Epidemiologists have great difficulty in applying well-known or standardized epidemiologic techniques in the context of great destruction, public fear, communal disruption, and the breakdown of the usual infrastructure for collecting and assembling data. The lack of time in which to organize an epidemiologic investigation, the reluctance of relief workers to keep records, the movement of populations from and within disaster areas, and many other factors work against accurate and complete observation; as a result, much valuable data has been lost. Furthermore, disaster-affected countries or regions may lack the people with epidemiologic expertise, the trained support staff, and the data-handling and communications equipment necessary to conduct rapid assessment surveys.

Most disaster epidemiologists have used cross-sectional survey methods to study the frequency of deaths, illnesses, injuries, and other adverse health effects of a disaster. Prevalence data resulting from such studies have been useful in estimating the strength of association, based on odds ratios, between particular disaster exposures and health outcomes. However, in the absence of well-defined population counts, the case-control design is the best method with which to identify risk factors, eliminate confounding, and study the interaction of multiple factors *(64)*. However, a faulty and indiscriminate use of this method may lead to wrong inferences and decisions that may be critical for the victims of disasters. Therefore, those implementing a case-control study in a disaster situation need to address several potential problems. First, they need to define clearly the outcomes of interest. In the vast majority of disasters, injuries are the most immediate outcome of concern. These need to be quantified and qualitatively defined. The quantification of injuries may lead to a study in which there are different levels of ''caseness.'' Although the existence of exposure may be easily determined in a disaster, the details of the exposure circumstances are essential for analysis. Although all case subjects and potential control subjects are by definition exposed (qualitatively) to the disaster, the differences between the two groups in circumstances and amount of exposure also need to be studied. The issues related to the selection of control subjects also need to be assessed clearly. In addition to establishing the internal validity of the observations, epidemiologists need to be concerned with the external validity of their findings (i.e., the degree to which their findings are generalizable to the entire affected population). Thus, control subjects have to be representative of the community under study. The case-control method could also be used in a sequential manner within the framework of the surveillance of long-term health problems of disaster victims.

Despite the importance of case-control studies, longitudinal studies are needed for documenting of incidence and thus for estimating the magnitude of risk. Observations of health effects in cohorts defined by type and level of exposure would also facilitate an assessment of dose-response relationships, of changing risks, and of the proportion of risk attributable to the disaster experience. Practically, however, such cohort and longitudinal studies are difficult to initiate and conduct in populations affected by disasters, because investigators often have trouble assembling the personnel, equipment, and supplies necessary to conduct sophisticated follow-up of affected individuals and appropriate nonexposed groups. Furthermore, epidemiologists must retrospectively identify the cohorts early in the postdisaster period in order not to miss medium-term effects of the exposure. Disasters in many developing countries occur in settings where following people long term is inherently difficult because of such problems as no census information, rapid changes in the population of disaster-affected areas, no universal health or social security coverage, few systems for tracking people who leave, no forwarding addresses from post offices, and many people with the same last name. In the absence of a continuous follow-up system, epidemiologists may generate longitudinal information based on periodic cross-sectional assessments of the same population over time as attempted by Lima *et al. (65)*. Despite the difficulty of conducting longitudinal studies, several disaster cohort studies of populations exposed to human-generated disasters (e.g., Hiroshima, Bhopal, Seveso) are currently in progress *(66, 67)*.

In disasters, the work of epidemiologists and government decision-makers must be coordinated. It is virtually impossible for epidemiologists to be successful in a postdisaster setting if they operate on their own, since they must rely on governmental relief authorities for access to transportation, communication, and often the very ability to gain entry to a disaster site.

Because the health issue is only one part of the broad disaster problem and perhaps not the major one, epidemiologic studies of disasters require the contributions of people from a wide diversity of fields. They also require the expertise of people from all branches within the discipline of epidemiology (e.g., communicable disease, chronic disease, and health care epidemiology) and the contributions of both medical and social epidemiologists. Unfortunately, most natural-disaster research has addressed the problem from the point of view of a single discipline, that of either epidemiologists, sociologists, or engineers. This lack of active collaboration between workers from different disciplines has been a major shortcoming of past research into the health effects of disasters. For example, structural engineering competence is necessary to understand the mechanisms of building failure in earthquakes or hurricanes, and epidemiologic expertise is necessary to understand the process of human injury caused by such building failure. Working alone, neither structural engineers nor epidemiologists can provide a complete description of the health effects of such disasters *(68)*.

Critical Knowledge Gaps and Research Priorities in Disaster Epidemiology

Research relating to disasters is often imprecise in identifying etiologic factors associated with increased morbidity and mortality. If epidemiologic approaches to the study of disasters are to be applied effectively, theoretical models must be developed further and research strategies must be refined (e.g., study design and sampling methods). The following are specific steps that epidemiologists can take to help make the results of disaster epidemiology more precise:

- Develop standardized protocols for gathering information to be used in decision-making during the immediate postdisaster period (e.g., develop validated ''indicators'' for rapid assessment). This includes identifying which type of information should be collected, developing data-collection methods that are simple and quick to use, and determining which techniques of data collection are best under adverse field conditions. The availability of standard questionnaires that can be modified quickly for each new disaster will make data collection faster and more efficient *(69)*.

- Standardize disaster terminology, technologies, methods and procedures, etc. These include types of emergency supplies, techniques of needs assessment, and methods of vulnerability analysis. Disaster workers in all parts of the world would benefit from such standardization because it would lead to better international understanding, improved coordination of relief management, and easier comparison of data collected on health effects *(70)*.

- To reduce problems associated with identifying, selecting, and distributing large quantities of unsolicited medical supplies, food, and clothing *(71)*, conduct operational research to determine what medical supplies are (1) actually needed (on the basis of number and nature of injuries and standard acceptable treatments), (2) most commonly requested at local and national levels, (3) provided by the national or international community.

- Conduct more-extensive evaluation studies designed to assess the efficiency and effectiveness of emergency interventions. Such studies might include comparisons of population groups who had interventions with those who did not, comparisons of different types of interventions, and comparisons of subjects' status before and after an intervention.

- Make greater use of existing disaster information systems (e.g., the American Red Cross, the National Weather Service, the insurance industry) and record linkages in order to establish databases suitable for epidemiologic research *(72, 73)*.

- Identify measures designed to prevent a particular type of injury from happening in the first place, or at least to prevent an injury from becoming worse than it already is.

- Identify measures designed to improve the delivery of appropriate medical care to disaster victims within an appropriate time frame. Such measures include conducting search-and-rescue operations, providing emergency medical services, importing skilled providers from nonimpacted areas, and evacuating the injured to underutilized medical facilities.

- Identify measures that facilitate the return of the existing health care system to its normal predisaster state.

- Institute a standardized definition of disaster-related injury and a uniform classification scheme. The current absence of such standardization hinders detailed comparisons of data from studies of different disasters and even of data from studies performed in different areas affected by the same disaster *(74)*.

- Further study the actual risk of increased disease transmission following disasters and the impact of sanitation and disease-control measures on that risk.

- Thoroughly study problems associated with the influx of large quantities of relief supplies and volunteer relief personnel from outside a disaster-affected area, and disseminate the results to disaster-relief organizations.

- Conduct further cost-benefit and cost-effectiveness analyses of disaster-relief operations.

Summary

The role of epidemiology in disaster situations has included the following broad framework of activities:

- predisaster activities such as hazard mapping, vulnerability analysis, education of the local community, and provision of guidelines for medical and rescue training
- rapid assessment of health and medical needs through surveys and investigations
- continuous monitoring and surveillance of the health problems faced by the affected population
- implementation of disease-control strategies for well-defined problems
- assessment of the use and distribution of health services following a disaster
- etiologic research on the causes of morbidity and mortality due to disasters, the findings from which can be used to identify strategies for effective injury- and death-prevention strategies
- development of long-term follow-up studies of populations affected by disasters focusing on the natural history of exposure and health effects

Epidemiology can provide much-needed information on which a rational, effective, and flexible policy for the management of disasters can be based. In particular, epidemiology provides the tools for rapid and effective problem solving during public health emergencies such as natural and technological disasters *(75)*. Results of epidemiologic studies of disasters have not only led to the scientific measurement and description of disaster-associated health effects, but have been used to identify groups in the population at particular risk for adverse health events, to help emergency managers match resources to needs, to monitor the effectiveness of relief efforts, to improve contingency planning, and to formulate recommendations for decreasing the adverse public health consequences of future disasters.

References

1. Lilienfeld AM, Lilienfeld DE. *Foundations of epidemiology*, 2nd ed. New York: Oxford University Press, 1980.
2. Foege WH. Public health aspects of disaster management. In: JM Last, editor. *Public Health and Preventive Medicine*. Norwalk, CT: Appleton-Century-Crofts, 1986:1879–1886.
3. Lechat MF. *Role and limits of epidemiology in disaster management*. Geneva: World Health Organization, 1991.

4. Noji EK. Disaster epidemiology: challenges for public health action. *J Public Health Policy* 1992;13:332–340.
5. Binder S, Sanderson LM. The role of the epidemiologist in natural disasters. *Ann Emerg Med* 1987;16:1081–1084.
6. Lechat MF. The epidemiology of disasters. London: *Proceedings of the Royal Society of Medicine* 1976;69:421–426.
7. Western K. *The epidemiology of natural and man-made disasters: the present state of the art* [dissertation]. London: University of London, 1972.
8. Logue JN, Melick ME, Hansen H. Research issues and directions in the epidemiology of health effects of disasters. *Epidemiol Rev* 1981;3:140–162.
9. Seaman J. Epidemiology of natural disasters. *Contributions to Epidemiology and Biostatistics* 1984;5:1–177.
10. Gregg MB, editor. *Public health consequences of disasters*. Atlanta: Centers for Disease Control, 1989.
11. Lechat MF. Updates: the epidemiology of health effects of disasters. *Epidemiol Rev* 1990; 12:192–197.
12. Sayler LF, Gordon JE. The medical component of natural disasters. *Am J Med Sci* 1957; 234:342–362.
13. Foege W, Conrad RL. *IKOT IBRITAM Nutritional Project: report to the International Committee of the Red Cross*. Atlanta: Center for Disease Control, 1969.
14. Boss LP, Toole MJ, Yip R. Assessments of mortality, morbidity, and nutritional status in Somalia during the 1991–92 famine: recommendations for standardization of methods. *JAMA* 1994;272:371–376.
15. Centers for Disease Control. A manual for the basic assessment of nutrition status in potential crisis situations. Atlanta: Centers for Disease Control, 1981.
16. Sommer AS, Mosley WH. East Bengal cyclone of November 1970. *Lancet* 1972;1:1029–1036.
17. Sommer AS, Mosley WH. The cyclone: medical assessment and determination of relief and rehabilitation needs. In: Chen LC, editor. *Disaster in Bangladesh*. New York: Oxford University Press, 1973:119–132.
18. Glass RI, Noji EK. Epidemiologic surveillance following disasters. In: Halperin WE, Baker EL, Monson RR, editors. *Public Health Surveillance*. New York: Van Nostrand Reinhold, 1992:195–205.
19. Seaman J. Disaster epidemiology: or why most international disaster relief is ineffective. *Injury* 1990;21:5–8.
20. de Ville de Goyet C, Del Cid E, Romero E, *et al.* Earthquake in Guatemala: epidemiologic evaluation of the relief effort. *PAHO Bull* 1976;10:95–109.
21. Glass RI, Urrutia JJ, Sibony S, *et al.* Earthquake injuries related to housing in a Guatemalan village. *Science* 1977; 197:638–643.
22. Bernstein RS, Baxter PJ, Falk H, *et al.* Immediate public health concerns and actions in volcanic eruptions: lessons from the Mt. St. Helens eruptions, May 18–October 18, 1980. *Am J Public Health* 1986;76(Suppl.):25–37.
23. Disaster epidemiology. *Lancet* 1990;336:845–846.
24. Noji EK, Passerini E, Gabel S. *Epidemiology of disasters: a topical bibliography*. Topical bibliography #18. Boulder, Colorado: Natural Hazards Research and Applications Information Center, University of Colorado, 1994:1–68.
25. Glass RI, Craven RB, Bregman DJ, *et al.* Injuries from the Wichita Falls tornado: implications for prevention. *Science* 1980;207:734.

26. French JG, Ing R, Von Allmen S, Wood R. Mortality from flash floods: a review of National Weather Service Reports, 1969–81. *Public Health Rep* 1983;98:584–588.

27. Armenian HK, Noji EK, Oganessian AP. Case control study of injuries due to the earthquake in Soviet Armenia. *Bull World Health Organ* 1992;70:251–257.

28. Philen RM, Combs DL, Miller L, *et al*: Hurricane Hugo-related deaths: South Carolina and Puerto Rico, 1989. *Disasters* 1992;16:53–59.

29. Centers for Disease Control: Injuries and illnesses related to Hurricane Andrew—Louisiana, 1992. *MMWR* 1993;42:243–246.

30. Toole MJ, Waldman RJ. Prevention of excess mortality in refugee and displaced populations in developing countries. *JAMA* 1990;263:296–302.

31. Noji EK, Baldwin R, Toole M, Glass R, Blake P. *The role of WHO in disaster epidemiology: operations, research and training.* Geneva: World Health Organization, 1991.

32. Centers for Disease Control and Prevention (CDC). *Disaster epidemiology research program* [pamphlet]. Atlanta: CDC, 1993.

33. Noji EK, Frumkin H. Disaster preparation course at the Emory University School of Public Health [letter]. *Am J Public Health* 1994;84:1341–1342.

34. Landesman LY. The availability of disaster preparation courses at US schools of public health. *Am J Public Health* 1993;83:1494–1495.

35. Lillibridge SR, Burkle FM, Noji EK. Disaster mitigation and humanitarian assistance training for uniformed service medical personnel. *Mil Med* 1994;159:397–403.

36. Sanderson LM. Toxicologic disasters: natural and technologic. In: Sullivan JB, Krieger GR, editors. *Hazardous materials toxicology: clinical principles of environmental health.* Baltimore: Williams & Wilkins, 1992: 326–331.

37. Centers for Disease Control: Rapid health needs assessment following Hurricane Andrew—Florida and Louisiana. *MMWR* 1992;41:696–698.

38. Hlady WG, Quenemoen LE, Armenia-Cope RR, *et al*. Use of a modified cluster sampling method to perform rapid needs assessment after Hurricane Andrew. *Ann Emerg Med* 1994; 23:719–725.

39. Guha-Sapir D, Lechat MF. Immediate needs assessment in acute disasters: some quick and dirty indicators. CRED working paper. Brussels: Center for Research on the Epidemiology of Disasters (CRED), Catholic University of Louvain, 1985.

40. Guha-Sapir D. Rapid assessment of health needs in mass emergencies: review of current concepts and methods. *World Health Stat Q* 1991;44:171–181.

41. Guha-Sapir D, Lechat MF. Information systems and needs assessment in natural disasters: an approach for better disaster relief management. *Disasters* 1986;10:232–237.

42. Guha-Sapir D, Lechat MF. Reducing the impact of natural disasters: why aren't we better prepared? *Health Policy and Planning* 1986;1:118–126.

43. Noji EK. The role of epidemiology in natural disaster reduction: an interdisciplinary approach. In: *Proceedings of the 2nd US–Japan Natural Disaster Reduction Workshop*, 23–27 September 1991, Karuizawa, Japan. Tokyo: Japan Science and Technology Agency, 1992:327–345.

44. Noji EK. Chemical hazard assessment and vulnerability analysis. In: Holopainen M, Kurttio P, Tuomisto J, editors. *Proceedings of the African Workshop on Health Sector Management in Technological Disasters, 26–30 November, 1990, Addis Ababa, Ethiopia.* Kuopio, Finland: National Public Health Institute, 1991:56–62.

45. Jones NP, Noji EK, Krimgold FR, Smith GS. Considerations in the epidemiology of earthquake injuries. *Earthquake Spectra* 1990;6:507–528.

46. Lillibridge SA, Noji EK, Burkle FM. Disaster assessment: the emergency health evaluation of a disaster site. *Ann Emerg Med* 1993;22:1715–1720.

47. Thacker SB, Berkelman RL. Public health surveillance in the United States. *Epidemiol Rev* 1988;10:164–190.
48. Spencer HC, Campbell CC, Romero A, *et al.* Disease surveillance and decision making after the 1976 Guatemala earthquake. *Lancet* 1977;2:181–184.
49. Bernstein RS, Baxter PJ, Falk H, *et al.* Immediate public health concerns and actions in volcanic eruptions: lessons from the Mt. St. Helens eruptions, May 18–October 18, 1980. *Am J Public Health* 1986;76(Suppl.):25–37.
50. Surmieda RS, Abad-Viola G, Abellanosa IP, *et al.* Surveillance in evacuation camps after the eruption of Mt. Pinatubo. In: *Public health surveillance and international health.* Atlanta: Centers for Disease Control, 1992:9–12.
51. Centers for Disease Control and Prevention. Morbidity surveillance following the Midwest flood—Missouri, 1993. *MMWR* 1993;42:797–798.
52. Woodruff B, Toole MJ, Rodriguez DC, *et al.* Disease surveillance and control after a flood: Khartoum, Sudan 1988. *Disasters* 1990;14:151–163.
53. Centers for Disease Control. Surveillance of shelters after Hurricane Hugo—Puerto Rico. *MMWR* 1990;39:41.
54. Lee LE, Fonseca V, Brett K, Mullen RC, *et al.* Active morbidity surveillance after Hurricane Andrew. *JAMA* 1993;270;591–594.
55. Lindtjorn B. Disaster epidemiology [letter]. *Lancet* 1991;337:116–117.
56. Brenner SA, Noji EK. Risk factors for death and injury in tornadoes: an epidemiologic approach. In: Church C, Burgess D, Doswell C, Davies-Jones R, editors. *The tornado: its structure, dynamics, prediction, and hazards.* Washington, D.C.: American Geophysical Union, 1993:543–544.
57. Glass RI, Craven RB, Bregman DJ. Injuries from the Wichita Falls tornado: implications for prevention. *Science* 1980;207:734–738.
58. de Bruycker M, Greco D, Lechat MF. The 1980 earthquake in Southern Italy: Morbidity and mortality. *Int J Epidemiol* 1985;14:113–117.
59. Roces MC, White ME, Dayrit MM, Durkin ME. Risk factors for injuries due to the 1990 earthquake in Luzon, Philippines. *Bull World Health Organ* 1992;70;509–514.
60. Staes CJ, Orengo JC, Malilay J, *et al.* Deaths due to flashfloods in Puerto Rico, January 5, 1992: implications for prevention. *Int J Epidemiol* 1994;23:968–975.
61. McDonnell S, Troiano RP, Hlady WG, *et al.* Long-term effects of Hurricane Andrew: revisiting mental health indicators. *Disasters* 1995;19:235–246.
62. Lechat MF, de Wals PM. *Evaluation of health intervention after a natural disaster.* Brussels: Centre for Research on the Epidemiology of Disasters, 1981.
63. Noji EK Evaluation of the efficacy of disaster response. *UNDRO News* 1987July/August:11–13.
64. Armenian HK. Methodologic issues in the epidemiologic studies of disasters. In: *Proceedings of the international workshop on earthquake injury epidemiology: implications for mitigation and response, Baltimore, July 10–13, 1989.* Baltimore: Johns Hopkins University, 1989:95–106.
65. Lima BR, Pai S, Toledo V, *et al.* Emotional distress in disaster victims: a follow-up study. *J Nerv Ment Dis* 1993;181:388–393.
66. Bertazzi PA. Epidemiology in the investigation of health effects of man-made disasters. *Progress in Occupational Epidemiology* 1988;3–14.
67. Velimirovic B. Non-natural disasters—an epidemiological review. *Disasters* 1980;4:237–246.
68. Jones NP, Noji EK, Krimgold F, Smith GS. Considerations in the epidemiology of earthquake injuries. *Earthquake Spectra* 1990;6:507–528.

69. Noji EK. Information requirements for effective disaster management. In: *Proceedings of the international conference on emergency health care development*. Washington, D.C.: Medical Care Development International, 1990:41–48.

70. Gunn SWA. The language of disasters. *Prehospital and Disaster Medicine* 1990;5:Special Report.

71. Autier P, Ferir M, Hairapetien A, *et al*. Drug supply in the aftermath of the 1988 Armenian earthquake. *Lancet* 1990;335:1388–1390.

72. Patrick P, Brenner SA, Noji EK, Lee J. The American Red Cross—Centers for Disease Control natural disaster morbidity and mortality surveillance system [letter]. *Am J Public Health* 1992;82:1690.

73. Lillibridge SA, Noji EK. The importance of medical records in disaster epidemiology research. *Journal of the American Health Information Management Association* 1992; 63:137–138.

74. Noji EK. Analysis of medical needs in disasters caused by tropical cyclones: the need for a uniform injury reporting scheme. *J Trop Med Hyg* 1993;96:370–376.

75. Armenian HK. In wartime: options for epidemiology. *Am J Epidemiol* 1986;124:28–32.

3

Surveillance and Epidemiology

SCOTT F. WETTERHALL
ERIC K. NOJI

Disasters disrupt normal or existing relationships between people and their environment, and social relationships among and within groups of people. These disruptions require action by public health officials to mitigate the resulting adverse health effects, to prevent as much damage as possible, and to restore delivery of public services to pre-disaster levels. To respond appropriately and effectively to the challenges and threats that disasters and their consequences pose to public health, everyone involved in relief efforts—policymakers, disaster managers, resource coordinators, field-workers, and the victims themselves—require timely and accurate information. Public health surveillance can identify health problems, establish priorities for decision-makers, and evaluate the effectiveness of relief activities.

Public health surveillance is the cornerstone of epidemiology. Epidemiology is the study in populations of the distribution of diseases, other adverse health events, and their determinants in populations. The past decade has seen the emergence of disaster epidemiology (1, 2); disaster epidemiologists apply descriptive and analytical techniques to the study of disasters. In recent years, epidemiologic techniques have become key components of many disaster-relief operations. Using these techniques, epidemiologists can define rapidly the nature and extent of health problems, identify groups in the population at particular risk for adverse health events, optimize the relief response, monitor the effectiveness of the relief effort, and recommend ways of decreasing the consequences of future disasters (3).

With descriptive epidemiology, the analysis of surveillance data involves characterizing the distribution of a health event by time, person, and place (*4*). Results of analytical studies (e.g., case-control studies to identify risk factors [*5, 6*] and longitudinal
studies to measure changes over time [*7*]) have provided disaster managers with important information for use in planning future prevention and relief efforts. People with
training and skills in epidemiology are usually most qualified to organize and operate
a public health surveillance system, but successful operation requires collaborating with
a variety of health workers and professionals from other disciplines.

Public health surveillance is the ongoing, systematic collection, analysis, and interpretation of data about specific health events (*8*). These data are used in planning,
implementing, and evaluating public health programs. Public health surveillance after
disasters is an iterative process in which simple health outcomes are constantly monitored and interventions assessed for efficacy (Fig. 3-1). Data on health events are analyzed, transformed into usable information, and disseminated to decision-makers for
action. Subsequent responses might influence or modify the events under surveillance,
resulting in the collection of additional data, the performance of additional analyses and
their dissemination, and further action. For greatest effectiveness, a surveillance system
must integrate epidemiologic, behavioral, laboratory, demographic, vital statistical, and
other types of data to provide information needed for policy development and action.

Disasters are routinely characterized as having three phases: preimpact, impact, and
postimpact (*9*). Information needs—as well as methods of data collection, analysis, and
dissemination—generally vary by phase. In this chapter, the term ''public health surveillance'' encompasses the broad taxonomy of assessment activities—those which link
data collection to public health action—that might be undertaken during the successive
phases of a disaster (Table 3-1).

The challenges to conducting public health surveillance in disaster settings include

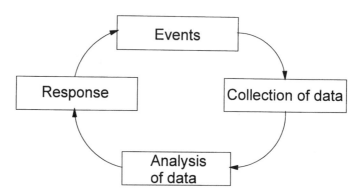

Figure 3-1. The surveillance cycle. *Source*: Foege WH. Public health aspects of disaster management. In: Last J, editor. Maxcy-Rosenau-Last: *Public health and preventive medicine*, 12th
ed. Norwalk, CT: Appleton-Century-Crofts, 1986:1879–1886. *(42)*

the following: (1) data must be collected rapidly under highly adverse conditions; (2) multiple sources of information must be integrated in a cohesive fashion; (3) circumstances and forces may exist that impede the flow from one step in the surveillance cycle to the next; and (4) the cycle from information to action must be completed rapidly, accurately, and repeatedly.

This chapter focuses primarily on conducting public health surveillance in natural-disaster settings. (See Chapters 15, ''Famine,'' and 20, ''Complex Emergencies,'' for descriptions of nutritional surveillance and surveillance in refugee camp settings, respectively). Here, we review the steps in planning a surveillance system, and we discuss the methodologic problems of postdisaster assessment and surveillance. We also review specific surveillance methods and survey techniques that have been applied in disaster settings, discuss critical gaps in knowledge, and offer suggestions for future research.

Planning a Surveillance System

The steps in developing a surveillance system are well established (*10–13*) and follow a logical sequence. In conducting public health surveillance in disaster settings, many of these steps should be undertaken simultaneously and may need to be modified to compensate for mitigating circumstances or to satisfy unique information needs.

Establish Objectives

Just as the purposes and objectives of any disaster-relief efforts must be clearly articulated and widely shared, the surveillance system that supports those relief efforts must have well-defined objectives. Clear objectives allow the system to operate more efficiently, particularly when time, personnel, and material resources are scarce. Traditionally, data from a surveillance system can be used in several ways (Table 3-2). For example, a rapid needs assessment after Hurricane Andrew in 1992 documented the proportion of households with acute needs (*14*). Nutrition surveys in refugee camps have documented that the very young are at increased risk for morbidity and mortality (*15*). Examination of age-specific mortality after an earthquake in Guatemala led to studies that linked age and birth order with risk for mortality (*16*). The objectives of the surveillance system and the anticipated uses of the information it generates should specify the type of system that is developed and determine the events that are monitored.

Develop Case Definitions

Case definitions permit the ''case,'' or adverse health event, to be characterized by using clinical, epidemiologic, or laboratory data. The elements of a case definition can be arrayed to convey the degree of certainty in the diagnosis; for example, a clinical

Table 3-1 Characteristics of Data Collection Methods in Disaster Settings*

Assessment Method	Requirements		Data-Gathering Techniques			
	Time	Resources	Indicators	Advantages	Disadvantages
1. Predisaster "background" data	Ongoing	Trained staff	Reporting from health facilities and practitioners	Provides baseline data for detecting problems and assessing trends	None
			Disease patterns and seasonability		
2. Remote: airplanes, helicopter, satellite	Minutes/hours	Hardware	Direct observation, cameras	Quick; useful when ground transport out; useful to identify area affected	Expensive; large objective error; minimal specific data
			Destroyed buildings, roads, dams, flooding		
3. On-site "walk-through" (ride through)	Hours/days	Transportation, maps	Direct observation, talks with local leaders and health workers	Quick; visible; does not require technical (health) background	Nonquantitative data; potential bias; high error rate; "most-affected" areas may be unreachable
			Deaths, homeless persons, numbers and types of diseases		

			Rapid surveys	Rapid quantitative data; may prevent mismanagement; can provide data for surveillance	Not always random samples; labor intensive; risk of overinterpretation
4. "Quick and dirty" surveys	2–3 days	Few trained staff	Deaths, no. hospitalized, nutritional status, (see also 3)		
5. Rapid health screening system	Ongoing (as needed)	Health workers; equipment depends upon data that are collected	Collect data from fraction of persons being screened Nutritional status, demography, hematocrit parasitemia	Can be established quickly; collects data and provides services (vaccines, vit. A, triage) in migrating populations	Minimal resource needs, useful for "closed populations" only; no information obtained on persons not screened
6. Surveillance system	Ongoing	Some trained staff; standard diagnoses; method of communicating data	Routine data collection in standardized manner Mortality/morbidity by diagnosis and age	Timely; expandable; can detect trends	Requires resources for operation; needs to be monitored continuously
7. Survey	Variable: hours/days	Experienced field epidemiologist or statistician; reliable field staff	Random or representative sample selection Varies according to purpose of survey	Large amount of specific data obtained in brief time	Labor intensive (needs epidemiologist and statistician for data interpretation)

Source: Adapted from Nieburg's Model for data collection methods in disaster situations, in *Health aspects and relief management after natural diasters,* Center for Research on the Epidemiology of Disasters, Bruxelles, Belgium, 1980.

Table 3-2 Objectives of a Surveillance System

- Estimate the magnitude of a health problem

- Identify groups at increased risk for adverse health outcomes

- Detect epidemics or other outbreaks

- Generate and test hypotheses regarding etiology

- Monitor changes in infectious agents

- Detect changes in health practices

- Identify research needs

- Evaluate control strategies

---

diagnosis may represent a "probable" case, whereas laboratory evidence might be required to establish a "confirmed" case. Case definitions can simplify and standardize reporting practices when multiple sources (e.g., physicians, hospitals, relief centers) are reporting data to the surveillance system (*17*). For example, case definitions have been developed for nationally notifiable diseases in the United States (*18*). Broad clinical categories of symptoms and signs (e.g., fever and cough, diarrhea) have frequently been used to classify cases of disease in surveillance of health facilities after disasters (*11, 12, 19*).

Determine Data Sources

The objectives of the surveillance system determine which data sources are most appropriate. Rapid assessments done immediately after a disaster's impact frequently must rely on remote aerial reconnaissance, brief on-site inspections, and limited field surveys (Table 3-1) (*12, 13, 20*). Facility-based surveillance of hospitals, emergency medical operations, and temporary shelters can provide information on people seeking care in the aftermath of a disaster. Compared with the routine practice of public health surveillance, surveillance in disaster settings may require using nontraditional sources of information (e.g., police, humanitarian aid agencies, civil defense organizations, religious officials, pharmacies).

Develop Data-Collection Instruments

Ideally, data-collection instruments for public health surveillance in a disaster setting should be developed, tested, and distributed well before a disaster occurs so that precious time is not wasted designing new instruments when standardized ones are available (*11, 12*). Data-collection instruments should be designed to collect only the minimal, most essential information in a clear and unambiguous fashion. When feasible, forms should be designed for ease of data entry. *Epi Info*, a public-domain software package developed by the Centers for Disease Control and Prevention (CDC), can be used to generate questionnaires as well as to enter and analyze data (*21*).

Field-test Methods

Under emergency conditions, there is little time to field-test data-collection methods. Whenever feasible, however, field testing should be done to determine if the data being collected will answer the questions being asked (*22*). Employing standard techniques, such as cluster sampling, that have been successfully applied in other settings will ensure greater confidence in the quality of the data. Similarly, training field-workers to follow standard protocols will improve data quality and might prevent problems that become apparent only during data analysis—long after corrective action can be taken.

Develop and Test Analysis Strategy

The analysis strategy should be established in conjunction with the development of the data-collection instrument and methods, rather than after the data have been collected and computerized. The analytical approach should answer the questions posed by the objectives of the system. When special surveys are planned, prior consultation with statisticians is desirable to ensure that appropriate analytical methods are used (*23*).

Develop Dissemination Mechanism

For the information to be useful, it must be disseminated through appropriate channels in a timely fashion. Whenever possible, before data collection begins, those conducting surveillance activities should establish linkages with the people and organizations who will be receiving and using surveillance information. Information should be disseminated to public health and other government officials, the media, other relief workers, and to people within the affected community. In particular, the public should always be informed about the risks and the occurrence or absence of disease in areas affected by the disaster. Radio, television, and other media should be used to inform affected populations about the activities and contributions of routine disease-control programs to disaster relief. Finally, those responsible for surveillance activities should provide feedback to the field-workers who assisted in data collection. Including in the feedback loop those people who collect or report data displays appreciation for the essential service they provide and enhances the likelihood that they will continue to participate.

Assess Usefulness of System

Surveillance systems, even temporary ones established for the duration of a disaster, should be evaluated to ensure that they are meeting their objectives (24). If the data from the surveillance system are not being used, then the system is not meeting its fundamental objective. Because the purpose of surveillance is to establish priorities for taking action, lack of a mechanism for acting upon the health data that are collected makes surveillance conducted after a disaster meaningless. In such a situation, the surveillance system should either be modified to meet the needs of decision makers or terminated.

Methodological Problems: Postdisaster Assessment and Surveillance

Although the steps in conducting postdisaster assessments and establishing surveillance systems are straightforward, their successful implementation under field conditions poses challenges that require multiple skills—in communications and public relations, management and administration, and public health, as well as in technical expertise in survey design, statistics, and epidemiology. The goal is to provide accurate information in a timely fashion on the health status of the affected population. Accomplishing this, however, entails facing recurrent and vexing methodologic problems (Table 3-3).

The need for timeliness and accuracy in the assessment supersedes other requirements for collecting and analyzing data. Unfortunately, simultaneously satisfying these needs

Table 3-3 Methodologic Issues in Postdisaster Assessment and Surveillance

- Compromise between timeliness and accuracy

- Competing priorities for information

- Logistical constraints

- Absence of baseline information

- Denominator data unavailable

- Underreporting of health events

- Lack of representativeness

- Resource costs of collecting and analyzing data

- Lack of standardized reporting mechanisms

usually requires trade-offs or compromises such as using less-than-ideal sampling methods (*11, 25*). Such a situation has prompted practical adages such as "being roughly right is generally more useful than being precisely wrong" (*26*).

Data and information needs must be prioritized. Unfamiliarity with the relationship between the nature and phase of the disaster and the need for specific types of information can cause essential resources to be misdirected (*27*). Assessment priorities should relate to the type of disaster and its anticipated effects (*28*). For example, sudden-impact disasters require that relief focus on providing basic needs such as water, food, fuel, and shelter. Gradual-onset disasters (e.g., famines) might also require emphasis on services such as providing vaccines or supplemental feedings. Similarly, the phases of a disaster—preimpact, impact, and postimpact—will influence the types and sources of information needed (*9*) (Table 3-1).

Logistical constraints will influence the collection, analysis, interpretation, and dissemination of surveillance data. Disasters might sever communications systems and impede normal transportation. The disaster can disrupt or destroy the public health infrastructure—hospitals and health departments and their personnel (*19, 29*). Such disruptions can necessitate employing untrained personnel as field-workers, thereby affecting the quality of the data collected. Recruiting outside workers to perform assessment and surveillance activities is an alternative, but the unfamiliarity of these workers with local languages and customs might compromise data quality (*30*) or impair the delivery of preventive services (*31*). If possible, at least one member of the assessment team should be familiar with local customs and conditions (e.g., cultural norms, practices).

Baseline information may be absent or unavailable. Public health officials need information on health status before the disaster to estimate the size of the population at risk, to identify groups that are particularly vulnerable, and to estimate the magnitude of the effect of the disaster. For example, in refugee camps, rapid migration of people often means that composition of the refugees by age and sex and their baseline nutritional status may be unknown. These uncertainties hamper targeting relief efforts appropriately and make early collection of this information through rapid assessment techniques a priority (*32, 33*). Baseline information is also needed to determine whether the health problems that are detected after the disaster represent true increases rather than improved case ascertainment. After Hurricane Andrew, for example, surveillance data gathered at emergency medical facilities were difficult to interpret because the expected proportion of visits to a clinic for a particular cause (e.g., diarrhea) was unknown before the disaster (*19*).

The size of the population at risk (also referred to as "denominators") might be difficult to obtain. Denominator data are required to calculate rates (e.g., the number of deaths from heatstroke per 100, 000 persons at risk) (*34*). Rates permit valid comparisons of morbidity and mortality between populations that differ in size and composition (e.g., distributions by age, race, and sex). Comparing absolute numbers of a health event in two groups may be misleading if the underlying populations at risk differ in size or other characteristics (*35*). In the United States, decennial census data (and more recent intercensal estimates) should be available to officials conducting surveillance after a disaster. However, because the impact of the disaster within a particular geographical area is frequently not uniform (*36*), more refined and localized estimates of the population at risk might be required.

Public health surveillance systems operating in disaster settings should have high sensitivity (i.e., they should have the ability to detect cases) to ensure that the health outcomes of interest are being ascertained and to provide early, although perhaps non-specific, warnings of unusual epidemiologic occurrences. Sensitivity refers to the capacity of the surveillance system to detect "true" cases of illness or injury (*24*). Yet, even under normal circumstances, the underreporting of communicable diseases by health care providers is well documented (*37, 38*). Reasons for underreporting include lack of knowledge, negative attitudes toward health departments, and misconceptions about the need for and use of surveillance information (*39*). Disruption of communications and transportation systems after a disaster can impede reporting and further diminish the sensitivity of the surveillance system. Events that occur outside the domain of the health care system might go undetected. For example, mortality rates in refugee camps might be underestimated because deaths might not occur in medical facilities (*11*).

Other factors, including the complexity of the case definitions that are used, can influence the sensitivity of the surveillance system. In many settings, even during non-disaster conditions, specific diseases (e.g., malaria or dysentery) are difficult to diagnose, particularly without laboratory confirmation. If the case definitions used in emergency settings require complex clinical criteria as opposed to simpler criteria (e.g., fever with rash or bloody diarrhea), underreporting may occur. In such circumstances, the level of training of the health care workers and the availability and sophistication of health care facilities will influence the sensitivity of the system. On the other hand, improving the efficiency of postdisaster public health surveillance can result in the reporting of an increased number of diseases. Although this increase can reflect greater disease transmission, it also can simply represent an increase in the number of reporting units or a heightened awareness and concern about communicable diseases after a disaster. Finally, the absence of reporting should not be equated with the absence of disease.

The information collected by a surveillance system might not be representative of the population at risk. Certain practices, such as focusing on the most affected areas rather than on the entire disaster area, could introduce sampling bias (*12*). Biased or nonrepresentative results are more likely to occur if the surveys rely on convenience samples (*36*). Similarly, surveys that must be conducted at specific times of the day or in specific locations because of logistical factors (e.g., the availability or safety of field-workers) or that use a particular methodology (e.g., telephone surveys) may overrepresent people who are present at those times or who have access to technology such as telephones. Even when more robust sampling procedures are employed in a survey, treating dissimilar sampling units (e.g., single-family dwellings and multifamily dwellings) as comparable can bias results (23). Moreover, using facility-based surveillance methods (e.g., interviewing people attending an emergency clinic or those living in a public shelter) will accurately represent those subgroups seeking treatment but will not provide information about people who do not seek care.

The trade-off between the cost and value of the information collected is usually unknown (25). Collecting surveillance information incurs an opportunity cost. In other words, developing and operating a surveillance system in a disaster setting could be perceived as diverting resources from other important relief programs and services that have been established (e.g., building shelters). Decision-makers, particularly those who are unfamiliar with public health or surveillance, may view such diversions as unacceptable unless those who develop the system can demonstrate that the benefits from collecting the information (e.g., having data to respond to community concerns) outweigh the costs (40).

Finally, reporting mechanisms are often unstandardized. Epidemiologists should develop methods to ensure that surveillance activities undertaken during a disaster are simple, flexible, and acceptable. Flexibility refers to the capacity of the surveillance system to be easily modified so that other health events of emerging importance can be monitored. An acceptable system is one in which the people responsible for providing information—hospital workers, other medical care providers, field-workers—freely participate. Acceptability also reflects the willingness of decision-makers to use the data that are collected. Standardized reporting mechanisms that include case definitions will improve the quality of the information that is collected and will increase the likelihood that it is used in a timely fashion. Standardization also will permit lessons learned in one setting to be applied to future situations.

Surveillance and Assessment: Selected Examples of Strategies and Methods

To provide useful information and to accommodate the nature, scope, and phase of the disaster, surveillance and assessment methods and activities frequently need modification. Information needs, including the type and amount of data and the frequency with which it is collected, change rapidly as a disaster evolves. Thus, the surveillance cycle must revolve many times: immediately—with "quick and dirty" assessments of problems using the most rudimentary techniques of data collection; in the short term—with assessments that involve establishing simple but reliable sources of data; and in the long term—with ongoing surveillance to identify continuing problems and to monitor responses to the interventions (3).

Disaster Planning

Disaster planning must include strategies and methods for rapidly implementing public health surveillance during and after a disaster. The preimpact stage is the period between recognition of an imminent hazard and its destructive effect on the population and its environment. Under ideal circumstances, disaster planning will be tested and implemented long before the preimpact stage begins (*26, 41*). During disaster planning, public health officials should develop a management system, command structure, and contingency plans for emergency communications (*41*). Additionally, the relationships and responsibilities among public health officials and other emergency response personnel (e.g., police, firefighters, rescue squads, Red Cross and civil defense workers) should be established (*13*). Those responsible for surveillance should assemble relevant baseline information—population data, location and capacity of health facilities, and other public services (*26*). Public health officials should ensure that mechanisms, channels, and target audiences for disseminating surveillance information are in place.

Rapid Epidemiologic Assessment

A rapid epidemiologic assessment is usually conducted shortly after impact (*11, 13, 26, 42, 43*). The purpose of this assessment is to estimate these factors:

- overall magnitude of the impact of the disaster (geographical extent, number of affected persons, and estimated duration)
- impact on health (e.g., number of casualties)
- integrity of health services delivery systems
- specific health care needs of survivors
- disruption of other service sectors (power, water, sanitation) that contribute to public health
- extent of response to the disaster by local authorities

Information collected during this rapid assessment should be used to plan and implement immediate responses. The emphasis of these assessments is to gather a small amount of relevant information quickly (usually 2 to 4 days after a sudden-impact disaster). This ''quick and dirty'' approach requires a multidisciplinary team (e.g., an epidemiologist, statistician, engineer, and health planner) (*36*) and relies on visual inspection, interviews with key personnel, and surveys (*13*). The health effects of a disaster can be measured by a series of indicators that permit objective assessment and are used to guide relief efforts (Table 3-4). Such indicators include mortality; morbidity; the number of damaged houses, homeless persons and nonfunctioning hospitals; and the status of community lifelines (e.g., water, electricity, gas, sewage disposal).

After sudden-impact disasters, time constraints and disruption of an area's infrastructure have frequently made it necessary to conduct rapid assessment surveys using non-

Table 3-4 Selected Health Status Indicators and Their Use in Natural Disaster Settings

DEATHS

A. Number of impact-related deaths in population of disaster area

- Assessing magnitude of the disaster
- Evaluating effectiveness of disaster preparedness
- Evaluating adequacy of warning system

B. Number of impact-related deaths by age and gender subgroups

- Identifying high-risk groups for additional contingency planning

C. Number of impact-related deaths in population within specific location or habitat

- Analyzing vulnerability of building structures
- Identifying locations for improving preventive measures

D. Number of deaths per number of destroyed houses

- Assessing adequacy of building structures

E. Number of impact-related deaths per unit of time after the disaster in population of disaster area

- Determining need for rescue measures
- Evaluating effectiveness of rescue measures
- Assessing self-reliance of affected community
- Evaluating community's predisaster rescue training

CASUALTIES

A. Number of deaths per number of casualties

- Calculating indices to estimate the number of casualties (and emergency supplies needed) in different disaster settings

B. Number of casualties per population of disaster area

- Evaluating predisaster planning and preparation
- Evaluating adequacy of warning system
- Estimating needs for emergency care and relief

C. Distribution of types of casualties

- Identifying risk factors to be addressed in predisaster planning and relief efforts
- Estimating needs for emergency care

MORBIDITY

A. Number of medical consultations in the surviving population

- Estimating type and volume of immediate medical relief needed
- Evaluating appropriateness of relief provided
- Identifying remote population groups affected by the disaster
- Assessing needs for further contingency planning

B. Time distribution of medical consultations

- Scheduling medical-relief efforts
- Identifying remote population groups affected by the disaster
- Assessing use of medical services by the affected population

C. Distributions of types of medical conditions

- Identifying critical services to be maintained in emergencies

Table 3-4 Selected Health Status Indicators and Their Use in Natural Disaster Settings (*Continued*)

D. Incidence of communicable diseases

- Identifying risk for communicable disease and need for contingency planning
- Assessing need for additional surveillance and control measures

E. Occupancy of hospital beds and duration of hospitalization

- Monitoring hospital service capacity
- Evaluating adequacy of hospital care

F. Geographical origin of hospitalized patients

- Assessing adequacy of relief supplies
- Evaluating need for field treatment sites and other additional facilities

---

Source: Adapted from Lechat MF. Disasters and public health. In: Guha-Sapir D, Lechat MF, editors. *A short compendium of basic readings for disaster epidemiology and management.* Brussels: Center for Research on the Epidemiology of Disasters, 1986:21–22.

probability sampling methods. These methods may produce biased results because they are often based on purposive, convenience, or haphazard selection of subjects for interview (*13, 44*). Recently, however, investigators demonstrated the use of a modified cluster-sampling method to perform a rapid needs assessment after a hurricane (*14, 45*). In the first survey conducted 3 days after Hurricane Andrew struck south Florida in August 1992, clusters were systematically selected from a heavily damaged area by using a grid that had been overlaid on aerial photographs. Survey teams interviewed seven occupied households in consecutive order in each selected cluster. Results were available within 24 hours of beginning the survey. Surveys of the same heavily damaged area and of a less severely affected area were conducted 7 and 10 days later, respectively.

Initial survey workers found few households with injured residents, but a large proportion of households were without telephones or electricity. The workers' findings convinced disaster-relief workers to focus on providing primary care and preventive services to residents rather than to divert resources in order to establish unnecessary mass-casualty trauma services. The cluster-survey method used in this rapid assessment was modified from methods developed by the World Health Organization's Expanded Programme on Immunization (EPI) to assess vaccine coverage (*46*). Although cluster surveys have been used in refugee settings to assess nutritional and health status (*32, 33, 47*), this activity represented the first use of the EPI survey method to obtain population-based data after a sudden-impact natural disaster.

Although cluster-survey techniques hold promise for providing information rapidly after a disaster, in certain settings these techniques may be less applicable. For example, epidemiologists who used a cluster-survey technique after the January 1994 earthquake in Northridge, California, found that the technique needed modification. Unlike the damage from hurricanes, which is generally uniform over a large geographical area and can thus support the use of cluster sampling, earthquake-related damage varies considerably, with some areas experiencing little destruction and others experiencing heavy destruction. The extent of damage after earthquakes depends on local soil conditions, the distance and rate of ground-shaking attenuation from the epicenter, and the quality of building construction. Therefore, using a cluster-sampling approach to assess damages after an earthquake may cause health authorities to miss seriously affected areas, and thus to underestimate overall damages (48).

Active Surveillance that Uses Existing Medical Facilities

In addition to conducting rapid assessments, health officials have implemented temporary or enhanced surveillance activities at existing medical facilities in order to characterize morbidity and mortality resulting from a disaster (49). These efforts, commonly referred to as short-term assessments (28), attempt to enumerate the number and characteristics of people who are ill, injured, or dead.

In August 1992, in Louisiana, for example, the state Office of Public Health (OPH) set up an active emergency surveillance system for obtaining information on injuries and illnesses associated with Hurricane Andrew (50). Officials contacted hospital emergency departments, coroners' offices, and public utilities in the 19 parishes that were in the path of the hurricane. The OPH created a case definition for hurricane-related fatal or nonfatal injury or illness and developed a questionnaire to obtain demographic information and data on the nature and cause of the injury or illness. OPH personnel made periodic telephone calls to stimulate reporting of hurricane-related events. Of the 42 hospital emergency departments contacted, 21 participated; 5 of 19 coroners' offices and 1 of 2 public utilities also participated in the system. Of the 17 fatal outcomes reported, 8 occurred before the hurricane reached landfall; the majority (86%) of the 383 nonfatal events were injuries, most commonly cuts and lacerations.

The operation of this system demonstrates the feasibility of collecting morbidity and mortality data from existing emergency medical facilities. The Louisiana experience also underscores several difficulties in operating such a system. Data on morbidity and mortality are available through many sources—hospital emergency departments, police and fire departments, the American Red Cross, medical examiners and coroners offices—but these sources frequently use different methods of defining, ascertaining, and reporting cases of injury or illness. Moreover, recruiting and training hospital personnel—who may be unfamiliar with public health surveillance—to complete reports is challenging and time-consuming. Developing easily modified surveillance questionnaires and guidelines for standardizing data-collection procedures should improve the efficiency and consistency of surveillance in existing medical facilities (51).

Active Surveillance Using Temporary Medical Facilities

A sudden-impact disaster can severely damage existing medical care facilities and interrupt other public health functions and operations. In such circumstances, attempts to characterize the needs of the affected population have prompted the use of public health surveillance in temporary shelters (*31, 52, 53*). Alternatively, active surveillance can be initiated in temporary medical facilities frequently established in the aftermath of the disaster.

After Hurricane Andrew struck south Florida in 1992, the medical system suffered severe damage. Many acute-care facilities and community health centers were closed and physicians' offices destroyed in the impact area (*29*). State and federal public health officials, the Red Cross, and the military established temporary medical facilities to care for the affected population and relief workers. During the 4 weeks after the hurricane struck, officials established active surveillance at 15 civilian free-care centers, at 8 emergency departments in and surrounding the impact area, and at 28 military free-care sites (*19, 29*). Public health workers reviewed medical logbooks and patient records daily, and tabulated the number of visits using simple diagnostic categories (e.g., diarrhea, cough, rash).

The purpose of the surveillance activity was to characterize the health status of the population affected by the hurricane and to evaluate the effectiveness of emergency public health measures. Data from the system indicated that injuries were an important cause of morbidity among civilians and military personnel but that most injuries were minor. The surveillance information was particularly useful in responding to rumors about the occurrence of outbreaks (and in avoiding widespread administration of typhoid vaccine) and in determining that large numbers of volunteer health care providers were not needed.

Although this active surveillance effort achieved its objectives, public health officials operating this system encountered several problems. First, various relief agencies needed to coordinate their efforts. Data from the civilian and military systems had to be analyzed separately because different case definitions and data-collection methods were used. Second, there was no baseline information available to determine whether health events were occurring with a frequency greater than expected. Third, rates of illness and injury could not be determined for civilians because the size of the population at risk was unknown. Although proportional morbidity (the number of visits for a particular cause divided by the total number of visits to the facilities) can be easily obtained, it is often difficult to interpret. For example, an increase in one category (e.g., respiratory illness) may result from a decline in another category (e.g., injuries), rather than from a true increase in the incidence of respiratory illness.

Despite these difficulties, establishing active surveillance at medical care facilities after a disaster can yield timely information for guiding relief efforts. Active surveillance, using standardized case definitions and data-collection protocols, can be implemented in several settings, including Red Cross shelters, medical facilities of other nongovernmental relief agencies, existing clinics and hospitals, and disaster field offices and assistance centers.

Sentinel Surveillance

Sentinel surveillance refers to collecting, analyzing, and interpreting information from a selected subset of potential data sources—hospitals, other health care facilities, laboratories, and individual providers—to monitor the health of a population. Sentinel surveillance may be useful in monitoring the incidence of disease and injury under the following circumstances: (1) there is no preexisting public health surveillance system; (2) the operation of the existing surveillance system has been disrupted; (3) information on the event of interest cannot be readily obtained by using existing surveillance systems; or (4) time and resource constraints prohibit collecting information through population-based surveys (*54*). Sentinel surveillance systems provide a limited amount of information in a timely fashion.

Sentinel surveillance has been used to monitor the health status of populations affected by natural disasters. For example, in the immediate aftermath of the eruption of Mount St. Helens on May 18, 1980, surveillance activities for respiratory and other illnesses related to ashfall were established in the 18 main hospitals located in the path of the ashfall east of the volcano (*55, 56*). Additional hospitals were recruited in western Washington after the eruption on May 25. Such rapid recruitment of reporting sites illustrates the flexibility of sentinel surveillance. In 1990, a major earthquake struck a widespread area in northern and central Luzon Island in the Philippines. Because of widespread destruction of medical facilities and disruption of communications, sentinel surveillance was established in each of the areas affected by the earthquake (*57*). These sentinel activities indicated that increases in measles or diarrheal illness did not occur after the earthquake, and this information was used to dispel rumors and reassure the public. After a flood in Khartoum, Sudan, in 1988, sentinel clinics in each of three urban districts collected surveillance data. The clinics were chosen on the basis of their accessibility to surveillance workers as well as on the presumed representativeness of their patients to the flood-affected population (*58*). Data obtained from such sentinel clinic surveillance indicated that diarrheal disease accounted for the greatest number of clinic visits, while malaria was the second most common reason for seeking medical attention.

Sentinel surveillance can also include surveillance by networks of individual physicians (*59*), although using physicians' offices in disaster settings has been limited. In the United States, sentinel physicians have monitored annual morbidity associated with influenza (*60*); in France, sentinel physicians, who are linked via a computer network, monitor seven communicable diseases; these physicians submit weekly electronic reports to France's Ministry of Health (*61*).

The advantages of using sentinel surveillance are its timeliness, flexibility, and acceptability, but establishing sentinel surveillance in disaster settings requires overcoming the same challenges and problems that are posed by other methods of surveillance (*62*). Recruiting and training participants—either personnel from sentinel facilities or individual health care providers—and standardizing data-collection procedures consume time and resources. Sentinel surveillance is an inefficient method for detecting rare events because the number of patient encounters with an individual practitioner or facility is limited. Finally, the representativeness of the sentinel system can be difficult to estimate. Nonetheless, sentinel surveillance might be a practical alternative for gathering information from a subset of facilities (shelters, disaster-assistance centers) during a disaster that has affected a large geographical area.

Investigation of Rumors

Rumors are defined as circulating reports that have unknown veracity or opinions that cannot be attributed to a discernible source. Rumors frequently circulate in disaster settings, and their rapid investigation and disavowal (or confirmation) is an important function of public health officials who are responsible for surveillance and other health-information activities.

Rumors arise in these settings for several reasons. First, disasters can disrupt normal modes of communication between affected populations and civil officials and other authorities. Uncertainty and perceived loss of control might engender fears and concerns in an affected population—as well as in relief workers—that heighten the susceptibility to rumors. Frequently, misconceptions circulate among the public, the media, and officials about specific health risks after a disaster. Thus, fears of epidemics of infectious diseases frequently emerge after a disaster (*63*). Health workers who lack appropriate experience misdiagnose common conditions as diseases with epidemic potential (e.g., they may mistake viral conjunctivitis for measles) (*58*). The press, equipped with advanced telecommunications equipment and arriving on the scene at the same time as relief workers, might interview people who have incomplete or anecdotal information and broadcast the interviewees' opinions as informed fact. Politicians or other authorities who are attempting to establish control may make unfounded statements on the basis of vague information or their personal agendas. Civil authorities and relief agencies might report differing estimates of the impact of the disaster, such as the number of casualties. Even small discrepancies in these numbers can generate public distrust and engender fears that authorities may be concealing or suppressing information.

Rumors should be investigated fully and rapidly to reassure people that public health officials are implementing appropriate control measures. By demonstrating a willingness to investigate rumors, public health and other relief workers will enhance their credibility. By investigating all significant rumors, health officials can assess accurately an evolving situation and validate the accuracy of their surveillance data. Authorities and relief workers will be encouraged to make decisions on the basis of sound information and thereby avoid unnecessary diversion of scarce resources.

Critical activities for effective rumor control are (1) establishing a clear chain of command for disaster-relief efforts, (2) designating a spokesperson for responding to inquiries and providing regular updates on information, and (3) using surveillance and epidemiologic methods to investigate each rumor. Adopting a clear command structure (*13, 41*) ensures that information moves through channels accurately and efficiently. A designated spokesperson who has updated surveillance data can disseminate consistent, authoritative, and educational information to the public, the press, and other government agencies and relief organizations. Through regular updates and briefings, the spokesperson can become a valuable resource for the media, which may then hesitate to broadcast unsubstantiated stories without first checking with authorities (see Chapter 7, "Effective Media Relations").

Rumors might come to the attention of public health officials from many different sources, including politicians, reporters, other relief workers, physicians, and disaster victims themselves. Information from the surveillance system should provide the background information (e.g., the number of casualties and the nature of their injuries and illnesses, the types of endemic diseases and their temporal trends) for initial evaluation of a rumor's plausibility (*7*).

The investigation of a rumor should follow the same stepwise approach that is used for investigating a potential outbreak (*64*). The investigator should focus on confirming the existence of the event ("confirming the diagnosis") by answering the following questions: Who reported the event? On what basis has the diagnosis been made? Has the event been confirmed by using reliable methods (e.g, laboratory confirmation or corroboration by multiple observers)? Have officials consulted other independent sources of information (records from hospitals or other relief agencies) available to confirm the existence of the event? By using a systematic approach, investigators can frequently dispense with rumors before their existence causes additional disruption of relief efforts.

Special Investigations

In addition to conducting rapid assessments and establishing temporary surveillance systems for monitoring morbidity and mortality, public health officials frequently must conduct focused and special investigations to deal with specific problems. These investigations might require laboratory support and the expertise of specialized personnel.

Ensuring safe drinking water and appropriate waste disposal are critical elements of relief efforts after many types of disasters (*11, 65*). Earthquakes, hurricanes, and floods can damage civil-engineering structures (e.g., water-treatment facilities and water mains) or cause power outages (*66*). Displacement might cause population shifts that overburden existing systems. Sanitarians and other environmental health experts must ensure the safety of drinking-water supplies by measuring levels of residual chlorine, coliforms, and nitrates (*66*). When supplies are contaminated, public advisories to boil water should be broadcast or alternative sources identified and provided.

A disaster will occasionally pose an unanticipated respiratory hazard that requires immediate investigation. For example, during the 2 weeks after the heavy ashfalls associated with the eruption of Mount St. Helens, samples of ash were collected by state and federal personnel and analyzed by the National Institute for Occupational Safety and Health (NIOSH) (55). Subsequently, industrial hygienists collected airborne samples in affected communities in Washington, Idaho, and Oregon. Results of these analyses led to recommendations that certain workers in the logging industry and agriculture use goggles and respirators. The analyses also indicated that the general population was not at increased risk for fibrotic or obstructive lung disease (55).

Appropriate response to emergency events involving hazardous substances requires identification of the substance and its anticipated effects (67, 68). According to the Hazardous Substances Emergency Events Surveillance System, from 1990 through 1992, 3,125 emergency events were reported from participating states (68). Substances released most frequently were volatile organic compounds, herbicides, acids, and ammonias. Nearly three-quarters (984) of the 1,353 injured people involved in these events were not using any personal protective equipment at the scene.

Although outbreaks of communicable diseases are uncommon following natural disasters, particularly in the United States (63), these diseases may be responsible for substantial morbidity and mortality in certain international settings (69). In camps for refugees and displaced populations, diarrheal diseases, measles, and acute respiratory illness are among the leading causes of death (11, 69). Thus, focused investigations that use appropriate laboratory methods will enhance surveillance activities by promoting efficient implementation and evaluation of control strategies.

Collection and laboratory testing of specimens serves several functions: (1) confirming the presence of a pathogen; (2) identifying subgroups or areas where scarce resources, such as vaccines, should be directed; and (3) improving case management by selecting appropriate antibiotics (12). For example, although clinical case definitions have been developed for dysentery (e.g., diarrhea with visible blood in the stool), reports of clinical cases of dysentery should be quickly confirmed by culture and the antibiotic susceptibility of isolates determined. If laboratory resources are limited, it is not necessary to culture a specimen from every person thought to have the disease once the diagnosis has been confirmed. At the same time, implementing control measures should not be delayed pending laboratory confirmation (11).

Results of laboratory studies have been used to guide vector-control efforts. For instance, in 1993, after extensive summer flooding in the upper midwestern United States, officials were concerned that large expanses of standing water would provide the habitat for mosquito species that transmit the arboviruses known to cause St. Louis encephalitis and western equine encephalitis (70). Public health authorities completed surveillance by trapping and testing mosquitoes for evidence of these arboviruses. Because results indicated that risk for mosquito-borne encephalitides was low, costly widespread prophylactic mosquito control (with application of insecticides) was not undertaken.

Veterinary services and laboratory investigations might be needed to evaluate health risks posed by animal populations. During the 3 weeks after the 1976 earthquake in Guatemala, the number of dog bites in Guatemala City increased substantially, and people feared a rabies epidemic (*71*). The Ministry of Health instituted a program of canine vaccination and elimination of stray dogs, and officials detected no increase in the number of cases of rabies in humans. Recommendations for animal rabies control and postexposure management of animals, including laboratory testing, have been developed (*72*).

Cluster Surveys to Estimate Health Service Needs

Information needs evolve during the days, weeks, and months after a disaster (*28*). Whereas initial efforts by public health and other relief workers might focus on rapid assessment—with the collection of information to minimize immediate morbidity and mortality and to provide basic services such as shelter and food—subsequent information-gathering efforts must begin to focus on the longer-term needs of the affected population. The information collected during secondary relief efforts and the rehabilitation phase of a disaster can be used to target health services and other public programs to assist the community in its recovery (*36*). Multidisciplinary teams can collect this information using community surveys, but population-based surveys can be expensive, time-consuming, and logistically difficult. Use of cluster surveys, adapted from methods originally used to estimate vaccine coverage in developing countries (*46*), holds promise as a timely and feasible method for measuring the service needs of a population during the rehabilitative phase of a disaster.

Two months after Hurricane Andrew struck Dade County Florida, health officials conducted a cluster survey to (1) determine the distribution of displaced persons in the county, (2) estimate health needs, (3) gauge access to health and social services, and (4) assess evacuation behaviors (*23, 73*). To establish a sampling frame, survey personnel divided Dade County into six zones on the basis of the damage sustained in each zone. In an attempt to make the survey results self-weighting (a statistical technique that simplifies calculation of survey estimates), the officials selected, with probability proportional to size, 30 census tracts in each of the 6 zones. Within each cluster, 10 households were consecutively selected by using a random start (*23*). The data were analyzed by using CSAMPLE, a software module of *Epi Info* (CDC, Atlanta, Georgia) that permits analysis of multistage survey data (*74*).

Results of the survey documented that overcrowding was highest in the Homestead, Florida, area (where the hurricane's impact was greatest) and decreased progressively the greater the distance from this area. The proportion of households in which at least one person had indicators of stress or anxiety was also highest in the Homestead area. Similarly, a larger proportion of households in the Homestead area reported inhabitants who had lost health insurance because of the storm (*25, 73*). The results of the survey were used to target additional mental health and other services for residents of the

Homestead area. Thus, cluster surveys can be used to direct resources appropriately during the rehabilitative phase of a disaster. However, using this method also poses several methodologic challenges. The destruction of an unknown number of dwellings within clusters makes sampling proportional to size difficult and necessitates simplifying assumptions that can then result in biased results (*23*). Therefore, assessment must be an ongoing process, with information collected throughout the postdisaster, rehabilitation, and reconstruction phases. Such a practice will encourage sustained feedback concerning changes in postimpact needs and will allow authorities and disaster-relief agencies to modify their response efforts.

Critical Knowledge Gaps

Public health surveillance comprises the collection, analysis, interpretation, and dissemination of information that leads to public health action—activities that are conceptually straightforward. Although numerous surveillance activities, from preimpact identification of vulnerable groups to postimpact rapid assessments, short-term surveys, and long-term monitoring of the population, have been undertaken in response to disasters, relatively few of these surveillance efforts have been evaluated in a systematic fashion (*75*). Criteria have been developed for evaluating surveillance systems (*24, 76*). Ultimately, every surveillance system should be judged by its usefulness (i.e., whether the information that was collected and disseminated met the objectives of the system). In assessing usefulness, certain attributes of the system, such as simplicity, flexibility, and timeliness, should be evaluated. All surveillance systems used in disaster settings should undergo an evaluation by public health officials. Identifying successful strategies and acknowledging shortcomings will yield critical information for developing better methods of surveillance that can be implemented when the next disaster strikes.

Standardized reporting methods should be developed. Unfortunately, standardized and widely accepted case definitions for disaster-related deaths or injuries do not exist (*77–80*). As a first step, case definitions of disaster-related illnesses and injuries should be developed, agreed upon by the various federal, state, and voluntary agencies that are involved in relief efforts, and disseminated to the public health and emergency management communities. Case definitions must be simple and readily understandable by those who use them to ensure that the surveillance system is sufficiently sensitive at detecting the adverse health events of interest. Reporting procedures and easily modifiable standardized forms that can be used in a variety of settings should be developed. Although the emphasis in standardizing forms and procedures should be on flexibility and simplicity, allowance should be made for gathering sufficiently detailed information, such as the cause and circumstances of certain injuries, to guide interventions and prevention efforts (*17*). Case definitions and standardized reporting procedures will help expand surveillance activities after a disaster to hospital emergency departments, outpatient medical clinics, first-aid shelters, and sentinel physicians.

Collecting baseline information should also be an integral step in disaster preparedness. Although rates of illness or injury are the preferred epidemiologic measures for identifying risk factors and high-risk subgroups, too often data on the population at risk (denominator data) are not available. Without this information epidemiologists must use other, less direct measures such as proportional morbidity to estimate risk (*19, 29*). To improve the use and interpretation of such data, public health officials should consider collecting baseline information, such as the distribution of types of illnesses and injuries at various health facilities, as a component of their preparedness activities. Finally, no standardized methods or indicators exist to determine rapidly the needs of disaster victims and communities. Assessment indicators and surveillance methods in disaster settings should possess all four of the attributes crucial to disaster-relief activity. They should be (1) simple to use, (2) timely, (3) collectable under adverse field conditions, and (4) useful.

Research Recommendations

These activities should be undertaken to improve the efficiency and usefulness of public health surveillance in all phases of a disaster:

- Develop and widely disseminate standardized case definitions of disaster-related morbidity (illnesses and injuries) and mortality.
- Develop standardized reporting forms and procedures that can be easily modified for use in various settings.
- Establish mechanisms for coordinating surveillance efforts between public health officials and the armed forces, who have considerable expertise in communications and logistics supply and can mobilize personnel to assist with relief operations.
- Use and modify cluster-sampling techniques for conducting rapid assessments and estimating health service needs.
- Investigate the use of existing electronic data systems, such as hospital patient discharge data, as potential sources of timely information on morbidity.
- Test the feasibility of establishing and maintaining networks of sentinel physicians and health care facilities, particularly in areas at high risk for recurrent disasters.
- Explore using the Internet and other forms of electronic communication for collecting and disseminating emergency surveillance data.

Research must be conducted to improve postdisaster assessment information systems; to define what information should be collected, including the methodology of assessment; and to improve techniques of data collection. We must identify information that realistically can be gathered in the field for rapid decision-making after a disaster. The objective should be to develop standardized procedures for collecting data that can be linked to operational decisions.

Summary

Public health surveillance is an effective tool that can be used to prepare for and respond to the disruption and destruction that disasters bring. Although the effective use of surveillance information in guiding relief efforts and developing preventive measures is recognized, the full potential for using surveillance in disaster settings has not been realized. To achieve this potential, several challenges must be overcome. Decision-makers must develop a broader appreciation for the variety of uses and types of surveillance data. Those people who conduct surveillance must recognize that disseminating and communicating information are as important as collecting and analyzing data. The capacity to conduct surveillance must be supported by training personnel at all levels of the health sector in the practice and application of epidemiology and surveillance. Gaps in surveillance methodology and data coverage must be recognized and closed. Surveillance systems must be subjected to rigorous evaluation to ensure that they are meeting their established objectives. As these steps are realized, public health surveillance and epidemiology will provide the quantitative information needed for setting priorities and establishing the basis for rational decision-making after disasters.

References

1. Noji EK. Disaster epidemiology: challenges for public health action. *J Public Health Policy* 1992;13:332–340.
2. Disaster epidemiology [editorial]. *Lancet* 1990;2:845–846.
3. Glass RI, Noji EK. Epidemiologic surveillance following disasters. In: Halperin W, Baker EL, editors. *Public health surveillance*. New York: Van Nostrand Reinhold, 1992:195–205.
4. Cates W, Williamson GD. Descriptive epidemiology: analyzing and interpreting surveillance data. In: Teutsch SM, Churchill RE, editors. *Principles and practice of public health surveillance*. New York: Oxford University Press, 1994:96–135.
5. Kilbourne EM, Choi K, Jones TS, Thacker SB. Risk factors for heatstroke. *JAMA* 1982; 247:3332–3336.
6. Armenian HK, Noji EK, Oganesian AP. A case-control study of injuries arising from the earthquake in Armenia, 1988. *Bull World Health Organ* 1992;70:251–257.
7. Elias CJ, Alexander BH, Sokly T. Infectious disease control in a long-term refugee camp: the role of epidemiologic surveillance and investigation. *Am J Public Health* 1990; 80:824–828.
8. Thacker SB, Berkelman RL. Public health surveillance in the United States. *Epidemiol Rev* 1988;10:164–190.
9. Binder S, Sanderson LM. The role of the epidemiologist in natural disasters. *Ann Emerg Med* 1987;16:1081–1084.
10. Teutsch SM. Considerations in planning a surveillance system. In: Teutsch SM, Churchill RE, editors. *Principles and practice of public health surveillance*. New York: Oxford University Press, 1994:18–28.

11. Centers for Disease Control. Famine-affected, refugee, and displaced populations: recommendations for public health issues. *MMWR* 1992;41 (No. RR-13):1–76.

12. Western KA. *Epidemiologic surveillance after natural disasters.* Washington, D.C.: Pan American Health Organization, 1982:(scientific publication no. 420).

13. World Health Organization. *Introduction to rapid health assessment.* Geneva, Switzerland: WHO Office of Emergency Preparedness and Response, 1990, ERO/EPR/90.1.1.

14. Centers for Disease Control and Prevention. Rapid health needs assessment following Hurricane Andrew—Florida and Louisiana, 1992. *MMWR* 1992;41:685–688.

15. Toole MJ, Waldman RJ. An analysis of mortality trends among refugee populations in Somalia, Sudan, and Thailand. *Bull World Health Organ* 1988;66:237–247.

16. Glass RI, Urrutia JJ, Sibony S, Smith H, Garcia B, Rizzo L. Earthquake injuries related to housing in a Guatemalan village. *Science* 1977;197:638–643.

17. Noji EK. Analysis of medical needs in disasters caused by tropical cyclones: the need for a uniform injury reporting scheme. *J Trop Med Hyg* 1993;96:370–376.

18. Centers for Disease Control. Case definitions for public health surveillance. *MMWR* 1990; 39;(No. RR-13):1–43.

19. Lee LE, Fonseca V, Brett KM, *et al.* Active morbidity surveillance after Hurricane Andrew—Florida, 1992. *JAMA* 1993;270:591–594.

20. Center for Research on the Epidemiology of Disasters. *Health and relief management following natural disasters.* Proceedings of the World Health Organization Course; Brussels, Belgium, 1980 Oct. 12–24. Brussels: Center for Research on the Epidemiology of Disasters, 1980.

21. Centers for Disease Control and Prevention. *Epi Info,* Version 6: a word processing, database, and statistics program for epidemiology on microcomputers. Atlanta: Centers for Disease Control and Prevention, 1994.

22. Centers for Disease Control and Prevention. *Iowa's flood disaster of 1993: public health implications and recommendations.* Atlanta: Centers for Disease Control and Prevention, 1993.

23. Barker ND, Stroup NE, Lopez GM, Massey JT. *Evaluation of methods employed in the assessment of health care needs and access to care in Dade County, Florida following Hurricane Andrew.* DHHS Publication No. (PHS) 94–1214. Atlanta: U.S. Department of Health and Human Services, Centers for Disease Control and Prevention, 1993.

24. Klaucke DN, Buehler JW, Thacker SB, et al. Guidelines for evaluating surveillance systems. *MMWR* 1988;37(SS-5):1–18.

25. Binkin N, Sullivan K, Staehling, Nieburg P. Rapid nutrition surveys: how many clusters are enough? *Disasters* 1992; 16:97–103.

26. Guha-Sapir D. Rapid assessment of health needs in mass emergencies: review of current concepts and methods. *World Health Stat Q* 1991;44:171–181.

27. Stephenson RS. *Disaster assessment.* UNDP/UNDRO Disaster management training program module. Madison, Wisconsin: University of Wisconsin, 1992:pp. 1–42.

28. Lillibridge SR, Noji EK, Burkle FM Jr. Disaster assessment: the emergency health evaluation of a population affected by a disaster. *Ann Emerg Med* 1993;22:1715–1720.

29. Fonseca V. Army medical surveillance after Hurricane Andrew. Walter Reed Army Institute of Research, *WRAIR Communicable Disease Report* 1993;4:(no.2)1–4.

30. Babille M, De Colombani P, Guera R, Zagaria N, Zanetti C. Post-emergency epidemiological surveillance in Iraqi-Kurdish refugee camps in Iran. *Disasters* 1994;18:58–75.

31. Surmieda MRS, Abad-Viola G, Abellanosa IP, et al. Surveillance in evacuation camps after the eruption of Mt. Pinatubo, Philippines. *MMWR CDC Surveillance Summaries* 1992; 41(No. SS-4):9–12.

32. Nieburg P, Berry A, Stekatee R, Binkin N, Dondero T, Aziz N. Limitations of anthropometry during acute food shortages: high mortality can mask refugees' deteriorating nutritional status. *Disasters* 1988;12:253–258.

33. Porter JDH, Van Loock FL, Devaux A. Evaluation of two Kurdish refugee camps in Iran, May 1991: the value of cluster sampling in producing priorities and policy. *Disasters* 1993;17:341–347.

34. Jones TS, Liang AP, Kilbourne EM, et al. Morbidity and mortality associated with the July 1980 heat wave in St. Louis and Kansas City, Mo. *JAMA* 1982;247:3327–3331.

35. Gregg MB. Surveillance and epidemiology. In: Gregg MB, editor. The public health consequences of disasters. Atlanta, GA: Centers for Disease Control, 1989:3–4.

36. Guha-Sapir D, Lechat MF. Information systems and needs assessment in natural disasters: an approach for better disaster relief management. *Disasters* 1986;10:232–237.

37. Vogt RL, Clark SW, Kappel S. Evaluation of the state surveillance system using hospital discharge diagnoses, 1982–1983. *Am J Epidemiol* 1986;123:197–198.

38. Kimball AM, Thacker SB, Levy ME. Shigella surveillance in a large metropolitan area: assessment of a passive reporting system. *Am J Public Health* 1980;70:164–6.

39. Konowitz PM, Petrossian GA, Rose DN. The underreporting of disease and physicians' knowledge of reporting requirements. *Public Health Rep* 1984;99:31–35.

40. Wetterhall SF, Pappaioanou M, Thacker SB, Eaker E, Churchill RE. The role of public health surveillance: information for effective action in public health. *MMWR* 1992; 41(Suppl.):207–218.

41. Waeckerle JF. Disaster planning and response. *N Engl J Med* 1991;324:815–821.

42. Foege WH. Public health aspects of disaster management. In: Last J, editor. Maxcy-Rosenau-Last: *Public health and preventive medicine*, 12th ed. Norwalk, CT: Appleton-Century-Crofts, 1986:1879–1886.

43. World Health Organization. *Rapid health assessment in sudden impact natural disasters.* Geneva, Switzerland: WHO Office of Emergency Preparedness and Response, 1990, ERO/EPR/90.1.6.

44. Sommer A, Mosley WH. East Bengal cyclone of November, 1970: epidemiological approach to disaster assessment. *Lancet* 1972;1:1029–1036.

45. Hlady WG, Quenemoen LE, Armenia-Cope RR, *et al.* Use of a modified cluster sampling method to perform rapid needs assessment after Hurricane Andrew. *Ann Emerg Med* 1994; 23:719–725.

46. Henderson RH, Sundaresan T. Cluster sampling to assess immunization coverage: a review of experience with a simplified sampling method. *Bull World Health Organ* 1982;60:253–260.

47. Wijnroks M, Bloem MW, Islam N, *et al.* Surveillance of the health and nutritional status of Rohingya refugees in Bangladesh. *Disasters* 1993;17:348–356.

48. Noji EK. Progress in disaster management. *Lancet* 1994;343:1239–1240.

49. Centers for Disease Control and Prevention. Morbidity surveillance following the Midwest flood—Missouri, 1993. *MMWR* 1993;42:797–798.

50. Centers for Disease Control and Prevention. Injuries and illnesses related to Hurricane Andrew—Louisiana, 1992. *MMWR* 1993;42:242–251.

51. Pan American Health Organization (PAHO). *Guidelines for health needs assessment in the Caribbean.* Antigua: PAHO, 1990.

52. Dietz VJ, Rigau-Perez JG, Sanderson L, Diaz L, Gunn RA. Health assessment of the 1985 flood disaster in Puerto Rico. *Disasters* 1990;14:164–170.

53. Centers for Disease Control. Surveillance of shelters after Hurricane Hugo—Puerto Rico. *MMWR* 1990;39:41–47.

54. Woodall JP. Epidemiological approaches to health planning, management, and evaluation. *World Health Stat Q* 1988;41:2–10.
55. Bernstein RS, Baxter PJ, Falk H, Ing R, Foster L, Frost F. Immediate public health concerns and actions in volcanic eruptions: lessons from the Mount St. Helens eruptions, May 18–October 18, 1980. *Am J Public Health* 1986;76(Suppl.):25–37.
56. Baxter PJ, Ing R, Falk H, *et al*. Mount St. Helens eruptions, May 18 to June 12, 1980: an overview of the acute health impact. *JAMA* 1981;246:2585–2589.
57. Centers for Disease Control. Earthquake disaster—Luzon, Philippines. *MMWR* 1990; 39:573–577.
58. Woodruff BA, Toole MJ, Rodriguez DC, *et al*. Disease surveillance and control after a flood: Khartoum, Sudan, 1988. *Disasters* 1990;14:151–163.
59. Green LA, Wood M, Becker L, *et al*. The Ambulatory Sentinel Practice Network: purposes, methods, and policies. *J Fam Pract* 1984;18:275–280.
60. Centers for Disease Control and Prevention. Influenza—United States,1989–90 and 1990–91 seasons. *MMWR* 1992;41:(No. SS-3):35–46.
61. Valleron A-J, Bouvet E, Gaernerin P, *et al*. A computer network for the surveillance of communicable diseases: the French experiment. *Am J Public Health* 1986;76:1289–1292.
62. Center for Research on the Epidemiology of Disasters (CRED). *Sentinal epidemiologic surveillance in Bangladesh*. CRED Working Document No. 78. Brussels: CRED, 1989.
63. Blake PA. Communicable disease control. In: Gregg MB, editor. *The public health consequences of disasters*. Atlanta, GA: Centers for Disease Control, 1989:7–12.
64. Goodman RA, Buehler JW, Koplan JP. The epidemiologic field investigation: science and judgment in public health practice. *Am J Epidemiol* 1990;132:9–16.
65. Turnbull RK. Laboratory services in a refugee-assistance program. In: Allegra DT, Nieburg P, Grabe M, editors. *Emergency refugee health care—a chronicle of the Khmer refugee-assistance operation*. Atlanta, GA: Centers for Disease Control, 1983:153–157.
66. Pan American Health Organization (PAHO). *Environmental health management after natural disasters*. Washington, D.C.: PAHO, 1982:(scientific publication no. 430).
67. Binder S. Deaths, injuries, and evacuations from acute hazardous materials releases. *Am J Public Health* 1989;79:1042–1044.
68. Centers for Disease Control and Prevention. Surveillance for emergency events involving hazardous substances—United States, 1990–1992. *MMWR* 1994:43:(No. SS-2):1–6.
69. Toole MJ, Waldman RJ. Prevention of excess mortality in refugee and displaced populations in developing countries. *JAMA* 1990;263:3296–3302.
70. Centers for Disease Control and Prevention. Rapid assessment of vectorborne diseases during the midwest flood—United States, 1993. *MMWR* 1994;43:481–483.
71. Spencer HC, Campbell CC, Romero A, *et al*. Disease surveillance and decision-making after the 1976 Guatemala earthquake. *Lancet* 1977;2:181–184.
72. Centers for Disease Control and Prevention. Compendium of animal rabies control, 1993. *MMWR* 1993;42(No. RR-3):1–8.
73. Centers for Disease Control and Prevention. Comprehensive assessment of health needs 2 months after Hurricane Andrew—Dade County, Florida, 1992. *MMWR* 1993;42:434–437.
74. Kalsbeek W, Frerichs R. CSAMPLE: analyzing data from cluster survey samples. In: Dean AG, Dean JA, Coulombier D, *et al*. *Epi Info*, Version 6: a word processing, database, and statistics program for epidemiology on microcomputers. Atlanta, GA: Centers for Disease Control and Prevention, 1994, 157–182.
75. Dufour D. *Rapid assessment and decision making in emergency situations* [dissertation]. London: Univ. of London, 1987.

76. Thacker SB, Parrish RG, Trowbridge FL. A method for evaluating systems of epidemiologic surveillance. *World Health Stat Q* 1988;41:11–18.

77. Centers for Disease Control. Earthquake-associated deaths—California. *MMWR* 1989; 38:767–770.

78. Centers for Disease Control and Prevention. Flood-related mortality—Georgia, July 4–14, 1994. *MMWR* 1994;43:526–530.

79. Centers for Disease Control. Medical examiner/coroner reports of deaths associated with Hurricane Hugo—South Carolina. *MMWR* 1989;38:754–762.

80. Centers for Disease Control and Prevention. Preliminary report: medical examiner reports of deaths associated with Hurricane Andrew—Florida, August 1992. *MMWR* 1992; 41:641–644.

4

Managing the Environmental Health Aspects of Disasters: Water, Human Excreta, and Shelter

SCOTT R. LILLIBRIDGE

In addition to causing immediate adverse health effects such as injury and death, disasters disrupt environmental health safeguards that are critical for a population's survival, including the assurance of potable water, the proper management of human excreta, and the provision of shelter *(1)*. When such safeguards are interrupted, populations may experience increased rates of communicable diseases and other harmful effects related to exposure to cold weather, heat, or rain *(2, 3)*. Health professionals must understand the interplay between the environmental conditions and the status of a population's health if they are to provide effective relief services to a disaster-stricken community. For example, diarrheal illness resulting from the consumption of polluted drinking water or improperly prepared rations may require immediate action to purify water supplies or to dispose of contaminated food. Cold stress to a displaced population whose homes have been destroyed or increased rates of respiratory illness among persons residing in overcrowded community shelters are also examples of health problems that must be remedied through immediate improvements in the physical environment. Consequently, directing limited disaster relief resources toward the consequences rather than toward the root causes of inadequate states of environmental health may not be the most effective public health strategy to pursue in disaster situations. The purpose of this chapter is to help professionals whose skills are primarily in fields other than environmental health develop a better understanding of this aspect of disaster response.

Water Management In Disasters

Potable water is the most important immediate relief commodity necessary for ensuring the survival of disaster-affected populations, particularly when they have been displaced to regions where the supporting public health infrastructure has been destroyed *(4, 5)*. The primary importance of safe water in disaster-relief operations is not surprising when the roots of public health are considered. For example, the main reason life expectancy in developed countries has increased since 1900 is due to advancements in public sanitation *(6)*. Many of these advances were brought to communities through improvements in the quality of public water. In addition to the immediate life-sustaining benefits associated with the delivery of potable water, having clean water available also promotes other important sanitary and public health activities, ranging from hand washing to the provision of oral rehydration therapy.

In disaster-affected communities or displaced-persons camps where public water-purification activities have been disrupted, the population will be at much greater risk for waterborne diseases. In some cases the effects of waterborne diseases can be catastrophic. For example, cholera spread by water contaminated with *Vibrio cholerae* is estimated to have killed more than 50, 000 Rwandan refugees in camps just inside Zaire during the first weeks of July 1994 *(7)*. At the peak of this epidemic, the high crude mortality rate (CMR) reached 28–41 deaths per 10, 000 persons per day in the surveyed refugee camps. This epidemic occurred at a time of greatly reduced sanitary conditions. Specifically, the use of contaminated sources of water for human consumption by Rwandan refugees was identified as a primary cause of this infectious disease outbreak. Had treating diseases and injuries been the only focus of the relief effort rather than rapidly correcting the environmental sources of the epidemic, it is likely that the outbreak would have been worse and lasted much longer, particularly if susceptible refugees had continued to arrive. In this case, the CMR continued to decline and remained low, highlighting the importance of ensuring safe drinking water for acutely displaced populations. In addition, it was also apparent that earlier emergency environmental health interventions to assure potable water for the population might have *prevented* or reduced the size of the epidemic.

General Principles of Emergency Water Management

To reduce public health threats associated with the human consumption of contaminated water at disaster sites, emergency water programs must satisfy certain conditions. First, they must provide adequate quantities of water for fluid replacement, personal hygiene, cooking, and sanitation. If potable water supplies are insufficient in quantity, it is likely that populations will supplement their intake with water from unsafe sources. Second, programs must provide water of sufficient quality to prevent the transmission of disease. Potential sources of water for human consumption may need to be evaluated and treated to ensure potability. Last, because the quality and quantity of public water are so closely related to the health status of a disaster-affected population, emergency water programs must be an integral part of the public health component of disaster response.

Although health professionals must labor under political, logistical, and cultural constraints that make each disaster response somewhat unique, certain common procedures should generally be followed by those responsible for water management for disaster-affected populations (8–10). When emergency sources of water are urgently needed, officials should conduct a rapid environmental survey in order to help public health authorities establish relief priorities related to water management and other urgent environmental health concerns (8). In planning such a survey, health professionals should identify diseases endemic to the area and other pertinent surveillance data that might help in assessing the biologic risks associated with water sources at the disaster site (11). Sites with potential sources of water for a population's needs should be evaluated to determine their patterns of surface drainage, proximity to local sewage systems, and potential for chemical contamination. When evaluating a potential source of water for a disaster-affected population, health professionals must also consider the daily volume of water produced, its reliability as a continual source of water, and the costs associated with proper development. The rapidity with which a potential water system can be brought into service is often of paramount importance, particularly when managing displaced populations affected by waterborne epidemics. Untreated seawater can be used for bathing, for flushing toilets, and for most other purposes except human consumption.

When a population's normal source of potable water is contaminated, immediate remedial actions should be directed toward correcting the disaster-related factors that are degrading the quality of the water supply. Rapid environmental health remedies may include taking steps to halt the infiltration of public water by damaged sewage lines or repairing the brims of damaged community wells. Because the devastation of municipal water systems in urban areas may result in the sudden loss of potable water for large populations, the rapid repair of water-pumping stations or other mechanical components of the community's usual purification process should be a high priority in any disaster response (12, 13). If no water system is available because of the magnitude of the disaster or because the population has been displaced to undeveloped locations, new sources of potable water and methods for water distribution will need to be immediately developed.

When developing new sources of potable water at disaster sites, the most important factor to consider is its source. Surface water may be readily available but is subject to ongoing contamination from sewage, chemicals, or debris. However, with proper treatment, such water may be rapidly developed as an emergency source of potable water for a disaster-affected population. Groundwater from springs and wells may have superior microbiologic qualities when compared to surface water. If springwater is to be developed for human consumption, it is good practice to provide a barrier at its source to protect against surface contamination through the construction of a ''spring box'' (6). Ground water from shallow dug wells may be easily contaminated from surface drainage or through extravasation of polluted water from septic systems or latrines if the wells are not properly maintained, situated, or "skirted." Water from deeper drilled wells is usually superior to surface water in terms of microbiologic quality but may have unesthetic and occasionally harmful properties related to dissolved minerals *(6, 8)*. Unfortunately, the construction of drilled wells at disaster sites may require too much time and expense to be of use as a source of potable water during the initial days of an emergency response. In certain regions, rainwater may be sufficient to augment potable water supplies. However, such water may be contaminated unless steps are taken to maintain water quality during the collection or storage process (e.g., discarding the initial flow, maintaining chlorine residual during storage) *(8, 14, 15)*. Rainwater is also less reliable than sources developed from rivers or aquifers, since it may be prone to extreme seasonal variation.

Water Quality

Potable water is defined as water that is free from microbiologic or toxicologic contamination that would adversely affect human health. In general, water quality is assessed by laboratory analysis of representative water samples. Water characteristics such as microbial content, turbidity, color, salinity, pH, and chemical contamination may require immediate testing. Under emergency conditions, water quality analysis may be limited to testing for the presence of coliform bacteria or determining whether treatment with a water-purification agent such as chlorine is adequate.

Coliform organisms are found both in the environment and in the feces of animals and humans. Such microbial indicators are evaluated to determine whether pathogens might be present in drinking-water supplies. When coliform bacteria are found in treated water supplies, it suggests inadequate treatment or contamination after treatment *(16)*. Table 4-1 provides emergency guidelines for appraising the quality of potential water sources at disaster sites on the basis of their levels of coliform bacterial contamination *(8)*. *Escherichia coli (E. coli)* is also used as a microbial indicator of water quality. Its presence in water is more specific for fecal contamination consistent with human or other warm-blooded animal sources. Such water is considered unsafe for public consumption *(16)*.

Table 4-1 Microbial Guidelines for Water Samples Collected at Disaster Sites

Coliforms per 100 ml of Water	Water Quality
0–10	Reasonable quality
10–100	Polluted
100–1,000	Dangerous
>1,000	Very dangerous

Source: United Nations Children's Fund (UNICEF). *Assisting in emergencies: a resource handbook for UNICEF field staff.* New York: UNICEF, 1992.

In disaster settings and also in other less urgent situations in which water quality has been diminished, public health recommendations to ensure the potability of water include boiling the water to improve quality. CDC and the U.S. Environmental Protection Agency (EPA) recommend that water be rendered microbiologically safe for drinking by bringing it to rolling boil for one minute *(17)*. Boiling in that manner will inactive all major waterborne bacterial pathogens (e.g., *Vibrio cholerae, Yersinia enterocolitica*, enterotoxigenic *Escherichia coli, Salmonella, Shigella sonnei, Campylobacter jejuni*, and waterborne protozoa such as *Cryptosporidium parvum, Giardia lamblia*, and *Entamoeba histolytica (17)*. Boiling may be extended by one minute for every 1,000 meters of elevation above sea level *(16)*. However, boiling is usually not a practical method of rapidly purifying water when emergencies involve large populations, and boiling also carries the added burden of requiring a fuel source for heating *(10)*.

Because of the immediate demand for large volumes of potable water for disaster-affected populations, water for human consumption is usually obtained from readily available sources (e.g., rivers, lakes) and requires some form of chemical treatment for disinfection. Water may be treated with iodine, potassium permanganate, or chlorine in order to reduce microbiologic contamination *(14, 15)*. Iodine has been most useful for short-term disinfection of individual supplies of drinking water such as canteens and is often distributed in the form of "water-purification tablets" *(6, 16)*. Potassium permanganate ($KMnO_4$) has been used to treat large quantities of water such as water from springs or water in storage tanks. However, $KMnO_4$ has the drawback of requiring a relatively long contact time to disinfect water when compared to chlorine and may not be effective against *Vibrio cholerae* organisms *(14)*. Commonly, some form of chlorine is used at disaster sites to treat drinking water because of factors related to cost, availability, and the relatively low level of technical training that is required to monitor its use in the field. For example, ordinary household bleach (5.25% sodium hypochlorite) has been recommended for the emergency chlorination of drinking water for individual families by adding 6–8 drops per gallon of water and letting it stand for approximately 30 minutes *(6, 18)*.

Some parasitic diseases such as *Cryptosporidium parvum* are highly resistant to chlorination and are not easily killed or eliminated from water supplies without filtration *(17, 19)*. Filtration may also be required to remove other protozoans such as amoebas, giardia, and schistosomes *(6)*. Suitable filter materials for water filtration include sand, diatomaceous earth, and sand-anthracite combinations *(6, 8, 20)*. Although slow (gravity-driven) sand filters can be improvised in the field, it is best to seek professional consultation if large volumes of water will require filtration on a regular basis.

In addition to needing chemical treatment and filtration, some water sources may require a period of settling (sedimentation) to remove suspended particulate matter (turbidity) and to reduce biologic hazards before effective treatment can be accomplished *(21)*. Settling water supplies in areas protected from further contamination for 48 hours will significantly reduce the risk for schistosomiasis *(16)*. Unfortunately, chemical contamination from certain metals, chemical compounds, or toxins may not be removed through routine sedimentation, filtration, or chlorination *(6)*. It is also important to note that freezing at normal refrigeration temperatures will not kill all microbiologic organisms and is therefore not a suitable method of purifying water. Ideally, water should be "settled" to reduce biologic contamination and turbidity and then filtered prior to chlorination *(8)*. The addition of a coagulant such as alum can dramatically increase the rate of sedimentation.

When chlorine compounds are used to purify water for human consumption at a disaster site, testing to ensure an adequate chlorine residual should be part of routine environmental health surveillance. In the absence of filterable pathogens and turbidity levels greater than 1 Nephelometric Turbidity Unit (NTU)—which is a standard unit of light scattered by suspended particles in a water sample—water with free-chlorine residual concentrations of 0.2 to 0.5 mg/L with at least 30 minutes of contact time and a pH between 6.5 and 8.5 may be considered safe *(6)*. If water must be delivered rapidly to disaster sites, WHO recommends that water in tanker trucks should be treated with sufficient chlorine to ensure a concentration of 0.5 mg/L for a minimum of 30 minutes *(16)*. Under field conditions, such "indirect" biological monitoring based on the presence of bacteriocidal levels of chemical disinfectants may be easier to manage than directly measuring bacterial contamination.

Chlorine has greater bacteriocidal activity in water as a purifying agent at higher temperatures (e.g., greater bacteriocidal activity at 68° F compared with 36° F) and at lower pH and turbidity levels *(6)*. The amount of chlorine needed to purify water increases with the degree of contamination. However, the taste of water with higher residual free-chlorine levels in the range of 0.6 to 1.0 mg/L may begin to limit its acceptability to the population *(16)*. Common forms of chlorine that can be used in large quantities during emergencies include calcium hypochlorite bleaching powder and "High Test Hypochlorite" solutions *(6)*.

In addition to the frequent need to deliver external drinking water to a disaster site, flooded (and presumably contaminated) wells may need to be disinfected. Rehabilitating bored or dug wells usually involves repairing seals, protecting the contents from further surface-water runoff, and chemical disinfection. Table 4-2 lists typical recommendations for chlorinating dug wells that have been flooded. Such calculations are based on estimated well-water volumes *(18)*. In addition, during the well-decontamination process, the chlorine solution should be brought in contact with the entire surface of the well and associated piping for periods of 6 to 24 hours *(8, 18)*. On the following day, the well should be pumped until the chlorine odor disappears or until test results indicate that the well water is within an acceptable microbial and chemical range for human consumption.

Regardless of the standard used to evaluate water quality or to purify water supplies at disaster sites, water thought to be responsible for disease outbreaks should be considered contaminated until it can be retreated or retested to confirm its potability. Even if water has been adequately treated at a central location to ensure its potability, distribution systems at disaster sites that have temporarily lost the water pressure necessary

Table 4-2 Well Disinfection

Diameter of Well (in feet)	Bleach Calculations for Dug Wells	
	Amount of 5.25% Laundry Bleach per Foot of Well Depth	Amount of 70% Chlorine Granules Per Foot of Well Depth
3	1.5 cups*	1 ounce**
4	3.0 cups	2 ounce
5	4.5 cups	3 ounce
6	6.0 cups	4 ounce
7	9.0 cups	6 ounce
8	12.0 cups	8 ounce
10	18.0 cups	12 ounce

*one cup = 0.24 liter

**one ounce = 30 milliliter

Source: Centers for Disease Control and Prevention. *Flood: A prevention guide to promote your personal health and safety.* Atlanta: Centers for Disease Control and Prevention, 1993. *(18)*

to maintain a positive head of pressure throughout the pipe network should be immediately suspect for contamination. In addition, water that is to be brought to disaster sites and distributed as part of the relief effort should meet the same standards as any water designated for human consumption. Unfortunately, ''bottled'' water from commercial vendors may not meet normal quality standards for human consumption and should not be considered potable merely due to a commercial bottling process. If bottled water is used during relief activities, health officials should assess its origin, quality, and handling during transport. However, water-quality standards should not be used to keep water from a disaster-affected population; instead, they should be viewed as guides to promote the development of the highest quality of water that can be made available to the affected population given the immediate resource limitations. Once the emergency needs for potable water for the population have been addressed, public water systems should return to a more comprehensive program of regular water-quality testing *(14)*.

Distribution of Potable Water at Disaster Sites

Once potable water is made available to a disaster-affected population, it is important to locate distribution points within a reasonable distance to residential units to facilitate access. When displaced persons are located in temporary camps, water-distribution points in a camp system should not require persons to travel more than 100 meters to obtain potable water, and one spigot should be available for every 200–300 persons to provide adequate access to the population *(8, 20)*. Other than maintaining the quality of treated water at distribution sites, the most common problem associated with the distribution of potable water is managing wastewater and the runoff at distribution points. Inappropriately managed wastewater will collect in low areas and create odor or vector problems *(22)*. In addition, water-distribution vehicles may not be able to traverse mud hazards created by poorly managed drainage. The proper management of wastewater at disaster sites may require the construction of specialized drainage pits or soakage fields to manage the effluent *(8, 23)*.

According to the United Nations Children's Fund (UNICEF), people should receive 15–20 liters of potable water per day (Table 4-3) *(8)*. The absolute minimum amount of potable water to ensure a persons survival is in the range of 3–5 liters per person per day. However, such volume restrictions may be associated with a decline in the population's public health due to limitations imposed on personal hygiene. Heat stress and physical activity can substantially increase the human daily requirements for potable water to levels that are many times normal *(4, 23)*. Special attention must be given to ensuring that clinical facilities, feeding centers, and personal hygiene areas are supplied with adequate amounts of potable water (Table 4-3). Disaster victims may also require appropriate containers to transport potable water from the distribution points and to store it within their temporary shelters *(24)*. A recent study in Malawi showed that coliform-free water collected by refugees at distribution points soon had fecal coliform levels of 140/100 ml within just a few seconds after they filled their buckets. The source of this contamination was found to be the hands of the refugees who had contaminated the buckets during a previous process of rinsing out the buckets. The placement of a simple fixed-lid on the buckets reduced most of this contamination (written communication, Les Roberts, June 1995).

Disposal of Human Excreta

The improper management of human wastes even during nondisaster periods adversely affects public health. Communicable diseases that can be transmitted through contact with human feces include typhoid, cholera, bacillary and amoebic dysentery, hepatitis, polio, schistosomiasis, various helminth infestations, and common gastroenteritis *(10, 25, 26)*. Although most environmental health concerns relate to the management of human feces, in areas where *Schistosoma haematobium* and typhoid are endemic, proper disposal of urine may be an important public health consideration *(8)*.

Emergency methods used to dispose of human excreta include burying, burning, and composting *(8, 20, 26)*. Without an adequate amount of water, ''wet systems'' for excreta disposal that require flushing are impractical. In urban areas or communities with significant residual environmental health infrastructure, the provision and maintenance of a system of portable chemical toilets may be sufficient to manage human

Table 4-3 Daily Potable Water Needs Per Person

Liters	Need to be Addressed
15–20	Individual (optimum)
3–5	Minimum for survival
40–60	Health centers (per patient)
20–30	Mass-feeding centers (per beneficiary)
35	Washing facilities (per beneficiary)

Source: United Nations Children's Fund (UNICEF): *Assisting in emergencies: a resource handbook for UNICEF field staff.* New York: UNICEF, 1992.

wastes (feces and urine). In undeveloped areas or in regions where the sanitation infrastructure has essentially been destroyed, most populations will require some expedient form of burial such as dug latrines to manage human wastes *(8, 9, 20)*.

Methods of Human Excreta Disposal

The immediate sanitary objectives for health professionals at disaster sites are to control local defecation and to encourage the concentration of human wastes into areas where it can be managed appropriately *(10)*. The purpose of this activity is to limit the spread of human excreta into the water system and soil in order to reduce its potential to spread communicable diseases *(8)*. Such emergency waste-management efforts usually require the organization and maintenance of a latrine system. In its most basic form, such a system may be characterized by shallow earthen trenches or pits and accompanying hand-washing stations. Practical considerations associated with the disposal of human excreta into pits or trenches include knowledge of local soil conditions, drainage patterns, and the availability of water *(8)*. Public health officials also need to consider cultural norms of the population to be served by the sanitation system. For example, a large portion of the world's population have never been exposed to, nor do they normally use, Western-style latrines *(9)*. Other cultural factors that must be considered in the management of human excreta in the field under emergency conditions include a population's method of anal cleaning, need for privacy, cultural taboos, and previous sanitation practices *(8)*. It may also be necessary to educate the population on the proper use of toilet facilities and the disease potential from improperly managed human feces and urine, particularly if the population is unfamiliar with the design of the emergency sanitation facility being provided. Table 4-4 summarizes common public health strategies that may be useful in encouraging disaster-affected populations to dispose of their excreta at appropriate locations.

Ideally, temporary sanitation systems must be designed according to the physical constraints of the local environment and resource limitations rather than in response to

Table 4-4 Strategies to Control Human Surface Defecation at Disaster Sites

Designate specific areas for defecation

Protect latrines from surface water drainage

Consider cultural factors in latrine design (e.g., need for privacy)

Educate the population

Ensure proper latrine maintenance

Facilitate the population's access to latrines

---

a collection of disaster victims. If a shallow-trench latrine system is used, UNICEF recommends that trenches be at least 30 centimeters wide and 90–150 centimeters deep and that for every group of 100 persons to be served by the system, 3–5 meters of length should be added (8). If the ground is hard or has unacceptable percolation qualities, septic tanks, acquaprivies, or some temporary catchment device (e.g., bucket or steel drum) may be required to manage human wastes (20, 23). An emergency latrine system should provide at least one toilet seat (or squatting access point) per 20 persons (8). On the average, sanitation facilities require an estimated 2–5 liters of water per beneficiary per day for purposes of personal hygiene and facility cleaning. Temporary latrines should not be located closer than 6 meters from dwellings, 10 meters from community feeding stations and health centers, and 30 meters and downhill from community wells (8). Latrines located in temporary camps should not be established closer than 30–50 meters from expedient shelters (20).

Maintaining a Sanitation System for Human Excreta

When pit or slit trench latrine systems are used to manage human wastes, the regular addition of soil, diesel oil, or ashes to the latrine floor may help control insect vectors and reduce odors (8). Since it is unlikely that populations will use such facilities if they are not kept in a reasonable state of cleanliness, the sanitary maintenance of these facilities should be a high priority during the emergency-response period (26). Maintenance may require special contractual arrangements with local officials or relief organizations and accompanying public health education programs to ensure their continued use by the population. In addition to ensuring proper cleaning, temporary latrine facilities also require an adequate source of lighting for night use and proper adjustments in size to facilitate use by children. The maintenance of such a system will also require repairs and should be inspected periodically by health authorities. Relief agencies or governments that want to assist at disaster sites may provide technical assistance in the form of sanitarians, environmental engineers, hydrologists, material for latrine construction and maintenance, and disinfection supplies (8).

Shelter Management for Populations Affected by a Disaster

Basic mitigation strategies such as evacuating a coastal population before a hurricane's impact should include plans for managing the shelter needs of the relocated population. Apart from food and water, shelter is perhaps the most immediate need of disaster-stricken populations, particularly in cold weather. When displaced populations are suddenly subjected to severe cold stress, mortality rates may increase rapidly if proper shelter is not made immediately available *(27, 28)*. Without good logistical planning, delays in obtaining external shelter commodities like tents or plastic sheeting are common. Due to the importance of providing emergency shelter for disaster-affected populations, various relief organizations have stockpiled shelter materials in various locations throughout the world as part of strategic disaster preparedness *(9)*. In addition to the obvious health-related benefits associated with the provision of adequate shelter for a disaster-stricken population, such emergency construction is also necessary in the recovery phase for the development of more sophisticated relief services such as schools and health clinics.

In certain situations, such as earthquakes, the population may not want to rebuild or return to their homes until the risk from aftershocks has decreased and the debris has been removed *(8)*. Consequently, the demand for temporary shelter (or shelter-management services) may be great even in highly urbanized areas with surviving residential units. Cultural factors are also important to consider when planning the shelter needs of an affected population. For example, ethnic differences may prevent diverse populations from sharing shelter accommodations or even remaining within the same relief camp. In addition, it may be necessary to maintain family or clan identities in certain regions while rapidly addressing a population's emergency shelter needs.

Public Health Considerations Associated with Sheltering

Human factors also predispose certain individuals to the adverse health effects of cold stress. For example, the risk of death from exposure to cold weather following natural disasters is highest among the young, the aged, and the infirm *(27)*. Other factors, such as alcohol consumption, also increase a person's risk for succumbing to cold exposure *(29)*. Standing or working in water that is colder than 75° F will cause rapid loss of body heat and may place emergency responders as well as victims at risk for cold injury *(30)* (see Chapter 13 "Cold Environments"). When large segments of the population are to be evacuated from a disaster site, emergency-response workers must give special consideration to the needs of the elderly and the disabled. For example, Hurricane Elena (1985) resulted in the evacuation of more than a million coastal residents in Florida *(31)*. American Red Cross shelters housed 84, 000 people and experienced increased demands related to the needs of elderly shelter occupants (average age, 51 years). Such demands included special diets, oxygen, and a range of medications to treat chronic diseases.

Shelters containing large numbers of displaced persons should be monitored by an expanded public health surveillance system that collects information on populations affected by disasters *(32)* (see Chapter 3, ''Surveillance and Epidemiology''). Infectious disease surveillance of shelter should focus on whether diarrheal illnesses, acute respiratory diseases, and vaccine-preventable illnesses are present. In shelters housing large populations, information should also be gathered during environmental surveys to determine the source(s) of potable water and method(s) for disposal of human excreta. Emergency housing should minimize the risk of communicable disease due to overcrowding. If communal buildings are to be used as shelters for displaced populations, the minimum floor space should be at least 3.5 square meters per person *(33)*.

Physical Issues Associated with Shelter Management

At a minimum, effective sheltering at disaster sites should provide the occupants with a roof *(8)*. Materials such as plastic sheeting can be used to make temporary repairs on damaged residential units; such repairs protect the inhabitants while preventing further structural damage from environmental exposure. Plastic sheeting also requires minimal training for proper implementation *(9)*. Tents and prefabricated housing units may also be used to provide temporary shelter to disaster victims. However, they are considerably more expensive and heavier to transport than plastic sheeting and other material that might be used to effect repairs on existing residential structures.

During the emergency phase of a disaster, if tent camps are to be developed to shelter the population, the arrangement of tents should be orderly to facilitate census activity and public health surveillance, and to facilitate orderly camp management. Ideally, temporary camps should be planned and established around the availability of water and roads, and in areas with adequate surface drainage and soil conditions, well before the arrival of the population *(26)*. Such camps should provide at least 30 square meters of space per person *(8)*. To reduce the risk of fire in refugee camps, a 50-meter-wide firebreak is recommended for every 300 meters of temporary housing *(20)*. It is also important to remember that disaster victims in temporary shelters may require groundsheets, blankets, and a source of heating to be fully protected from the environment.

Conclusion

Populations affected by disasters often require emergency environmental health programs during the initial emergency response phase. Although this chapter has focused on the emergency management of water, human excreta, and shelter, other environmental health activities are also vital to the health of the population. Such activities include vector control, solid-waste management, injury prevention, personal hygiene, and proper food preparation and distribution. Emergency environmental health programs should begin with a rapid environmental survey to determine the needs of the disaster-affected population and the availability of local natural resources such as suitable land for emergency settlement. Health professionals must ensure that all disaster victims have access to a source of potable water, a system of sanitation, and adequate shelter. To achieve the greatest benefit for a disaster-affected population, coordinated environmental health activities should be an integral part of the overall emergency public health response.

References

1. Sidel VW, Onel E, Geiger HF, Leaning J, Foege WH. Public health responses to natural and human-made disasters. In: Last J, Wallace R, editors. *Maxcy-Rosenau-Last public health and preventive medicine*, 13th edition. Norwalk, CT: Appleton and Lange, 1992:1173–1185.
2. Blake PA. Communicable disease control. In: Gregg MB, editor. *Public health consequences of disasters*. Atlanta, GA: Centers for Disease Control, 1989:7–12.
3. Kilbourne EM. Cold environments. In: Gregg MB, editor. *Public health consequences of disasters*. Atlanta, GA: Centers for Disease Control, 1989:63–68.
4. Toole MJ, Waldman RJ. Prevention of excess mortality in refugee and displaced populations in developing countries. *JAMA* 1990;263:3296–3302.
5. Toole MJ, Waldman RJ. Refugees and displaced persons: war, hunger, and public health. *JAMA* 1993;270:600–605.
6. Salvato JA. *Environmental engineering and sanitation*, 4th ed. New York: John Wiley & Sons, 1992.
7. The Goma Epidemiology Group. Public health impact of the Rwandan refugee crisis: what happened in Goma, Zaire July 1994. *Lancet* 1995;345:339–343.
8. United Nations Children's Fund (UNICEF): *Assisting in emergencies: a resource handbook for UNICEF field staff*. New York: UNICEF, 1992:34–365.
9. Office of US Foreign Disaster Assistance (OFDA): *Field operations guide for disaster assessment and response*. Washington, D.C, OFDA, United States Agency for International Development (USAID), 1994.
10. Centers for Disease Control. Famine-affected, refugee and displaced populations: recommendations for public health issues. *MMWR* 1992;41(No. RR-13):1–74.
11. Armed Forces Medical Intelligence Center. *Disease and environmental alert reports* DST-1810H-227–92. Frederick, MD: Defense Intelligence Agency, 1992.
12. Centers for Disease Control. Public health consequences of a flood disaster—Iowa, 1993. *MMWR* 1993;42:653–656.
13. O'Carroll PW, Friede A, Noji EK, *et al*. The rapid implementation of a statewide emergency health information system during a flood disaster: Iowa, 1993. *Am J Public Health* 1995; 85:564–567.
14. Pan American Health Organization (PAHO). *Environmental health management after natural disasters*. Washington, D.C.: Pan American Health Organization, 1982.
15. Kozlicic A, Hadzic A, Hrvoje G. Improvised purification methods for obtaining individual drinking water supply under war and extreme shortage conditions. *Prehospital and Disaster Medicine* 1994;9:S25–S28.
16. World Health Organization (WHO). *Guidelines for drinking-water quality: recommendations*, Volume 1, 2nd ed. Geneva: World Health Organization, 1993:1–29.

17. Centers for Disease Control and Prevention. Assessment of inadequately filtered public drinking water—Washington, D.C., December 1993. *MMWR* 1994;34:667–669.
18. Centers for Disease Control and Prevention. *Flood: A prevention guide to promote your personal health and safety.* Atlanta: Centers for Disease Control and Prevention, 1993:1–11.
19. Panosian CB. Parasitic diarrhea. *Emerg Med Clin North Am* 1991;9:337–355.
20. Simmonds S, Patrick V, Gunn SW. Environmental health. In: *Refugee community health care*. New York: Oxford University Press, 1983.
21. Moeller DW. Water and sewage. In: *Environmental Health*. Cambridge, MA: Harvard University Press, 1992:54–79.
22. Lillibridge SR, Conrad K, Stinson N, Noji EK. Haitian mass migration: uniformed service medical support—May 1992. *Mil Med* 1994;159:149–153.
23. Department of the Army: *Field hygiene and sanitation. FM 21–10.* Washington, D.C.: Department of the Army, 1988:1–129.
24. Hoque BA, Sack B, Siddiqi M, *et al.* Environmental health and the 1991 Bangladesh Cyclone. *Disasters* 1994;17:143–152.
25. Morgan MT. Chronic and communicable diseases. In: *Environmental health*. Madison, WI: Brown & Benchmark, 1993:32–48.
26. Feachem RG, Bradley DJ, Garelick H, *et al. Sanitation and disease: health aspects of excreta and wastewater management.* New York: John Wiley & Sons, 1983.
27. Seaman J. Environmental exposure after natural disasters. In: Seaman J, editor. *Epidemiology of natural disasters.* Basel: Karger, 1984:87.
28. Centers for Disease Control. Public health consequences of acute displacement of Iraqi citizens—March–May 1991. *MMWR* 1991;40:443–446.
29. Abramowicz M. The treatment of hypothermia. *The medical letter on drugs and therapeutics.* 1994;36:116–117.
30. Centers for Disease Control and Prevention (CDC). *Extreme cold: a prevention guide to promote your personal health and safety.* Atlanta: Centers for Disease Control and Prevention, 1995:11.
31. Gulitz E, Kurtz A, Carrignton L. Planning for disasters: sheltering persons with special health needs. *Am J Public Health* 1990;80:879–880.
32. Centers for Disease Control. Surveillance of shelters after Hurricane Hugo—Puerto Rico. *MMWR* 1990;39:37–47.
33. Llewellyn CH. Public health and sanitation during disasters. In: Burkle FM, Sanner PH, Wolcott BW, editors. *Disaster medicine.* Hyde Park, NY: Medical Examination Publishing Co. Inc., 1984:133–168.

5

Communicable Diseases and Disease Control

MICHAEL J. TOOLE, M.D.

One of the most common myths associated with disasters is that epidemics of communicable diseases are inevitable. This myth is often perpetuated by the media and by local politicians who demand mass vaccination campaigns immediately following natural disasters such as hurricanes, earthquakes, and floods. The public's perception that disease outbreaks are imminent often derives from its exaggerated sense of the risk posed by dead bodies that remain exposed after an acute natural disaster. The truth is that communicable disease epidemics are relatively rare after rapid-onset natural disasters unless large numbers of people are displaced from their homes and placed in crowded and unsanitary camps *(1–3)*. On the other hand, numerous studies have shown a severe increase in the risk of epidemics during and after complex emergencies involving armed conflict, mass population displacement, relief camps, and food shortages *(4)* (see Chapter 20, ''Complex Emergencies'').

Causative Factors

Pathogens in the Disaster-Affected Area

If the pathogens that cause a disease are not present in the affected area and are not introduced after the disaster, then that disease will not occur even if environmental conditions are ideal for transmission. Outbreaks of communicable diseases after rapid-

79

onset disasters are more likely in developing countries than in industrialized countries. Risk factors in developing countries include poverty, poor access to clean water, poor sanitation, and low immunization coverage. Nevertheless, one cannot assume that specific pathogens do not exist in an area simply because there have been no published reports of disease caused by those pathogens. For example, toxigenic *Vibrio cholerae* 01 apparently persisted along the Gulf Coast of the United States *(5)* and in some waterways of Queensland, Australia, for years before being detected (G. Murphy, M.D., Queensland Department of Health, unpublished data). Other pathogens, such as *Shigella dysenteriae* type 1, *Neisseria meningitidis,* and the hepatitis E virus have been revealed as significant causes of epidemic disease in certain African countries only after outbreaks occurred in emergency settings *(6–8)*. In addition, certain diseases have only recently spread to previously disease-free regions; for example, cholera has emerged as a serious risk in Latin America only during the past 4 years *(9)*.

Population Displacement

The displacement of large populations rarely occurs as a result of acute natural disasters. Nevertheless, in 1973, floods in Nepal displaced many thousands of people, and in 1988, severe flooding in Khartoum, Sudan, destroyed the shanties of hundreds of thousands of *already displaced* southern Sudanese, creating the need for large, temporary camps. Following the Mount Pinatubo volcanic eruption in the Philippines in 1991, more than 100, 000 residents were displaced from their homes and placed in more than 100 evacuation camps *(10)*. In the United States, population displacement following acute natural disasters has been limited. Evacuation shelters, when established, have tended to be temporary; for example, the highest number of persons residing in shelters on any one day following the 1993 Midwest flood was 702 *(11)*.

The major cause of mass migration during the past 20 years has been civil war, in many cases complicated by famine. Almost 50 million people worldwide are currently refugees or internally displaced persons; many are living in camps where water, sanitation, and hygiene are inadequate *(12)*. Extensive epidemics of enterically transmitted diseases, including cholera, bacillary dysentery, and infection by the hepatitis E virus, have been common in these settings. Crowding, which is also a common characteristic of these camps, increases the risk of person-to-person transmission of measles, meningococcal meningitis, and acute respiratory infection (ARI).

Furthermore, mass migration may lead to epidemics of communicable diseases when populations residing in areas of low disease endemicity pass through or into areas of high endemicity during the course of their migration. Examples of explosive outbreaks of malaria among refugees with low levels of acquired malaria immunity include Cambodian refugees in eastern Thailand (1979), Afghan refugees in Pakistan (1980), Ethiopian refugees in eastern Sudan (1985), and Bhutanese refugees in Nepal (1992) *(4, 13)*. Refugees in Somalia and Sudan were exposed for the first time to schistosomiasis and leishmaniasis, respectively, when they moved into camps. The most recent pathogen whose transmission may be significantly affected by migration is the human immuno-deficiency virus (HIV). During the late 1980s, for example, many young male refugees from areas of southern Sudan, where the prevalence of HIV infection was low, migrated to areas of western Ethiopia where the HIV prevalence rate was relatively high. In the absence of active prevention programs, the HIV prevalence rate in this once largely unaffected group grew to 7% by 1992 (W. Brady, M.P.H., CDC, 1992, unpublished data).

Environmental Changes

Acute natural disasters may lead to an increase in the number of various disease vectors. Floods and hurricanes, for example, may lead to an increase in breeding sites for mosquitoes and thus to an increased mosquito population and an increased incidence of mosquito-borne diseases such as malaria, dengue, yellow fever, St. Louis encephalitis (SLE), Japanese B encephalitis, and *Wucheria bancrofti* filariasis in areas in which the pathogens are endemic. Dengue fever has been steadily increasing in incidence in many regions of the world during the past 10 years; the vector, *Aedes aegypti*, can be found in many areas that were previously free of the disease, including the Caribbean, South and Central America, and the southeastern United States. Sudden changes in mosquito breeding patterns following acute natural disasters may lead to unexpected epidemics of dengue and dengue hemorrhagic fever.

Disease vectors may have greater access to people who have lost their housing and are exposed to the environment (mosquitoes), are crowded together in camps (lice), or are brought into contact with rodents (fleas). In the United States, vector surveillance following Midwest floods in 1993 and Hurricane Andrew in 1992 documented no substantial increases in normal seasonal mosquito population densities; however, biting rates by nuisance mosquitoes increased because of damage to housing *(14, 15)*. Following both Hurricane Andrew and the 1993 Midwest flood, surveillance in affected states for vector-borne diseases such as SLE, dengue fever, and malaria showed no increase in seasonal incidence rates *(14, 15)*.

Epidemics of malaria followed Hurricane Flora in Haiti (1963) and flooding in Sudan in 1988 *(16, 17)*. Louse-borne relapsing fever and louse-borne typhus can pose a threat in areas with a reservoir, crowded living conditions, and heavy infestations with lice, but there are only a few such areas worldwide. A high prevalence of body lice has been reported among displaced persons and refugees in camps in Ethiopia, Somalia, Bosnia-Herzegovina, and Zaire. Outbreaks of louse-borne relapsing fever have been reported in refugee camps in Somalia (1986) and in transit camps for prisoners of war being transferred from Eritrea to Ethiopia in 1991 *(18, 19)*. Despite common fears of louse-borne typhus, few outbreaks have been reported since World War II; not a single case of typhus has been confirmed in the former Yugoslavia since the onset of war in 1991. The number of domestic flies may increase as a result of their breeding in feces, garbage, and dead animals and humans; flies may be able to transmit enteroviruses, *Shigella*, and conjunctivitis.

Other diseases spread by arthropods—such as leishmaniasis and murine and scrub typhus—are unlikely to occur as outbreaks after natural disasters. The recent outbreak of leishmaniasis in southern Sudan has been associated with mass population displacement due to war and the collapse of basic medical services in the region. The number of people bitten by dogs was observed to increase after an earthquake in Guatemala in 1976. Thus rabies may be a concern, although it would generally pose a serious threat only in areas in which domestic animals are the principal reservoir of the virus.

Floodwaters may spread the organisms that cause leptospirosis, typhoid fever, and a host of other potentially waterborne diseases. However, these diseases are more likely to be contracted through contaminated water supplies than through direct contact with floodwaters. Leptospirosis, which can be transmitted directly from contaminated water to skin and mucous membranes, appears to be an exception. Seaman *et al.* cite examples of outbreaks of leptospirosis following floods in Portugal (1967) and Brazil (1975) *(1)*.

An unusual environmentally related disease outbreak occurred in Ventura County following the 1994 southern California earthquake. During the 2 months after the earthquake, 170 people were diagnosed with acute coccidioidomycosis, an infection caused by the fungus *Coccidioides immitis*, which grows in soil *(20)*. During all of 1993, only 52 cases were reported in the county. This outbreak was associated with exposure to increased levels of airborne dust in the wake of the earthquake.

Loss of Public Utilities

Damaged or disrupted public water supplies, sewage systems, and power supplies may contribute to disease transmission following a disaster. The discontinuation of water services may lead people to use unclean water sources. A decrease in the quantity of water available may contribute to a deterioration in personal hygiene and lead to increased transmission of certain diarrheal diseases, including bacillary dysentery. The contamination of a large municipal water system, whether caused by breaks in the line, decreased pressure that allows sewage to enter the line, or a disruption to water treatment, can lead to the rapid transmission of pathogens to large numbers of people. One example that was not related to a natural disaster occurred in Sangli Town, Maharashtra State, India, in 1975 and 1976, when an estimated 9,000 cases of typhoid fever followed the failure of the municipal water system *(21)*.

Public utilities have been severely damaged during conflict-related emergencies in urban settings. For example, since the war began in Bosnia and Herzegovina in 1992, the quantity and quality of urban water supplies have deteriorated as a result of diverted water sources, cracked water pipes, a lack of diesel fuel to run water pumps, and frequent losses of water pressure that caused cross-contamination by sewage. In August 1993, piped water supplies in the capital, Sarajevo, were restricted to an average of 5 liters per person per day. (The Office of the United Nations High Commissioner for

Refugees [UNHCR] recommends a daily minimum water provision of at least 15 liters per person *[22, 23]*). Consequently, in Sarajevo between January and June 1993, the incidence of hepatitis A increased 5-fold, the diarrhea incidence increased 7-fold, and the dysentery incidence increased 12-fold. In contrast, active surveillance for typhoid fever in West Beirut and Sidon, Lebanon, between 1980 and 1982 showed a decrease in cases, despite an intensification of the conflict that resulted in interruptions in fuel supplies, water distribution, and environmental sanitary control measures during that time *(24)*.

Well-documented instances of waterborne disease outbreaks following natural disasters are unusual unless there are other complicating factors such as population displacement. In 1992, following extensive flooding in the war-ravaged Central Asian republic of Tajikistan, damage to water pipes caused the loss of 60% of the water supply in the affected districts, and the flooding of sewage treatment plants led to the contamination of river water. Despite these risk factors, surveillance revealed no significant increase in the seasonally adjusted incidence of diarrheal diseases (D. Koo, M.D., CDC, unpublished data, 1992). In contrast, flooding in the Sudanese capital of Khartoum in 1988 led to extensive contamination of wells and to a large increase in the proportion of morbidity that health facilities reported as being due to watery diarrhea *(17)*. One reason that waterborne disease epidemics are rare after natural disasters is that the risk is usually well recognized, and the provision of clean water is almost always a top priority. For example, although severe flooding in Iowa and Missouri in 1993 led to the disruption of public water and sewer systems in several counties, no increase in cases of diarrheal illness was reported in those or other affected counties *(25, 26)*.

Another reason why enteric disease outbreaks have been rare following acute natural disasters is that many disasters have occurred in areas that have no large, municipal water systems; instead, wells, streams, and springs are the primary water sources, and each usually serves a relatively small number of people. Such small water sources are unlikely to suffer additional contamination by human excrement after a disaster, and even when a source is contaminated, only a few persons are likely to be infected. One exception to this generalization occurred in 1971 in Truk District, Trust Territories of the Pacific, after a typhoon disrupted catchment water sources and forced people to use many different sources of groundwater that were heavily contaminated with pig feces. Consequently, there was an outbreak of 110 cases of balantidiasis (a disease caused by *Balantidium coli*, an intestinal protozoan whose principal natural reservoir is swine) (CDC, unpublished data). Other confirmed postdisaster outbreaks of waterborne disease include limited outbreaks of typhoid fever in Puerto Rico following Hurricane Betsy in 1956 *(27)* and in Mauritius following a cyclone in 1980 *(28)*.

Disruption of Basic Health Services

After disasters, routine public health services are often disrupted by the direct effects of the disaster and sometimes by ill-conceived efforts to divert routine health services into emergency relief programs. In developed countries, control programs for vector-borne and vaccine-preventable diseases may have achieved a level of coverage sufficiently high that temporary interruptions in routine programs may have minimal impact on the transmission of these diseases. In the United States, for example, basic health services were disrupted in wide areas in 1992 when Hurricane Andrew destroyed or damaged hospitals and health centers. However, free clinics were established almost immediately by the U.S. military and local health departments; surveillance showed no significant increase in morbidity due to communicable diseases *(29)*. In Bosnia and Herzegovina, many essential prevention programs have collapsed since the beginning of the war because health services have been diverted toward treating the war injured. In addition, the conflict has prevented much of the population from reaching health facilities, many of which have also been destroyed or heavily damaged. Consequently, antenatal care and child immunization programs have been severely curtailed. Only 22% to 34% of children in Sarajevo, Zenica, Bihac, and Tuzla have been immunized against measles; an average of only 49% against polio; and an average of only 55% against diphtheria and whooping cough *(22)*. Outbreaks of these diseases had not yet been reported by late 1994; however, they are inevitable if vaccination rates remain low.

In developing countries, the disruption of basic medical services because of disasters may have a greater public health impact. Even a brief interruption of preventive programs may be sufficient to give the pathogens an opportunity to spread rapidly. Inadequate clinical management of acute infectious diseases will contribute to an expansion of the reservoir of infection, thus promoting transmission in the area and high case fatality rates (CFRs) for particular diseases, especially malaria and dysentery. The risks may be increased by other postdisaster conditions, such as an increased number of mosquito breeding sites, population movements, and increased population density. The longer the disruption of basic medical services, the greater the risk of communicable disease outbreaks. Prolonged interruption of medical services is most likely to occur as a result of complex emergencies involving a degree of civil conflict. For example, civil war in Somalia from 1991 through 1993 led to the total collapse of the public health infrastructure; hospitals and clinics were destroyed or abandoned; and preventive programs, such as childhood immunization, ceased altogether. This collapse led to high mortality rates caused by extensive epidemics of measles and diarrheal diseases, including dysentery caused by *Shigella dysenteriae* type 1 and cholera. Community surveys in several districts of south-central Somalia in late 1992 indicated that 25% to 34% of deaths were due to measles *(30)*. A further 19% to 56% of deaths were attributed to diarrheal disease.

Impact of Food Scarcity and Hunger

Many types of disasters are associated with subsequent food shortages, especially in developing countries. Hurricanes and floods have destroyed crops and led to agricultural deficits several months later; for example, in 1974 in Bangladesh, extensive flooding that followed a hurricane led to famine and high death rates *(31)*. The intentional use of food as an instrument of war has been a common tactic in recent African civil conflicts, increasing the risk of famine; for example, wars in Mozambique (1984), Ethiopia (1985), Sudan (1988, 1993), Liberia (1990), Somalia (1992), and Angola (1993) have led to high prevalence rates of acute malnutrition among affected civilian populations *(4, 32)*. In most of these situations, elevated death rates were associated with increased rates of communicable diseases, including measles, malaria, ARI, and diarrheal diseases *(4)*. The relationship between malnutrition and communicable diseases is well known: diseases such as measles and diarrhea induce malnutrition, especially in young children, and malnutrition is associated with high CFRs for communicable diseases. Although malnutrition may not affect the incidence of communicable diseases, in disaster settings where the risk of malnutrition is high, one should expect high death rates related to endemic communicable diseases.

Specific Diseases Associated with Disasters

Communicable diseases reported in disaster settings have included (1) diseases transmitted person-to-person, including certain vaccine-preventable diseases; (2) enterically transmitted diseases; (3) vector-borne diseases. Most examples given here have been drawn from complex emergencies, where population displacement has been a major risk factor and high prevalence rates of acute malnutrition have contributed to high death rates. Tables 5-1 and 5-2 summarize outbreaks of communicable diseases attributable to acute natural disasters and to complex emergencies detected during the course of investigations by CDC since 1970.

Diseases Transmitted by Person-to-Person Contact

Measles
Few outbreaks of measles have been reported after acute natural disasters. One exception followed the volcanic eruption of Mount Pinatubo in the Philippines in 1991. More than 100, 000 people were displaced into evacuation camps; most of the displaced were members of the Aeta tribe who had lived on the slopes of the volcano. During the 3 months following the eruption, more than 18, 000 cases of measles were reported in the camps, representing 25% of all morbidity recorded in clinics *(10)*. Measles was associated with 22% of the deaths reported during the same period. Predisaster vaccination coverage levels in the Aeta tribe were very low, and attempts to vaccinate displaced children against measles were strongly resisted by tribal elders.

Outbreaks of measles within refugee camps were common prior to 1990 and caused many deaths. Low levels of immunization coverage, coupled with high rates of under-

Table 5-1 Outbreaks of Communicable Disease Attributable to Rapid-Onset Natural Disasters Detected in Postdisaster Investigations by the Centers for Disease Control and Prevention

Year	Country/State	Type of Disaster	Communicable Disease Outbreaks
1970	Peru	Hurricane	None
	U.S.A. (Texas)	Earthquake	None
1971	Truk District	Typhoon	Balantidiasis
1972	U.S.A. (S. Dakota)	Flood	None
	U.S.A. (Pennsylvania)	Flood	None
	Nicaragua	Earthquake	None
1973	Pakistan	Flood	None
1974	Sahel (W. Africa)	Drought/Famine	None
1976	Guatemala	Earthquake	None
1978	Zaire	Famine	None
	U.S.A. (Texas,	Tornado	None
	Oklahoma)		None
	Trinidad	Volcanic eruption	
	Dominica	Hurricane	None
	Marshall Islands	Flood	Respiratory infection
1980	Marshall Islands	Typhoon	None
	Mauritius	Cyclone	Typhoid fever
	U.S.A. (Washington)	Volcanic eruption	None
	U.S.A. (multiple states)	Heat wave	None
	U.S.A. (Texas)	Hurricane	None
1982	Chad	Drought, famine	None
	U.S.A. (Illinois)	Tornado	None
1983	Bolivia	Flood	None
1984	Mauritania	Drought, famine	None
	Bolivia	Drought, famine	None
1985	Puerto Rico	Flood	None
	Colombia	Volcanic eruption	None
1987	Somalia	Drought	None
1988	Bangladesh	Floods	None
	Sudan	Floods	Diarrheal disease, malaria
1989	France	Floods	None
	Puerto Rico	Hurricane	Acute respiratory infection
1990	Haiti	Drought	None
1991	Argentina	Volcanic eruption	None
	Bangladesh	Cyclone	None
	Philippines	Volcanic eruption	Measles
1992	U.S.A. (Florida,	Hurricane	None
	Louisiana)		None
	Nicaragua	Volcanic eruption	
	Tajikistan	Floods	None

Table 5-1 (*Continued*)

Year	Country/State	Type of Disaster	Communicable Disease Outbreaks
1993	Egypt	Earthquake	None
	Nepal	Floods	None
	U.S.A. (multiple states)	Floods	None
1994	Egypt	Floods	None
	U.S.A. (California)	Earthquake	Coccidioidomycosis
	U.S.A. (Georgia)	Floods	None

Sources: For 1970–1985: Ms. Nancy Nay, M.P.H., International Health Program Office, CDC, and Ms. Janis Videtto, Epidemiology Program Office, CDC; for 1986–1994: Eric K. Noji, M.D., National Center for Environmental Health, CDC, and International Health Activities Reports, ed. Virginia Sturwold, International Health Program Office, CDC.

nutrition and vitamin A deficiency, played a critical role in the spread of measles and the subsequent mortality within some refugee camps. Measles has been one of the leading causes of death among children in refugee camps; in addition, measles has contributed to high malnutrition rates among those who have survived the initial illness. Measles infection may lead to or exacerbate vitamin A deficiency, thus compromising immunity and leaving the patient susceptible to xerophthalmia, blindness, and premature death. In early 1985, the measles-specific death rate among children under 5 in one eastern Sudan camp was 30/1, 000/month; the CFR based on reported cases was almost 30% *(33)*. Large numbers of measles deaths were also reported in camps in Somalia, Bangladesh, Sudan, and Ethiopia *(34)*. Since 1990, however, mass immunization campaigns have been effective in reducing the measles morbidity and mortality rates in refugee camps (e.g., in Zaire, Tanzania, Burundi, and Malawi). Measles outbreaks, however, did not occur during other major refugee emergencies (e.g., among Somalis in Ethiopia in 1989 and among Iraqis in Turkey in 1991), probably because immunization coverage rates were already high in those refugee populations prior to their flight *(35)*.

Meningitis
The crowding associated with refugee camps places refugees in endemic areas at high risk for meningococcal meningitis, particularly those in countries within or near the traditionally described ''meningitis belt'' of sub-Saharan Africa *(7)*. Outbreaks have been reported in Malawi, Ethiopia, Burundi, and Zaire; however, mass immunization has proved to be an effective epidemic control measure in these situations, and meningococcal morbidity and mortality rates have been relatively low.

HIV and Other Sexually Transmitted Diseases
While not usually associated with natural disasters, the spread of HIV and other STDs may be associated with complex emergencies, especially when routine medical services

Table 5-2 Outbreaks of Communicable Disease Attributable to Complex Emergencies (Civil war, Refugees, and Famine)*

Year	Country	Type of Emergency	Communicable Disease Outbreaks
1979	Thailand	Refugees	Malaria
1980	Somalia	Refugees	Measles
1984	Mozambique	Civil war, famine	None
1985	Ethiopia	Civil war, famine	Meningitis, cholera
	Sudan	Refugees	Cholera, measles
1986	Somalia	Refugees	Hepatitis, non-A, non-B, Relapsing fever
1988	Malawi	Refugees	Cholera
1990	Ethiopia	Refugees	Hepatitis, non-A, non-B, pertussis
	Guinea	Refugees	None
	Malawi	Refugees	Cholera, measles
1991	Iraq/Turkey	Displaced persons	Cholera, dysentery
	Kenya	Refugees	Hepatitis E
1992	Azerbaijan	Civil conflict	None
	Bangladesh	Refugees	Diarrheal disease
	Ethiopia	Refugees	HIV
	Georgia	Civil conflict	None
	Nepal	Refugees	Measles, cholera, dysentery, Japanese B encephalitis
	Somalia	Civil war, famine	Measles, dysentery
	Zimbabwe	Refugees	Measles
1993	Angola	Civil war	Dysentery, cholera
	Armenia	Refugees	None
	Bosnia and Herzegovina	Civil war	None
	Burundi	Civil war	Dysentery
	Somalia	Civil war	Cholera
	Sudan	Civil war, famine	Measles, leishmaniasis
	Swaziland	Refugees	Cholera
	Tajikistan	Civil war, refugees	Cholera
1994	Angola	Civil war	Meningitis, hepatitis E
	Burundi	Refugees	Dysentery, cholera
	Rwanda	Civil war	Dysentery
	Sudan	Civil war	None
	Zaire	Refugees	Cholera, dysentery, meningitis

*Detected in the Course of Investigations by the Centers for Disease Control and Prevention.

Sources: For 1970–1985: Ms. Nancy Nay, M.P.H., International Health Program Office, CDC; for 1986–1994: International Health Activities Reports, ed. Virginia Sturwold, International Health Program Office, CDC.

break down. Several recent mass population migrations have taken place in areas where prevalence rates of HIV infection are high, such as Burundi, Rwanda, Malawi, Ethiopia, and Zaire. The HIV prevalence was 7% among adult male Sudanese refugees in western Ethiopia, one of the few refugee populations studied for this disease; the prevalence of infection among commercial sex workers living in the vicinity of the camp was greater than 40% (CDC, unpublished data, 1992). Serological surveys in this population also revealed high rates of previous infection with syphilis and chancroid. The contribution of HIV infection to morbidity and mortality among refugees has not been documented, but it may be significant. In the former Yugoslavia, there have been many reports of sexual assault and increasing prostitution; in addition, high rates of violence-related trauma have increased the rate of blood transfusions *(36)*. In this setting, where shortages of laboratory reagents to test blood for HIV are widespread, the risk of increased transmission of HIV is high, though such an increase has not yet been confirmed by studies.

Tuberculosis

Tuberculosis has not been associated with acute natural disasters; however, because the treatment of patients with active tuberculosis may be inadequate or incomplete during complex emergencies in which basic health services are disrupted, tuberculosis transmission may be increased in affected communities. Since the war began in Bosnia and Herzegovina in 1991, the incidence of new cases of tuberculosis has reportedly increased 4-fold *(36)*. Likewise, in Somalia during the civil war and famine of 1991–1992, routine case-finding, treatment, and follow-up of tuberculosis patients almost ceased. Consequently, there was a marked increase in both the incidence of new cases and the tuberculosis-related CFR *(37)*. Tuberculosis is well recognized as a health problem among refugee and displaced populations. The crowded living conditions and underlying poor nutritional status of these populations may foster the spread of the disease. Although not a leading cause of mortality during the emergency phase, tuberculosis often emerges as a critical problem once measles and diarrheal diseases have been adequately controlled. For example, in 1985, 26% of the deaths among adult refugees in Somalia and 38% of those among adult refugees in eastern Sudan were attributed to tuberculosis *(4)*. The high prevalence of HIV infection among many African refugee populations may contribute to the high rate of transmission.

Enterically Transmitted Diseases

Diarrheal Diseases

Diarrheal disease outbreaks have followed hurricanes and flooding in Bangladesh, Sudan, and Nepal; however, these disasters were complicated by significant population displacement, which seems to be the more significant factor in such outbreaks. Diarrheal diseases have emerged as the most lethal public health threat to refugees and internally displaced persons, whatever the cause of their displacement; for example, more than 70% of the deaths among Kurdish refugees in 1991 were associated with diarrhea *(38)*. Cholera epidemics have occurred commonly among refugees during the past decade; since 1985, cholera has been reported in camps in Somalia, Sudan, Ethiopia, Malawi, northern Iraq, Nepal, Bangladesh, Burundi, Rwanda, and Zaire *(4, 39)*. In most refugee settings, the CFR for cholera has been between 2% and 5% *(4)*. However, when cholera occurred among almost one million Rwandan refugees in the small Zairian town of Goma in July 1994, facility-based CFRs were as high as 22% during the early days of the epidemic *(39)*. Once adequate relief personnel arrived and treatment resources were obtained, the CFR dropped rapidly to 2%–3%. During the first month after the influx of refugees into Zaire, almost 50, 000 refugees died, an estimated 90% of the deaths being due to diarrhea or dysentery *(39)*. In addition, epidemic dysentery caused by *Shigella dysenteriae* type 1 has caused high morbidity and mortality rates among refugees in central and east Africa since 1992. Major dysentery epidemics have been reported among refugees in Burundi, Rwanda, Tanzania, and Zaire *(39, 40)*, as well as among displaced persons in Angola (P. Blake, M.D., personal communication, June 1994). CFRs for dysentery have been as high as 10% among young children and the elderly *(40)*.

Hepatitis

Outbreaks of hepatitis E infection among refugees in Somalia (1986), Ethiopia (1989), and Kenya (1991) have led to high overall attack rates and to CFRs among pregnant women as high as 17% *(8, 41)*. Because this disease has only recently been introduced to Africa, most adults have not yet been exposed to it. Because previous exposure to hepatitis A and B is relatively common in this region, any epidemic of hepatitislike illness in Africa with high attack rates among adults is likely to be caused by infection with the hepatitis E virus. The virus is enterically transmitted and is often associated with contamination of water supplies; the role of person-to-person spread is not yet clear, but it may not be an important mode of transmission.

Vector-Borne Diseases

Malaria

In 1963, in Haiti, an explosive malaria epidemic that followed Hurricane Flora caused more than 75, 000 cases of *Plasmodium falciparum* malaria; this outbreak was associated with a disruption of routine insecticide spraying and with changes to mosquito breeding sites caused by the hurricane *(16)*. Malaria has caused high rates of morbidity and mortality among refugees and displaced persons in countries where malaria is endemic, such as Thailand, eastern Sudan, Somalia, Kenya, Malawi, Zimbabwe, Burundi, Rwanda, and Zaire *(4, 39)*. Malaria-specific mortality rates have been especially

Table 5-3 Theoretical Risk of Acquiring Communicable Disease, by Type of Disaster

Disaster Type	Person-to-Person*	Water-borne†	Food-borne‡	Vector-borne§
Earthquake	Medium	Medium	Medium	Low
Volcanic eruption	Medium	Medium	Medium	Low
Hurricane	Medium	High	Medium	High
Tornado	Low	Low	Low	Low
Heat wave	Low	Low	Low	Low
Cold wave	Low	Low	Low	Low
Flood	Medium	High	Medium	High
Famine	High	High	Medium	Medium
Civil war/refuges	High	High	High	Medium
Air pollution	Low	Low	Low	Low
Industrial accident	Low	Low	Low	Low
Fire	Low	Low	Low	Low
Radiation	Low	Low	Low	Low

*Shigellosis, streptococcal skin infections, scabies, infectious hepatitis, pertussis, measles, diphtheria, influenza, tuberculosis, other respiratory infections, giardiasis, HIV/AIDS, other sexually transmitted diseases, meningococcal meningitis, pneumonic plague.

†Typhoid and paratyphoid fevers, cholera, leptospirosis, infectious hepatitis, shigellosis, campylobacteriosis, Norwalk agent, salmonellosis, *E. coli* (enterohemorrhagic, enterotoxigenic, enteroinvasive, and enteropathogenic), amebiasis, giardiasis, cryptosporidiosis.

‡Typhoid and paratyphoid fevers, cholera, infectious hepatitis, shigellosis, campylobacteriosis, salmonellosis, *E. coli* (enterohemorrhagic, enterotoxigenic, enteroinvasive, and enteropathogenic), amebiasis, giardiasis, cryptosporidiosis.

§Louse-borne typhus, plague, relapsing fever, malaria, dengue, viral encephalitides.

high when refugees from areas of low malaria endemicity have fled through, or into, areas of high endemicity. The severity of malaria outbreaks in Africa has been exacerbated by the rapid spread of chloroquine resistance during the 1980s. While the theoretical risk of other vector-borne diseases is high following disasters, few outbreaks of diseases such as dengue, SLE, Japanese B encephalitis, and yellow fever have been reported. Outbreaks of louse-borne relapsing fever have been reported from refugee camps in Ethiopia and Somalia.

Table 5-3 summarizes the theoretical risk of acquiring various types of communicable diseases following different types of disasters.

Public Health Measures

Appropriate measures to prevent and control communicable disease after disasters include sanitary measures (sanitation, provision of clean water, and vector control), medical measures (vaccination, laboratory services, and case management), and public health surveillance.

Sanitary Measures

Providing adequate quantities of relatively clean water is probably more effective than supplying small quantities of microbiologically pure water. UNHCR and WHO recommend that each displaced person be supplied with at least 15–20 liters of water per day *(23)*. In addition, adequate sanitation facilities should be provided, as well as an adequate supply of soap and appropriate hygiene education. Among children less than two years of age, breast-feeding will provide considerable protection against communicable diseases, including diarrhea; attempts to introduce or distribute breast-milk substitutes and infant feeding bottles should be strongly opposed in an emergency situation. Food protection and vector control are two other important interventions in certain settings. Efforts to control vectors may be extremely expensive and should not be automatic responses; action should be based on knowledge of diseases and specific vectors in the disaster area. Surveillance following the Midwest floods in 1993 showed almost no evidence of SLE activity among mosquito vectors in South Dakota, Iowa, and Illinois; therefore, contingency plans for large-scale mosquito adulticiding were not implemented. Mosquitoes and lice are usually the primary targets because flies and rodents are much more difficult to control and present less of a health hazard. The goal of postemergency sanitation measures should be restoring the predisaster levels of environmental services rather than attempting to improve on the original levels.

After an acute natural disaster, political leaders and public health officials are often under considerable pressure to take action to control communicable diseases. This pressure may come from the public, the news media, overseas donors, and volunteer relief workers, as well as from politicians themselves who want to do something visible to help. Unfortunately, political leaders and public health officials at the scene of a disaster may have had no experience dealing with emergencies and may believe communicable diseases to be a major threat when they are not. It is essential that these fears be addressed by establishing a surveillance system that is simple, accurate, and timely, and by convincing concerned officials that decisions regarding communicable disease control should be made in response to the data generated by the surveillance system. The public perception that epidemics follow disasters often centers on concern about the presence of many bodies on the streets and in public places. In reality, corpses of previously healthy people do not harbor dangerous pathogens; they pose no threat to the health of the living, other than being aesthetically disagreeable and possibly contributing to a larger fly population.

Medical Measures

Vaccination

Public pressure for action to control communicable disease following a disaster often focuses on the perceived need for mass vaccination, in particular against cholera and typhoid, diseases that the public commonly associates with disasters. Because the possibility of food and water being contaminated with human excrement often increases after a disaster, the risk of typhoid fever and cholera may well be greater than usual. In the case of refugees and displaced persons living in camps where water and sanitation facilities are inadequate, the elevated risk has been well documented. However, for the following reasons, mass vaccination against cholera and typhoid fever is not usually indicated:

- If the organism is not present in the area and has not been introduced after the disaster, the disease poses no threat regardless of environmental conditions. Thus, where the organism is not present (e.g., typhoid fever in the United States, cholera in Western Europe), it is highly unlikely to pose a problem even if water supplies are contaminated. At present, cholera may be a threat following disasters in Africa, Asia, much of Latin America, and parts of the former Soviet Union, such as the Central Asian republics and the Caucasus.
- The most practical and effective strategy to prevent waterborne cholera and typhoid is to provide clean water in adequate quantities and adequate sanitation. Sufficient soap and hygiene education will further prevent the transmission of waterborne diseases.
- A mass vaccination campaign cannot provide protection against typhoid at the time of greatest risk from contaminated water because multiple doses are required to achieve adequate immunity. Currently, the most affordable vaccine for developing countries (parenteral, heat-phenol-inactivated vaccine) has relatively low efficacy, requires two serial doses 1–4 weeks apart, and has severe side effects. The newer oral, live-attenuated vaccine (Ty21) has higher efficacy; however, it is expensive and must be administered in four serial doses *(42)*.
- The traditional parenteral cholera vaccine often used in epidemic settings in the past was only 50% effective in preventing cholera and is no longer recommended by WHO *(43)*. Of the two newer and potentially effective vaccines currently available, one requires two doses and does not induce immunity until 7–10 days after the second dose; the other, a single-dose, oral, live vaccine, has never been subjected to testing under field conditions and its use in disaster-affected populations would be controversial.
- Receiving a dose of vaccine may give people affected by disasters a false sense of security and lead them to fail to take elementary precautions such as boiling water or adequately reheating leftover food.
- Adverse reactions to both cholera and typhoid vaccines are frequent and sometimes severe, merely adding to the misery of disaster-affected communities.

On the other hand, disasters that cause significant displacement of populations into crowded camps create a high risk of *measles* transmission, especially in areas where immunization coverage rates are low. Measles immunization is the single most cost-effective public health intervention among children in developing countries. All children between the ages of 6 months and 12 years should be immunized against measles soon after their arrival in a refugee camp. Children 6 to 8 months of age should have a second dose of measles vaccine as soon as they reach 9 months of age *(34)*. One dose of vitamin A should be administered simultaneously with the vaccination, but only in children aged 9 months or older.

In areas where epidemics of *meningococcal meningitis* are known to occur, such as in Africa's "meningitis belt," surveillance for meningitis should be established. In the event of an outbreak, vaccination should be considered if (1) the presence of meningococcal disease is laboratory confirmed and (2) serogrouping indicates the presence of group A or group C organisms. If it is logistically feasible, the household contacts of people identified as cases should be checked and those needing immunizations should be given them. In some instances, however, organizing a mass immunization program may be simpler. Because cases of meningococcal meningitis are likely to cluster geographically within a refugee camp, it may be most efficient to focus the vaccination campaign on the affected area(s) first. The vaccination of children and young adults 1 to 25 years old will generally cover the at-risk population *(7)*.

Tetanus has not been common after disasters, and mass tetanus vaccination programs are not indicated. However, tetanus boosters may be indicated for previously vaccinated people who sustain open wounds or for other injured people, depending on their tetanus immunization history. Passive vaccination with tetanus immune globulin (Hypertet) is useful in treating wounded people who have not been actively vaccinated and those whose wounds are highly contaminated, as well as those with tetanus. *Gas gangrene* was an important problem for people with deep penetrating wounds, avulsions, open fractures, and crush injuries after the eruption of the Nevado del Ruiz volcano in Columbia in 1985; however, gas gangrene equine antitoxin is of little use against the disease, both because its efficacy is unknown and because allergic reactions to it may be severe.

Chemoprophylaxis

Mass chemotherapy to prevent diseases such as cholera and meningitis is usually not recommended. However, to prevent reinfection during outbreaks of meningococcal meningitis in refugee camps, health personnel should simultaneously administer chemoprophylaxis with rifampicin to all members of a household where a case has been diagnosed *(7)*. Recovering patients should also be administered chemoprophylaxis to eliminate carriage of the organism. Mass chemoprophylaxis has not proved to be an effective cholera control measure and is not recommended. If resources are adequate, health personnel might consider providing a single dose of doxycycline to immediate family members of patients with diagnosed cases. In some instances, chemoprophylaxis may be indicated for refugees arriving in an area with endemic malaria, especially if targeted to vulnerable groups such as young children and pregnant women. However, since *Plasmodium falciparum* malaria is resistant to chloroquine in most areas of the world, the use of newer drugs may be prohibitively expensive and may lead to relatively frequent adverse reactions.

Case Management

The most effective management of acute watery diarrhea, including cholera, is oral rehydration therapy (ORT) supported by adequate nutrition, including continued breast-feeding (44). Health workers need to be well trained in how to clinically assess dehydration, provide oral rehydration therapy in supervised settings, and treat severe diarrheal illness with intravenous therapy, appropriate antibiotics, or both. In the event of an outbreak of *cholera*, early case finding will allow treatment to begin rapidly. Aggressive case finding by trained community health workers should be coupled with community education to prevent panic and to promote good domestic hygiene. Treatment centers should be easily accessible. If the attack rate for cholera is high, health officials may need to establish temporary cholera wards to handle the patient load. Health centers should be adequately stocked with ORS, IV fluids, and appropriate antibiotics. Although rehydration efforts should be aggressive, they also must be carefully supervised, especially when children are rehydrated with intravenous fluids, in order to prevent fluid overload. Antibiotics, which should be administered orally, have been shown to reduce the volume and duration of diarrhea in cholera patients. Tetracycline is the antibiotic of choice if the pathogen is sensitive, although single-dose doxycycline can be used when available. In recent outbreaks in emergency settings, *Vibrio cholerae* 01 has been resistant to multiple antibiotics; in such situations, especially in developing countries, the use of more expensive antibiotics may not be indicated, and treatment efforts should focus on rehydration *(44)*.

Dysentery caused by *Shigella dysenteriae* type 1 has become increasingly common in African disaster settings. Appropriate treatment with antimicrobial drugs both decreases the severity and duration of dysentery caused by all species and serotypes of *Shigella*, and reduces the duration of pathogen excretion. The choice of a first-line drug should be based on knowledge of local susceptibility patterns. If patients do not respond within 2 days, the antibiotic should be changed to another recommended for shigellosis in the area. Patients showing no improvement after a further 2 days of treatment should be referred to a hospital or at least a laboratory where stool microscopy may be performed. Case management of dysentery has been complicated by the increasing resistance of *S. dysenteriae* type 1 to common, affordable antibiotics *(6)*. In the Zaire outbreak, the organism was resistant to all antibiotics except ciprofloxacin, which was used to treat those patients at high risk of mortality (young children, pregnant women, the elderly, and the severely ill). The emergence of dysentery caused by antibiotic-resistant strains of *Shigella dysenteriae* type 1 as a major public health problem among refugee populations in central Africa indicates the need for operational research to develop more effective prevention and case management strategies.

In disaster areas where malaria is endemic, a thorough epidemiologic assessment should be performed to assess the morbidity and mortality load due to malaria. Because health personnel are rarely able to have a microscopic examination of blood smears conducted for all patients, they need to establish the proportion of febrile illness attributable to malaria. Standard treatment policies also need to be developed, with clinical case definitions and drug regimens based on local chemosensitivity patterns.

Tuberculosis

During the early phase of any emergency relief operation, tuberculosis activities should be limited to the treatment of patients who present themselves to the health care system and in whom tubercle bacilli have been demonstrated. Although ensuring patient compliance with a protracted chemotherapy regimen may be easier in the confined space of a refugee camp, the personnel needed to supervise treatment may not be available. In addition, the uncertain duration of the refugees' stay, frequent changes of camp locations, and poor camp organization may hinder tuberculosis treatment programs. Therefore, tuberculosis control programs should not be established until other, more critical priorities have been adequately addressed (45).

Laboratory Services

Laboratory services are important but may be overused; not every person with a communicable disease needs to have laboratory confirmation of that fact. However, to control communicable diseases, emergency workers do need laboratory services to help them determine the causative agent and its antibiotic sensitivity in representative cases so that they can take appropriate control measures, provide effective treatment, and subsequently document that the pathogen has been controlled. These services are particularly critical in establishing whether cholera, typhoid fever, meningococcal meningitis, bacillary dysentery, and malaria are present. Laboratories that can do simple tests may be established in or near the disaster area; for more sophisticated tests, specimens need to be transported (in appropriate containers and conditions) to reference laboratories.

Communicable Disease Surveillance

Perhaps the most important element in the control of communicable diseases after disasters is the establishment of effective surveillance (4). When no reliable information is available on the occurrence of infectious disease, rumors fill the void, panic may result, and political and public health leaders may be forced to waste resources on unwise and unneeded control measures. On the other hand, when the leaders are confident that they have current and reasonably comprehensive information on the occurrence of infectious diseases, they are able to reassure the public with facts and can plan rational control measures as needed. To be effective, a surveillance system for the purposes of communicable disease control should be led by one person (preferably a national epidemiologist) or one agency whose primary responsibility is to maintain the surveillance system. It should also have the capacity to perform the following functions:

- Identify and focus on the communicable diseases of public health importance most likely to appear in the disaster-affected area.
- Establish reliable transportation and communications to the area(s) where communicable diseases are either being reported or most likely to occur.
- Identify an appropriate reference laboratory and develop a system for storing and transporting relevant specimens from the field to the laboratory.
- Standardize routine (or sentinel site) morbidity and mortality surveillance, including standard case definitions and reporting forms. (Diseases may be reported in terms of symptom complexes, such as fever with cough, watery or bloody diarrhea, and fever and rash. Reporting forms should be simple and the number of diseases reported should be kept to a minimum in order to ensure cooperation and compliance by clinic workers and to avoid overwhelming the various reporting levels with a large amount of unnecessary data.)
- Promptly investigate any unusual events detected by the surveillance system. (Differentiating disaster-related disease rates from predisaster baseline levels may be difficult because disease ascertainment may be significantly improved after a disaster; apparent increases in disease rates may be due to better reporting.)
- Promptly investigate reports or rumors of communicable disease outbreaks. (Political sources, unofficial community sources, reports from relief workers, and newspaper accounts should be taken seriously, since these informal sources may contain information on disease problems that have not been detected by the established surveillance system. Serious investigation of these reports will build confidence among the public that health officials are reacting responsibly.)
- Report daily to the central level until the situation stabilizes, and then report weekly. (Daily reports should include the absence of any cases of certain communicable diseases—such as cholera and measles—about which the public is likely to be especially concerned.)
- Analyze and disseminate surveillance reports in a timely manner to all persons and agencies who have an interest in the information. (Secrecy or slowness will breed distrust and seriously detract from the credibility of the surveillance system. Tabulation and analysis should not be so complex as to overwhelm the epidemiologists and prevent them from conducting field investigations and disease-control activities. When population denominators are not available, morbidity due to communicable diseases may be presented in terms of proportional morbidity. Surveillance reports should be disseminated as regularly as possible [e.g., weekly] in the form of a routine newsletter or bulletin.)

- Continue the surveillance until well after the emergency phase, even though enthusiasm may wane rapidly. (Outbreaks of communicable diseases may be quite late sequelae of disasters because exposure to the agents may be delayed [e.g., mosquito populations may not increase until some time after the initial disaster] or because the incubation period may be long [e.g., hepatitis].)

Conclusion

Although outbreaks of communicable diseases may occur after rapid-onset natural disasters, very few such outbreaks have been observed during the past few decades. In contrast, complex emergencies related to armed conflict, population displacement, crowded relief camps, and famine have been followed by numerous epidemics of communicable diseases, including cholera, dysentery, measles, and meningitis. Factors associated with many kinds of disasters may contribute to the transmission of communicable diseases; therefore, the establishment of public health surveillance and the implementation of appropriate sanitary and medical measures should be routine elements of the response to disasters.

Acknowledgement

The format of this chapter and much of the text is based on Chapter 3, "Communicable Disease Control," by Paul Blake, M.D., M.P.H., in *The public health consequences of disasters, 1989.* Atlanta: Centers for Disease Control, 1989.

References

1. Seaman J, Leivesley S, Hogg C. *Epidemiology of natural disasters.* New York: Karger, 1984.
2. World Health Organization. Communicable diseases after natural disasters. *Wkly Epidemiol Rec* 1986;11–14;79–81.
3. de Ville de Goyet C. Maladies transmissibles et surveillance epidemiologique lors de desastres naturels. *Bulletin de l'Organization mondiale de la Sante* 1979;57:153–165.
4. Centers for Disease Control and Prevention. Famine affected, refugee, and displaced populations: recommendations for public health issues. *MMWR* 1992;41:RR–13.
5. Blake PA. Cholera—a possible endemic focus in the United States. *N Engl J Med* 1980; 302:305–309.
6. Ries AA, Wells JG, Olivola D, *et al.* Epidemic *Shigella dysenteriae* type 1 in Burundi: pan-resistance and implications for prevention. *J Infect Dis* 1994; 169:1035–1041.
7. Moore PS, Toole MJ, Nieburg P, *et al.* Surveillance and control of meningococcal meningitis epidemics in refugee populations. *Bull World Health Organ* 1990;68:587–596.
8. Mast EE, Polish LB, Favorov MO, *et al.* Hepatitis E among refugees in Kenya: minimal apparent person-to-person transmission, evidence for age-dependent disease expression, and new serological assays. In: Kishioka K, Suzuki H, Michiro S, Oda T, editors. *Viral Hepatitis and Liver Disease* Tokyo: Springer-Verlag, 1994:375–378.

9. Centers for Disease Control and Prevention. Update: cholera—Western Hemisphere, 1992. *MMWR* 1993;42:89–91.

10. Centers for Disease Control and Prevention. Surveillance in evacuation camps after the eruption of Mt. Pinatubo, Philippines. *MMWR* 1992;41(Special Suppl. No. 4):9–12.

11. Centers for Disease Control and Prevention. Morbidity surveillance following the Midwest flood—Missouri, 1993. *MMWR* 1993;42:797–798.

12. U.S. Committee for Refugees. *World Refugee Survey, 1994.* Washington, D.C.: U.S. Committee for Refugees, 1994.

13. Marfin AA, Moore J, Collins C, *et al.* Infectious disease surveillance during emergency relief to Bhutanese refugees in Nepal. *JAMA* 1994;272:377–381.

14. Centers for Disease Control and Prevention. Emergency mosquito control associated with Hurricane Andrew—Florida and Louisiana, 1992. *MMWR* 1993;42:240–242.

15. Centers for Disease Control and Prevention. Rapid assessment of vectorborne diseases during the Midwest flood—United States, 1993. *MMWR* 1994;43:481–483.

16. Mason J, Cavalie P. Malaria epidemic in Haiti following a hurricane. *Am J Trop Med Hyg* 1965;14:533–539.

17. Woodruff BA, Toole MJ, Rodriguez DC, *et al.* Disease surveillance and control after a flood: Khartoum, Sudan, 1988. *Disasters* 1990;14:151–162.

18. Brown V, Larouze B, Desve G, *et al.* Clinical presentation of louse-borne relapsing fever among Ethiopian refugees in northern Somalia. *Ann Trop Med Parasitol* 1988;82:499–502.

19. Sundnes KO, Haimanot T. Epidemic of louse-borne relapsing fever in Ethiopia. *Lancet* 1993; 342:1213–1215.

20. Centers for Disease Control and Prevention. Coccidioidomycosis following the Northridge earthquake—California, 1994. *MMWR* 1994;43:194–195.

21. Sathe PV, Karandikar VN, Gupte MD, *et al.* Investigation report of an epidemic of typhoid fever. *Int J Epidemiol* 1983;12:213–219.

22. Centers for Disease Control and Prevention. Status of public health—Bosnia and Herzegovina, August–September 1993. *MMWR* 1993; 42:973, 979–982.

23. United Nations High Commissioner for Refugees. *Water manual for refugee situations.* Geneva, Switzerland: United Nations High Commissioner for Refugees, 1992.

24. Armenian H. Perceptions from epidemiologic research in an endemic war. *Soc Sci Med* 1989; 28:643–647.

25. Centers for Disease Control and Prevention. Public health consequences of a flood disaster—Iowa, 1993. *MMWR* 1993;42:653–656.

26. Centers for Disease Control and Prevention. Morbidity surveillance following the Midwest flood. *MMWR* 1993;42:797–798.

27. Masi AT, Timothee KRA, Armijo R. Estudio epidemiologico de un brote hidrico de fiebre tifoidea. *Bol San Pan* 1958;45:287–293.

28. Centers for Disease Control. *Typhoid fever outbreak in Cite Roche Bois, Port Louis, Mauritius.* Internal memorandum. EPI-80–45-2, May 10, 1982. Atlanta, GA: Centers for Disease Control, 1982.

29. Lee LE, Fonseca V, Brett K, *et al.* Active morbidity surveillance after Hurricane Andrew—Florida, 1992. *JAMA* 1993;270:591–594.

30. Moore PS, Marfin AA, Quenemoen LE, *et al.* Mortality rates in displaced and resident populations of central Somalia during 1992 famine disaster. *Lancet* 1993;41:913–917.

31. Curlin GT, Hossain B, Chen LC. Demographic crisis: the impact of the Bangladesh war (1971) on births and deaths in a rural area of Bangladesh. *Population Studies* 1976; 330:87–105.

32. Macrae J, Zwi AB. Food as an instrument of war in contemporary African famines: a review of the evidence. *Disasters* 1993;16:299–321.

33. Shears P, Berry AM, Murphy R, Nabil MA. Epidemiological assessment of the health and nutrition of Ethiopian refugees in emergency camps in Sudan, 1985. *BMJ* 1987;295:314–318.

34. Toole MJ, Steketee RJ, Waldman RJ, Nieburg P. Measles prevention and control in emergency settings. *Bull World Health Organ* 1989;67:381–388.

35. Toole MJ, Waldman RJ. Refugees and displaced persons: war, hunger, and public health. *JAMA* 1993;270:600–605.

36. Toole MJ, Galson S, Brady W. Are war and public health compatible? *Lancet* 1993;341:935–938.

37. Sudre P. *Tuberculosis control in Somalia*. Report EM/TUB/180/E/R/5.93. Geneva, Switzerland: World Health Organization, 1993.

38. Yip R, Sharp TW. Acute malnutrition and high childhood mortality related to diarrhea. *JAMA* 1993;270:587–590.

39. Goma Epidemiology Group. Public health impact of Rwandan refugee crisis: what happened in Goma, Zaire, July 1994. *Lancet* 1995;345:339–344.

40. Centers for Disease Control and Prevention. Health status of displaced persons following civil war—Burundi, December 1993–January 1994. *MMWR* 1994;43:701–703.

41. Centers for Disease Control. Enterically transmitted, non-A, non-B hepatitis—East Africa. *MMWR* 1987;36:241–244.

42. Centers for Disease Control and Prevention. Typhoid immunization. Recommendations of the Immunization Practices Advisory Committee. *MMWR* 1990;39(RR-10):1–5.

43. World Health Organization. *Guidelines for cholera control*. Report WHO/CDD/SER/80.4, Second Revision. Geneva, Switzerland: World Health Organization, 1990.

44. World Health Organization. *The treatment of acute diarrhea*. Report WHO/CDD/SER/80.2, First Revision. Geneva, Switzerland: World Health Organization, 1984.

45. Rieder HL, Snider DE, Toole MJ, *et al. Tuberculosis control in refugee settlements*. Tubercle 1989;70:127–134.

6

Mental Health Consequences of Disasters

ELLEN T. GERRITY
BRIAN W. FLYNN

The mental health consequences of exposure to a natural or technological disaster have not been fully addressed by those in the field of disaster preparedness or service delivery. Although the effects of exposure to trauma and disaster are viewed with various degrees of horror, sympathy, and fear by the general population and the media, a pervasive societal belief continues to exist that money can heal any psychological wounds resulting from the trauma and loss that disaster victims experience. When the wounds do not heal quickly, the phenomenon of blaming the victim can emerge. In this phenomenon, the victim's situation is viewed as unique or rare or is tied to personal characteristics or responsibility, and thus, is not deserving of large-scale or long-term support from society. This phenomenon, based in large part on fear of their own potential victimization, allows people who did not experience the disaster to view both the disaster and the victim's reactions as aberrations that are somehow individually caused, and thus separated from and unrelated to normal life.

Yet experiencing a disaster is often one of the single most serious traumatic events a person can endure, and this experience can have both short- and long-term effects on mental health and functioning, such as dissociation, depression, and post-traumatic stress disorder. To understand these effects, we must first grasp the nature of trauma, understand what happens to people when they experience it and then try to cope, and acknowledge what works and what does not in the process of recovery. Large-scale preparedness and emergency response programs need to consider the behavioral and emotional factors underlying the responses of people to such trauma, responses that can lead to the ultimate success or failure of disaster-relief and -preparedness programs.

Historical Perspectives

Summary of Disaster Mental Health Research

What do we already know about the mental health consequences of disasters? Several recent reviews (*1–4*) have summarized the scientific research literature for the strongest findings about how adults and children are affected by exposure to disasters. Research in this field has generally focused on questions related to the nature of mental health problems, the identification of specific groups who may be most at risk, and what factors in the environment or in the individual may modify the effects of exposure.

Although many people continue to believe that exposure to natural and technological disasters does not lead to psychological problems, strong evidence exists to the contrary. Research shows that mental health problems can result from exposure to natural and technological disasters (*2, 5–13*). These psychological problems include post-traumatic stress disorder (PTSD), depression, alcohol abuse, anxiety, and somatization. Other kinds of problems, including physical illness; domestic violence; and more general symptoms of distress, daily functioning, and physiological reactivity, have also been documented. These problems have been shown to occur when people experience a variety of natural disasters, such as volcanoes, fires, tornadoes, floods, and mudslides, as well as technologic disasters, such as the Three Mile Island nuclear reactor disaster, dam-break disasters, and building collapses (*1, 4*).

In a comprehensive review of the literature, Meichenbaum (*3*) compiled an extensive list of factors that appear to make people more vulnerable to the development of psychological problems, including the following:

- objective and subjective characteristics of the disaster, such as proximity of the victim to the disaster site, the duration of the disaster, the degree of physical injury, and the witnessing of grotesque scenes
- the characteristics of the postdisaster response and recovery environment, such as community cohesion, secondary victimization, and the disruption of social support systems
- the characteristics of the individual or group; for example, vulnerability to psychological problems has been shown to be greater among the elderly, the unemployed, single parents, children separated from their families, those with a history of psychological problems, and those for whom marital or marital discord existed before the disaster.

How long these reactions last is an important concern for crisis-counseling programs, and to date our knowledge about this is dependent upon the duration of research studies investigating the mental health consequences of disaster. Longitudinal studies are relatively rare and generally still somewhat restricted in duration (usually lasting at most about 2 years); the information is scarce about effects lasting beyond that time period. Within this time frame, however, a pattern of early recovery is emerging—with resolution of problems for many people within 16 months, but with problems persisting for some people for as long as 3 to 10 years after exposure to technological disasters. These kind of controlled studies allow us to obtain critical information about the mental health consequences of disasters; however, it is often difficult to conduct a scientifically sound study in a disaster-affected community.

Methodological Problems of Disaster Studies

Often, disaster researchers have been trained and are experienced in conducting field or community research, but during disasters, they will be conducting research under crisis conditions in which most aspects of community life are in a state of extreme flux, if not chaos. In general, practical issues such as the safety and health of the victims are paramount, and frequently research issues (e.g., obtaining access to victims, finding space and equipment, obtaining funding and local support) have a low priority. The practical details of disaster research are much more difficult to overcome, particularly with the design and timing issues linked so closely to the data-collection process and the scientific questions being pursued.

Because predisaster baseline data is virtually impossible to obtain, except in those rare instances when a disaster occurs in a specific community not long after a comparable mental health study has been completed (*11*), a direct causal link between disasters and mental health consequences is difficult to determine. Researchers rely on appropriate methodologies and statistical analysis techniques to develop models and determine relationships among key variables. Such methods and techniques include the use of using comparison or control groups, collecting retrospective data, and relying on early data collection during the acute phase of recovery to examine these questions. Norris and Kaniasty (*14*) have reviewed the reliability of retrospective data.

Despite difficulties, the inherent importance of the questions motivates disaster researchers to continue their efforts. Disaster and other trauma researchers often appreciate the value of crisis situations as a unique window through which the psychological mechanisms of human survival can be viewed most clearly. Both the positive and negative extremes of human behavior that occur in crisis situations underscore the normal process of human development and change. In addition, participating in research projects can become an avenue in which meaning can be created from an otherwise meaningless event; for researchers, providing that opportunity can be rewarding. Funding support for acute response research, by the National Institute of Mental Health (the RAPID program) and the National Science Foundation (the Quick Response Program), has also helped to alleviate the practical problems of getting started (see Footnotes 1 and 2).

Training Issues for Disaster Research and Service Providers

Within the specialty area of traumatic stress research, investigators are conducting disaster research with ever-increasing levels of scientific sophistication and sensitivity to human concerns. The number of research studies has increased and the focus on key questions, such as treatment methods, acute-response issues, and the variations in response among ethnic and racial groups, has direct implications for recovery and service delivery.

However, without appropriate training, researchers new to traumatic stress research may approach the field of disaster research with a naïveté that can lead to problems at a disaster site. For example, inexperienced researchers may make demands regarding access to victims during the early periods of disaster response, thus interfering with critical recovery efforts. Social science researchers who want to enter the field of disaster research must prepare themselves thoroughly by obtaining the necessary training to conduct research appropriately. Even trauma researchers from non-disaster-related traumatic stress specialties (e.g., domestic violence, combat trauma) should carefully consider how the nature of the trauma may affect how data can be collected, analyzed, and understood.

Those conducting training programs for mental health service providers face similar issues. Generally, recruiting mental health professionals to participate in disaster-recovery programs is not difficult, particularly during the acute phase. However, the challenge still remains to orient inexperienced mental health professionals to this work before, during, and after a disaster strikes. Academic programs in the traditional mental health disciplines generally contain little crisis-intervention training, and although these courses provide clinicians with skills to diagnose and treat mental illness, clinicians are rarely taught how to provide support for or enhance mental health, particularly during a crisis. Nearly all disaster mental health intervention training occurs outside of traditional university-based clinical training programs; most occurs after disaster strikes. Clearly, more training and more research on effective training methods is needed.

1. RAPID Program, Program Announcement #PA-91-04; Contact: The National Institute of Mental Health, Violence and Traumatic Stress Research Branch, Parklawn Building, Room 10C-24, 5600 Fishers Lane, Rockville, Maryland 20857.

2. National Science Foundation Quick Response Grants; Contact: Ms. Mary Fran Myers, Natural Hazards Research and Applications Information Center, Campus Box 482, University of Colorado, Boulder, Colorado 80309-0482.

Providing Mental Health Services in Disasters Before Disaster Strikes

Responding effectively to the psychological needs of people after a disaster depends on advance planning. Unfortunately, governments and other groups have seldom emphasized the psychological consequences of disaster as a critical part of disaster preparedness, even when plans to deal with other issues are in place. Without planning, key questions go unanswered or will have to be answered in the midst of the crisis. For example, what groups will respond to the acute needs of survivors? What training do they have or need? What are their specific responsibilities? What are the priorities for service delivery? How will human resources be coordinated, monitored, and evaluated?

Careful attention to these and other key issues can help ensure that qualified people provide critical, timely, and appropriate psychological services. Planning also helps to ensure that the mental health service community can combat problems created by the uncontrolled and often unsolicited offers of assistance that often follow large-scale disasters. Such assistance may be well-intentioned but can also be of dubious quality.

Effective response by mental health service professionals can be enhanced by incorporating mental health planning into disaster-preparedness activities at all levels. Individual mental health agencies should have a disaster plan in place. Although hospitals usually have general disaster plans as a requirement for hospital accreditation, they seldom consider their specific institutional role in providing mental health services or the impact of a large-scale disaster on the mental health of their employees. Additionally, county, state, and federal mental health authorities need to work closely with their governmental counterparts who are responsible for general emergency preparedness for their region.

In recent years, disaster response has become an increasingly formal and structured activity. For the mental health community to be a full participant in this response effort, it must learn (or establish) its role and know the roles of others before disaster strikes. These various key players and their roles in responding to disasters, as well as the role mental health agencies can play, have been thoroughly described in an excellent overview by Myers (*15*).

System-Level Response to Mental Health Needs

Initial Response: What Do We Know?

During small-scale, non-federally-funded responses to emergencies, the individual mental health provider or local mental health agency may have no established role in the official response by authorities and may receive little assistance from government or other agencies. However, the greater the severity of a disaster and the more it begins to overwhelm local and state resources, the greater the likelihood that communities will find that outside assistance in the form of consultation and funding is available to them. If the mental health community is fully involved in disaster planning, it will be prepared to determine what outside assistance or funding it needs to respond rapidly and appropriately to the disaster. Preplanning and full involvement in local emergency preparedness are essential to rapid and coordinated mental health response.

The American Red Cross usually offers assistance in the aftermath of all disasters, regardless of their size or severity. This organization responds to events ranging from a single family emergency (such as a house fire) to a catastrophic disaster (such as the Hurricane Andrew disaster in Florida in 1992). Furthermore, in 1992, the Red Cross fully implemented its Disaster Mental Health Services Program (*16–17*). This program, which trains licensed mental health professionals to extend disaster mental health services on site to Red Cross workers and primary victims (*18*), is designed to work closely with local mental health agencies.

During a relatively smaller-scale local emergency such as a train or plane crash, little or no government assistance is available to mount a public health response that addresses the psychological consequences of disasters. Local mental health providers rely heavily on their own established programs and resources, as well on resources available through the Red Cross and other voluntary groups.

When the needs created by a disaster exceed the resources of the local and state governments, a state's governor may request a Presidential Disaster Declaration. Should this declaration be made and have included within it provisions for services to people as well as state agencies, states then become eligible to apply for funding to support crisis counseling and training programs and public information and education services through the Robert T. Stafford Disaster Relief and Emergency Assistance Act (P.L. 100–707). This Act is administered by the Federal Emergency Management Agency (FEMA). The crisis-counseling program provisions in the Act (Section 416) are administered through an interagency agreement by the Emergency Services and Disaster Relief Branch (ESDRB) in the Center for Mental Health Services (CMHS), which is part of the Substance Abuse and Mental Health Services Agency (SAMHSA), of the U.S. Public Health Service (*19*). A full description of this program can be obtained from the ESDRB (see Footnote 3). Through the crisis-counseling programs, short- and long-term funding programs are available; when combined, these programs provide funding for services very quickly (within fourteen days of the presidential declaration) until one year after the disaster.

The crisis-counseling program has been providing funding for mental health services for the last 20 years and has accumulated a wealth of experience and knowledge about the delivery of mental health services after disasters. Because research has not been a component of this program, systematic data collection and program evaluation have not been routinely performed. Nevertheless, the practical experience gained at the local and national level has been enormously useful in handling each succeeding disaster. The Stafford National Disaster Relief legislation has helped fund crisis counseling programs

3. Emergency Services and Disaster Relief Branch, Center for Mental Health Services, Parklawn Building, Room 16C-26, 5600 Fishers Lane, Rockville, Maryland 20857.

in 35 states and territories, with the number of programs growing steadily over the years. In 1994, nearly $60 million was awarded for crisis counseling services in the wake of disasters in the United States.

Impediments to System-Level Response

The most significant impediment to organized disaster response in the public sector has been the changing nature of the public mental health system. Comprehensive community mental health centers, the cornerstone of the federal mental health services initiative during the 1960s and 1970s, are increasingly rare. Today, in most areas of the country, the public mental health system is largely (and often exclusively) oriented to serving people with severe and persistent mental illness. More broad-based programs, such as general client outpatient services, school programs for children, specialized programs to serve the elderly, and consultation and education programs, which are similar in structure and function to that of disaster crisis counseling programs, are nearly nonexistent. Because of changes in the public mental health system, one often finds that the foundation upon which to build a crisis-counseling program no longer exists.

As a result, public community mental health agencies, which remain the primary sponsors of crisis-counseling programs, often face a significant mission conflict as they find themselves in the awkward position of being called upon to provide essential broadbased services after disasters. After years of effort to define agency functions for specific populations and relatively narrow programs within their communities, directors of community health programs now must respond to very different demands from their communities and governmental funding sources, who will expect them to respond rapidly and with a much broader organizational orientation during and after a disaster.

Positive Outcomes of System-Level Response

In addition to whatever else disasters may be, they are always political events. No matter how clearly circumscribed an agency's role may be in normal times, its ability to respond rapidly and appropriately to human and community needs during and after a disaster will have an impact on its standing and reputation. Many community mental health agencies have found that successful leadership in disaster mental health programs has solidified the organization's political and funding status in their communities. The perception remains in most communities that, regardless of the specific population normally served by community mental health agencies, individuals will look to these agencies for overall leadership and guidance in times of disasters.

Ironically, while the established organizational mission of community mental health agencies often appears to be antithetical to the mission of crisis-counseling programs, the recently developed case management model (now an integral part of most mental health provider agencies) has much in common with what disaster crisis counselors do. Many community mental health programs have found that a crisis-counseling program has been instrumental in the creation of strong new relationships with other health and social services agencies. These new relationships then become a resource for providing services to their established clientele long after the disaster response is over.

Characteristics of Mental Health Services, Service Recipients, and Service Providers

Effective mental health services dealing with disasters are different from traditional mental health services in several important ways. These differences result from distinctive points of view regarding (1) who the service recipient is and (2) how best to provide assistance.

Service Recipients

While recognizing that there will be individuals and groups with special needs, the overarching principle of mental health services after disasters is that the recipients of services are normal people, responding normally, to a very abnormal situation. Inherent in this perspective is the belief that the people served have a history of successful coping, even if they may be temporarily unable to cope with what they have experienced. It is assumed that, given appropriate assistance, including education about what they are going through emotionally and otherwise, most individuals will return to normal functioning.

Most disaster survivors who experience psychological sequelae after a disaster have never been recipients of mental health services and usually do not see themselves as candidates for psychotherapy or other treatment. For this reason, as well as because of their assumed absence of psychopathology, it is critical that a psychological diagnosis not be assigned indiscriminately or prematurely. Because the stigma of mental illness still exists in our society, a strong psychiatric or diagnostic approach might be inappropriate and potentially harmful when applied during crisis-intervention efforts. Since traditional mental health services, on the other hand, may be inclined to take such a position, it is important that mental health service providers receive appropriate crisis-intervention training.

Necessary and Appropriate Service

The federal disaster mental health program is based on a crisis-counseling model. Crisis-counseling programs are designed to provide relatively short-term interventions with individuals and groups experiencing psychological reactions to large-scale disasters. The goals of this type of intervention are (1) to assist people in understanding their current situation and reactions; (2) to assist in their review of options; (3) to provide emotional support; and (4) to encourage and support connection with other individuals and agencies who may assist the individual. This kind of assistance is focused on helping the person deal with an actual current situation and rests on the assumption that the individual is capable of resuming a productive and fulfilling life following the disaster experience. The person's efforts to resume a normal life are supported by the offer of assistance and information at a time and in a manner appropriate to his or her experience, education, developmental stage, and ethnicity. Individuals are helped to cope with the psychological aftermath of the disaster, to mitigate additional stress or psychological harm, and to develop coping strategies that the individual may be able to call upon in the future. The programs have an outreach orientation and strive to bring the services directly to the people in need.

Crisis counseling should not be perceived or defined as mental health "treatment." "Treatment," as typically defined in the mental health community, implies some type of psychological disorder or disease. This diagnosis of a disorder or disease is made following a psychological assessment conducted by a licensed mental health professional. Treatment interventions vary widely in techniques, philosophy, goals, and duration, and include various forms of psychotherapy ("talk" therapies) and psychopharmacology (drug treatment). This kind of treatment may involve a variety of goals and techniques not found in crisis counseling. These include, but are not limited to, efforts to develop insight into a wide variety of historical and current life experiences, resolution of unconscious conflicts, personality reconstruction, and long-term treatment of mental disorders.

Written documentation is incomplete and sometimes inconclusive, but throughout the 20 years of the federal crisis-counseling program, many service providers report that, in general, while large numbers of people may demonstrate some of the symptoms associated with some psychological disorders (most notably depression, anxiety, and post-traumatic stress disorder), relatively few develop a diagnosable mental disorder significant enough to warrant treatment as described above.

Experienced providers involved with disaster crisis-counseling programs over the years have also observed that the needs and psychological sequelae of disaster survivors are neither neatly categorized nor straightforward. During the disaster-recovery period, some individuals may benefit greatly from brief psychotherapy in addition to crisis-counseling services. Providers in the traditional mental health system and the disaster crisis-counseling programs should coordinate their efforts to provide optimal mental health services after disasters for their more seriously affected clients. Furthermore, individuals with a preexisting mental disorder can also experience new disaster-related problems and should be able to avail themselves of the services and expertise of the disaster crisis-counseling program in addition to their regular treatment.

Because of the mental health competence of most disaster survivors, the service provider should attempt to determine the personal and psychological strengths of the person and elicit a discussion of coping mechanisms successfully used by the individual in the past. Although similar to other kinds of psychosocial history-taking in clinical settings, the focus of this history in crisis counseling is on emotional trauma history and the management of earlier crisis situations so that the individual can be assisted in reestablishing coping mechanisms that have been beneficial in the past.

Outreach Services

Because of factors like the "normalcy" of the disaster population and the enduring negative stigma associated with mental health treatment, people seldom seek assistance for their psychological problems following a disaster; therefore, nearly all successful mental health programs must bring these services directly to people where they are during this time of crisis, such as shelters, new or temporary homes, churches, or schools.

The Natural Helping Network

Following disasters, people tend to turn to their traditional sources of support and assistance, such as the extended family, the church, the school, and the primary care physician. It is important to recognize the key role that such individuals and groups can play in effective disaster stress education and intervention. All members of natural helping networks should be included in community education and/or training efforts. It is also important to remember that these individuals (or someone close to them) may also be primary victims; some providers may also become secondary victims—that is, they may experience additional disaster-related problems as a result of their multiple roles as victim and provider.

Active and Directive Caregiving

Many mental health professionals have been trained in nondirective caregiving techniques—that is, techniques that focus on reflection, fairly passive support, and the development of insight. These techniques, however, appear to be both inadequate and inappropriate for most recent disaster victims. For most victims, the disaster experience is an extraordinarily new one. Disaster survivors may have difficulty seeing a relationship between their past and their current experience. In addition, especially in the first days and weeks following a disaster, survivors are overwhelmed by the sheer magnitude and complexity of the tasks facing them and the new organizations with which they must now interact (e.g., FEMA, Red Cross, insurance companies). Thus, survivors often seem to respond best to directive caregiving—that is, very concrete suggestions regarding how to organize and prioritize tasks, and how to manage their stress and respond to the needs of their loved ones. Techniques that are less directive, although effective in long-term therapy, work less well in crisis counseling.

Services Providers

The 20-year history of the federally funded crisis-counseling experience indicates that effective crisis counselors do not necessarily require the background and credentials of licensed mental health professionals. They do need:

- sound training in disaster mental health theory, crisis-counseling techniques, screening and identification of persons who may be in need of mental health treat-

ment, stress management and coping strategies, and sensitive and active listening skills
- comfort with nontraditional helping roles
- comfort in using outreach methods such as participation in community meetings, and working with people at home, church, school, or local businesses, rather than relying on the more usual office appointment structure
- knowledge of the culture, structure, and resources of the community

Furthermore, in order to use trained nonprofessionals, these disaster mental health programs must have:

- provisions for supervision of nonprofessionals by licensed mental health professionals who have specialized disaster mental health training
- an established and well-functioning referral system for seriously affected individuals who may require extensive treatment

These suggestions are not intended to eliminate mental health professionals from providing disaster-related psychological services; such professionals can and often do provide such services very effectively. At the same time, having training and experience as a mental health professional does not ensure that any particular individual has the skills and characteristics necessary to be an effective disaster mental health provider. Additional training may be needed. The test of the match includes the following factors:

- the extent to which mental health professionals can integrate alternative conceptualizations, ones that may be very different from their prior training and work experiences (e.g., absence of diagnosis, interventions in very nontraditional settings, role ambiguity)
- degree of comfort in working with paraprofessionals or trained nonprofessionals
- directive caregiving skills
- ability to incorporate crisis counseling theory and practice into the theoretical framework that usually guides the practitioner's interventions (e.g., psychoanalytical, cognitive/behavioral, insight-oriented approaches)

Similarities to Traditional Mental Health Services

Although this chapter thus far has focused on the uniqueness of services provided to disaster survivors, there are many ways in which the skills used in traditional mental health treatment positively transfer to disaster work. These include the practitioner's abilities to

- understand the history and cultural context in which the individual operates
- practice active listening
- assess the support systems which exist(ed) for the individual

Sequence and Nature of Human Response

It is widely accepted that human psychological response to disaster follows a sequence (*18, 20–21*). While the specific characteristics of this sequence may vary, in most instances the psychophysiological sequence includes a progression that moves from activated defenses, through early stage responses, to an anger and frustration phase, and finally to some level of resolution. At the community level, an analogous progression of change also occurs. In comparing these two spheres of experience—psychophysical and sociocultural—the stages of the sequential changes in each depends to some extent on the characteristics of the specific disaster, such as the suddenness of impact, duration of the event, and probability of reoccurrence. Furthermore, because the pattern of change for human and community responses is neither straightforward nor simple, and because individual behavior may vary widely, these variables also influence the nature of individual and community recovery. Table 6-1 illustrates these patterns of change.

Table 6-1 The Sequence of Psychological Response to Disaster

Event Sequence .		*Psycho/Physical Sequence*		*Socio/Cultural Sequence*
Warning (long/short/none)	→	**Defenses activated** (fight/flight, trauma history)	→	**Varied** (family/community preparedness)
Alarm (may not exist)	→	**Heightened anxiety** (various psychophysiological reactions)	→	
Impact (confined/ widespread)	→	**Stun reaction**	→	**Heroism** (extraordinary feats/ leadership)
Inventory/Rescue (assess the impact, care for injured)	→	**Mood and attitude extremes** (joy/relief/disillu- sionment/frustration)	→	**Honeymoon** (celebration of survival)
Recovery (short/protracted)	→			
Reconstruction	→	**Ambivalence** (reality of loss/salvage sets in)	→	**Disillusionment** (reality of loss, frustration with government)
	→	**Varied Responses** (learning/growth, long-term health/psychological effects)	→	**Reconstruction** (new social and political patterns)

Psychological Response

Individual and community responses to disaster are numerous and have been explored in a variety of ways by disaster researchers (*9, 12–13, 15, 21–24*). Within the typical range of psychological responses soon after a disaster, a number of indications of disaster-related stress are seen. These reactions are often categorized as (1) psychophysiological, (2) behavioral, (3) emotional, and (4) cognitive.

- Psychophysiological signs include fatigue, nausea, fine motor tremors, tics, profuse sweating, chills, dizziness, and gastrointestinal upset.
- Behavioral signs include sleep and appetite changes, increased substance abuse, hypervigilance, ritualistic behavior, gait change, and crying easily.
- Emotional signs include anxiety, depression, grief, irritability, and feeling overwhelmed.
- Cognitive signs are decision-making difficulties, confusion, impaired concentration, and reduced attention span.

Long-term effects of disaster-related stress may include nightmares, intrusive thoughts, decreased libido, anxiety, depression, domestic violence, and decreased job performance.

Reaching and Serving Special Groups

Although most disaster-response programs are organized for assistance to a general population, most programs make attempts to reach special groups that may be at high risk of developing more serious psychological problems as well as groups that may have special difficulties fully utilizing psychosocial resources. These groups include, but are not limited to, the following:

- children
- frail elderly
- people with serious mental illness
- racial and ethnic minorities
- families of people who die in a disaster
- other demographic and special needs groups

Children

Children are particularly at risk because they have not yet developed adult coping strategies and do not yet have the life experiences to help them understand what has happened to them. In addition, most young children depend on routine and consistency in their environment, relationships, and home life for a sense of security and identity. These domains of a child's life are often significantly disrupted following a disaster. Several references are particularly helpful in understanding the psychological impact of disasters on children (25–28), and a few others provide examples of interventions with children as well (29–31).

Problems of children can also emerge at school (32–33) and at the doctor's office (34). These settings should be an integral part of any community mental health disaster plan. Teachers and health care professionals are also appropriate recipients of disaster mental health training and consultation.

Frail Elderly

The elderly are best prepared for disaster on the basis of life experience; they have seen and survived more than younger victims. At the same time, elderly victims often have health problems, making them vulnerable to disaster stress, and they may also lack a strong support system to aid in recovery. Strong emotional attachments to long cherished property and mementoes lost or destroyed in disasters can be an additional and significant source of distress for the elderly.

People with Serious Mental Illness

With today's expanded community-based care, people with serious mental disorders rely heavily upon a multifaceted support system in order to live in a community setting. This support system may be seriously compromised following a disaster.

A working group of planners, health care providers, and consumers recognized the critical need for including the provision of appropriate assistance to people with serious mental illness as an important component of the overall community response to a disaster (35). Programs developed for this special group by disaster professionals should take into account the important point that people with serious mental illness can also experience "normal" disaster stress; a previous diagnosis should not overshadow what may be a very normal reaction to a disaster.

Racial and Ethnic Minorities

The community support structures for racial and ethnic minorities may be quite different from those of other groups in disaster-affected communities. Service needs and problems may vary considerably because there may be a higher representation of minority groups in lower socioeconomic strata, there may be a need for non–English language materials, and there may be a variation in the acceptance of mental health services by these groups, as well as access to community mental health services. Some ethnic groups may have culturally determined beliefs regarding psychosocial intervention, the acceptability of expressing feelings, and the appropriateness of discussing personal problems. It is important to determine the specific needs of these groups and the ways in which the beliefs and needs may affect recovery and service delivery.

Families of People Who Die in a Disaster

Families in which a person dies as a result of the disaster have clearly different support needs from those of the general population. In addition to the physical, economic, and social stability losses that affect most disaster victims, this group must cope with the grief that attends the death of a loved one. A bereaved family member may feel guilty for causing or failing to prevent the death. Individuals in this group appear to be further isolated and psychologically assaulted during the early "honeymoon" phase following disasters when so much individual, community, and media attention is devoted to giving thanks for those who survived and asserting how "it could have been so much worse." For those who lose loved ones in a disaster, it is already much worse, and every T-shirt proclaiming "I survived the ____ disaster" is a reminder of the loss of one who did not survive.

Other Demographic and Special-Needs Groups

The needs of all demographic groups represented in a particular disaster-affected region should be addressed in any mental health disaster response plan. Recent examples of special groups that have been included in federally sponsored crisis-counseling programs are military families, commercial fishers, farm families, and migrant workers.

Other "special needs" groups that may require specialized programs include people with visual and hearing impairment, people with limited mobility (e.g., people confined to wheelchairs), people who are developmentally disabled and their families, and people diagnosed with HIV and other serious and chronic illnesses.

The Catastrophic Disaster

In the United States, truly catastrophic disasters—those that cause widespread massive destruction, destroy major portions of the community infrastructure, and cause pervasive acute medical and public health problems and disruption in sheltering, food, and water supplies—are rare. However, in 1992, both Hurricane Andrew in Florida and Hurricane Iniki in Hawaii fell within this category. Catastrophic disasters include features such as:

- serious and prolonged damage to community infrastructure
- large-scale and protracted family dislocation and relocation
- prolonged sensory exposure to disaster consequences
- cumulative stress
- protracted recovery periods
- threat or reality of reoccurrence resulting in failure of adaptive defense mechanisms

Because catastrophic disasters are rare, the differential mental health impact of catastrophic disasters has not yet been fully researched. However, recent trends suggest that unique patterns of behavior are linked to this more serious and prolonged catastrophe. In general, psychological sequelae seem to last longer, services provided by public health agencies are more likely to be disrupted for an extended period of time, "secondary disasters'' seem to be more widespread (e.g., unemployment, long-term economic decline, changes in community structure and composition), and the incidence of domestic violence increases. In these situations, one can anticipate the likelihood of increased numbers of referrals to long-term psychological counseling.

At the present time, the full implications of catastrophic disasters for crisis-counseling programs are being reviewed at the federal level, and it would be premature to draw definitive conclusions. However, it does appear that the need for a different type of program, both in terms of duration and scope, may be emerging from these recent major disaster experiences.

Disaster Worker Stress

> Whoever fights monsters should see to it that in the process he does not become the monster. And when you look long into the abyss, the abyss looks into you.
>
> —Nietzsche

Sources of Stress

No discussion of mental health consequences of disaster would be complete without a review of the special stresses experienced by emergency and disaster workers. This group, broadly defined, includes workers who routinely deal with emergencies but who, in a disaster, experience events on a larger and more intense scale. This group includes first responders (e.g., police, fire and rescue personnel, and emergency room workers) as well as workers whose jobs routinely include disaster response, such as emergency management or civil defense workers. Other specialized workers affected by disasters include utility crews, military personnel, and people who must handle large numbers of dead bodies.

Three primary sources of disaster worker stress as described by Hartsough & Myers (*36*) include (1) event stressors: the physically adverse environment that characterizes much of disaster work; (2) occupational stressors: stress related to factors such as very heavy responsibility and conflicting roles; and (3) organizational stressors: factors such as organizational conflict and individual status within the organization.

Signs of Stress

Disaster workers may show any or all of the more common indications of disaster-related stress described earlier (such as trouble concentrating, fatigue, irritability) but also may display several relatively unique symptoms of stress, including:

- depersonalization—a defense mechanism intended to dehumanize the victim or survivor in order to reduce or eliminate identification with the victim

- "gallows" or "black" humor—another mechanism to depersonalize the victim or survivor
- hypervigilance
- excessive unwillingness to disengage from the disaster or the helping role (manifested by a refusal to stop work at the end of a shift)

Interventions

Numerous intervention techniques for disaster worker stress have been developed. Several approaches derive from the military experience (*13, 26, 37*). One approach includes "Critical Incident Stress Debriefing" (CISD) (*38*). Although CISD has been widely utilized, few systematic studies have been conducted to establish its effectiveness in disasters (*39*). The American Red Cross has developed a multiple stressor debriefing model (*40*), but no formal evaluations have been completed regarding its effectiveness. Without question, more research is needed on the efficacy of all interventions for reducing disaster worker stress.

Most programs focusing on reducing worker stress fail to address the role of the disaster worker's employer or employing organization. Any effective stress mitigation program must address the mental health needs of disaster workers before, during, and after disasters. The well-being of emergency response staff and other workers should be a major component of both predisaster planning and postdisaster organizational review.

Stress management should begin before a disaster occurs. There should be in every disaster-relief program a serious organizational commitment to worker well-being, careful matching of employee skills with appropriate disaster-related work, promotion of stress management as a job skill, encouragement of interpersonal support among all staff members, and the development of a disaster mental health trauma program for workers consisting of a variety of intervention and educational opportunities.

Stress-management activities include (1) identification and assignment of appropriate staff to monitor stress-related problems during the disaster; (2) establishing procedures to ensure access of the mental health staff to key decision-makers at the disaster site who have authority to take actions to address the causes of this increased stress; and (3) educating staff, during their debriefing interviews when their deployment to a disaster area ends, about the importance of addressing their stress. After a disaster, a variety of resources, types of interventions, and organizational supports should be made available to disaster-relief workers (*41*).

Critical Knowledge Gaps

Critical gaps in knowledge still remain. We must discover the answers to these questions about the mental health consequences of disaster:

- What is the effect of the type and size of the disaster on the severity of mental health consequences? For example, is a catastrophic disaster markedly different from a smaller disaster, requiring a different type and quality of disaster mental health response?
- What are the risk factors for long-term mental health problems after disasters? What specific characteristics of individuals, organizations, or communities can contribute to or mitigate the mental health effects of a disaster?
- What interventions are most effective in the early stages of disaster response to help prevent long-term mental health problems? What are the most critical and effective characteristics of ''debriefing'' interventions that can lead to positive change?
- What are the most effective interventions for the alleviation of acute and long-term mental health problems for both primary victims and for emergency workers.

Although most researchers and service providers believe that social support can facilitate post-disaster recovery among victims, more research is needed to examine the nature of this support and what characteristics of relationships can lead to better recovery (*42*).

Research Recommendations

Studies should be conducted to:

- examine the effectiveness of debriefing and other interventions conducted during early response, for emergency workers and for primary victims
- examine risk factors for understudied populations experiencing any particular disaster—for example, family research, ethnicity studies, and investigations that focus on the severely mentally ill patients, those who are developmentally disabled, and individuals living in rural areas
- examine the long-term mental health effects of catastrophic disasters among and across individuals, families, communities, organizations, and states
- replicate past research to determine the generalizability of currently accepted findings—for example, a cross-site study that utilizes similar methods, sampling techniques, and research questions across communities
- develop and refine models of organizational change under crisis conditions within disaster-response teams or organizations
- explore the specific role of social support in modifying the overall frequency, severity, and course of psychological disorders; explore the importance of personal vulnerability and prior psychopathology in the occurrence of such disorders. (Specific groups particularly dependent on social support, such as children, the elderly, and the physically ill, should be included.)

- investigate the differential experience of facing a trauma as an individual or as part of a group

Much of the research on the mental health effects of disaster has been conducted among Western populations. To expand our understanding of the mental health effects of disaster, it is imperative to include a cross-cultural approach, and to conduct research with populations from developing countries who are so often affected by natural and human-caused disasters. This research will allow the study of cross-cultural variations in frequency, symptomatology, course, and treatment needs, and will clarify the moderating effect of culture on problems and disorders (*42*).

References

1. Baum A, Fleming I. Implications of psychological research on stress and technological accidents. *Am Psychol* 1993;48(6):665–672.
2. Green BL. Psychosocial research in traumatic stress: An update. *J Traum Stress* 1994; 7(3):341–362.
3. Meichenbaum D. *Disasters, stress, and cognition.* Paper presented for the NATO Workshop on Stress and Communities, Chateau da Bonas, France, June 14–18, 1994.
4. Solomon S, Green BL. Mental health effects of natural and human-made disasters. *PTSD Res Quart* 1992;3:1:1–7.
5. Baum A, Gatchel RJ, Schaeffer MA. Emotional, behavioral, and physiological effects of chronic stress at Three Mile Island. *J Consult Clin Psychol* 1983;51:565–572.
6. Bravo M, Rubio-Stipec M, Canino GJ, Woodbury MA, Ribera JC. The psychological sequelae of disaster stress prospectively and retrospectively evaluated. *Am J Community Psychol* 1990;18:661–680.
7. Bromet EJ, Parkinson DK, Schulberg HC, Dunn LO, Gondek PC. Mental health of residents near the Three Mile Island reactor: A comparative study of selected groups. *J Prev Psych* 1982;1:225–274.
8. Green BL, Grace MC, Lindy JD, Glesser GC, Leonard AC, Kramer TL. Buffalo Creek survivors in the second decade: Comparison with unexposed and nonlitigant groups. *J Applied Soc Psychol* 1990;20:1033–1050.
9. Norris FH, Murrell SA. Prior experience as a moderator of disaster impact on anxiety symptoms in older adults. *Am J Community Psychol* 1988;16:665–683.
10. Shore JH, Tatum EI, Vollmer WM. Psychiatric reactions to disasters: The Mount St. Helens experience. *Am J Psych* 1986;143:590–596.
11. Smith EM, Robins LN, Pryzbeck TR, Goldring E, Solomon SD. Psychosocial consequences of disaster. In: Shore J, editor. *Disaster stress studies: new methods and findings.* Washington, D.C.: American Psychiatric Press, 1986:49–76.
12. Steinglass P, Gerrity E. Natural disaster and post-traumatic stress disorder: Short-term versus long-term recovery in two disaster-affected communities. *J Applied Soc Psychol* 1990; 20:1746–1765.
13. Ursano RJ, McCaughey B, Fullerton CS. *Individual and community responses to trauma and disaster: The structure of human chaos.* Cambridge, U.K.: Cambridge University Press, 1994.

14. Norris FH, Kaniasty K. Reliability of delayed self-reports in disaster research. *J Trauma Stress* 1992;5(4):575–588.

15. Myers D. *Disaster response and recovery: A handbook for mental health professionals.* DHHS Publication No. (SMA) 94–3010. Rockville, MD: Center for Mental Health Services, 1994.

16. American Red Cross Disaster Mental Health Services. *Disaster service regulations and procedures.* American Red Cross Publication 3050M. Washington, D.C.: American Red Cross, 1991.

17. Morgan J. Providing disaster mental health services through the American Red Cross. *Nat Ctr PTSD Clin Quart* 1994;4(2):13–14.

18. American Red Cross. *Disaster mental health services I.* American Red Cross Publication 3077. Washington (DC): American Red Cross, 1993.

19. Flynn BW. Mental health services in large scale disasters: An overview of the Crisis Counseling Program. *Nat Ctr PTSD Clin Quart* 1994;4(2):11–12.

20. Farberow NL, Frederick CJ. *Training manual for human service workers in major disasters* (DHEW Publication No. (ADM) 90–538). Rockville, MD: National Institute of Mental Health, 1978.

21. Cohen RE, Ahearn FL. *Handbook for mental health care of disaster victims.* Baltimore, MD: The Johns Hopkins University Press, 1980.

22. Drabek TE. *Human system responses to disaster: An inventory of sociological findings.* New York, NY: Springer-Verlag, 1986.

23. Figley CR. *Trauma and its wake: Traumatic stress, theory, research, and practice.* New York, NY: Brunner/Mazel, 1988.

24. Ursano RJ, Fullerton CS. Cognitive and behavioral responses to trauma. *J Applied Soc Psychol* 1990;20(21):1766–1775.

25. Farberow NL, Gordon NS. *Manual for child health workers in major disasters* (DHHS Publication No. [ADM] 86–1070). Rockville, MD: National Institute of Mental Health, 1981.

26. Pynoos RS. Grief and trauma in children and adolescents. *Bereavement Care* 1992;11(1):2–10.

27. Pynoos RS, Nader K. Prevention of psychiatric morbidity in children after disasters. In: Pynoos R, Nader K: *Prevention of mental health disorders, alcohol and drug use in children and adolescents* (Office of Substance Abuse Prevention, Prevention Monograph-2). DHHS Publication No.98–1646. Washington, D.C.: U.S. Government Printing Office, 1989:225–271.

28. Saylor CF. *Children and disasters.* New York: Plenum Press, 1993.

29. Pynoos RS, Nader K. Psychological first aid and treatment approach to children exposed to community violence: Research implications. *J Trauma Stress* 1988;1(4):445–473.

30. Emergency Services and Disaster Relief Branch. (1992a). *Children and trauma: the school's response* [videotape].

31. Emergency Services and Disaster Relief Branch. *Hurricane Blues* [videotape]. Rockville, MD: Center for Mental Health Services (CMHS), Substance Abuse and Mental Health Services Agency (SAMHSA), 1992.

32. La Greca AM, Vernberg EM, Silverman WK, *et al. Helping children prepare for and cope with natural disasters: A manual for professionals working with elementary school children.* Coral Gables, FL: University of Miami, 1994.

33. Nader K, Pynoos R. School disaster: Planning and interventions. *J Soc Beh and Pers* 1993; 8:1–21.

34. Emergency Services and Disaster Relief Branch and the American Academy of Pediatrics. *Psychosocial consequences of disasters: A handbook for primary health care providers.*

Rockville, MD: Center for Mental Health Services (CMHS), Substance Abuse and Mental Health Services Agency (SAMHSA), 1996.

35. Emergency Services and Disaster Relief Branch. *Responding to the needs of people with serious and persistent mental illness in times of major disaster.* Rockville, MD: Center for Mental Health Services (CMHS), Substance Abuse and Mental Health Services Agency (SAMHSA), 1996.

36. Hartsough DM, Myers DG. *Disaster work and mental health: Prevention and control of stress among workers.* Rockville, MD: National Institute of Mental Health, 1985.

37. Ursano RJ, Fullerton CS. *Exposure to death, disasters and bodies* (DTIC: A203163). Bethesda, MD: Uniformed Services University of the Health Sciences, 1988.

38. Mitchell JT. When disaster strikes . . . The Critical Incident Stress Debriefing process. *J Emerg Med Serv* 1983;8(1):36–39.

39. Hiley-Young B, Gerrity ET. Critical Incident Stress Debriefing (CISD): Value and limitations in disaster response. *Nat Ctr PTSD Clin Quart* 1994;4(2):17–19.

40. Armstrong K, O'Callahan WT, Marmar CR. Debriefing Red Cross disaster personnel: The multiple stressor debriefing model. *J Trauma Stress* 1991;4(4):581–593.

41. Flynn BW. *Returning home following a disaster. Prevention and control of stress among emergency workers: A pamphlet for workers.* Rockville, MD: National Institute of Mental Health, 1987.

42. World Health Organization Division of Mental Health. *Psychosocial consequences of disasters: Prevention and management.* Geneva: World Health Organization, 1992.

7

Effective Media Relations

R. ELLIOTT CHURCHILL

During a disaster, rapid communication and favorable relationships with the news media are essential components of responsible public health practice. Whether correctly or wrongly, individuals and groups usually turn to the news media as their first, best, and undisputed source of information about what to do in preparation for disasters, what has happened in a disaster, and what they should do after a disaster. In late 1990, an unfounded prediction of an earthquake in the central United States led to earthquake anxiety for millions of people, hundreds of thousands of student-days of absences from schools, and over $100 million spent on earthquake insurance premiums. This episode demonstrated that the public would benefit from an early, coordinated effort by scientists and the media to provide clear and accurate information. It is particularly important that this authoritative information be provided to the media and to emergency-preparedness personnel in a timely manner.

Most of CDC's experience working with the media to disseminate information rapidly has not been associated with major natural disasters in the United States. Rather, our communications with the media, the public, and health professionals have resulted from national health crises such as the outbreak of Legionnaires' disease in 1976, Guillain-Barré syndrome associated with the swine influenza immunization program in 1976, the chemical exposures in Love Canal in New York in 1979, toxic shock syndrome in 1980, and acquired immunodeficiency syndrome (AIDS). Nevertheless, the same procedures (e.g., management of information dissemination) and the same relationships with the media apply whether for a natural disaster or a nationwide health crisis.

When we speak of "the media," we generally mean the channels through which we convey information and attempt to communicate with groups of people. The office telephone, for example, is a communications medium or channel, but it is primarily designed to allow one person to make voice contact with one other person. It has little amplification capability over a face-to-face discussion between two people. Commercial television, on the other hand, is a medium or channel through which one person has the potential to reach millions of other people—verbally and visually and in a current time frame. Television is an excellent example of a "mass communications" medium. Other mass media currently in widespread use include radio, print, and computer-based telecommunications.

Science and the Media

For several reasons, people in public health—indeed, people in science in general—are often reluctant to deal with representatives of the mass media. First, scientists as a group prefer controlled, measured settings and processes. The more people involved in a situation, the less predictable the outcome becomes. For more or less complete predictability, a scientist is safest in the research laboratory—surrounded by machines and established protocols.

Second, scientists spend a great deal of time and effort learning their discipline. With their understanding comes an entire system of jargon—terms, expressions, and descriptions that they and other scientists in their field understand readily. It is not necessarily easy to translate the language of science into everyday language. Most scientists prefer to "talk science" to other scientists, because the effort they must expend in conveying their messages is considerably less than that required to make their information understandable to people outside their particular field of science.

Third, the primary goal of mass media is to convey information in such a way that they make a financial profit. Media representatives are salespeople, and they are in an extremely competitive business throughout the world. Many scientists have had disappointments in their dealings with the media because of misquotation, distortion, interviews that appear to be personal or professional attacks, broken promises to publish or broadcast a message, and the like. At least sometimes, those disappointments reflect the unfortunate consequences of the scientist and the reporter having conflicting priorities.

Although these concerns and the many others that may apply in the scientist's dealing with media representatives are valid, the fact remains that we live in an era of mass communications. CNN International is viewed around the world. Electronic mail and other telecommunications devices connect even remote areas with the mainstream of information with which the world is being bombarded.

Public Health and the Media

For science in general—and public health science in particular—to get its messages about control and prevention of illness, disability, and death to the people who need to hear them, it must use current communications technology effectively. The gatekeepers of that technology from a messenger's point of view are the media representatives— the all-powerful and dreaded producers, editors, and reporters of information.

At the receiving end of the information are the target audiences—those of public health and those of the media. A target audience is that subgroup of a population for which a particular message is believed to have the most relevance. A message may also be directed at secondary or even tertiary target audiences, but one must determine the primary target audience for every public health message to ensure that the message is crafted appropriately, timed for greatest impact, and conveyed through the medium most likely to reach that audience.

Another important concept in managing the creation and dissemination of public health messages is the single overriding communications objective (''SOCO''), which is the essence of the message that needs to be conveyed. The SOCO needs to be simply and clearly stated so that the media and the target audience reached through the media have no problem in understanding what the SOCO means. Major reasons for communicating health information include the following:

- to elicit immediate action
- to promote a long-term change in behavior
- to help the target audience understand why certain actions have been taken
- to solicit support for or participation in projects or programs
- to report on scientific findings or other program accomplishments

Public health scientists are finally beginning to appreciate that the reporting units of science and of the mass media are different. Scientists report in—because they deal in—facts. Mass media report in messages, because messages are units that are crafted in such a way as to allow for persuasion—for selling.

Not only must scientists learn to deal with media representatives, but public health scientists, at least, must learn to seek out and deal with the media. They must become proactive rather than remain reactive, and they must learn to operate on a positive and straightforward basis in order to retain control of the agenda and the content and tone of the messages they want conveyed.

When preparing to work with the media in conveying a health message to a target audience, the public health practitioner needs to ask the following questions:

- What do I want to say? (Content and SOCO)
- To whom do I want to say it? (Audience)

- What is the most effective way to say what I want to say? (Approach)
- What is the best means (and time) for getting my message across? (Medium)
- What do I want to have people in the target audience do as a result of hearing (reading) my message? (Impact)

Actually, the practice of proactive interaction with the media contributes to meeting the goals of both public health and the media. More news or other types of health information, provided on a timely (and agreed-upon) basis, as part of a comprehensive campaign of "health information for action" will provide the media with the raw material from which they make their living. At the same time, it will get the public health messages to the target audiences and allow them to react and make needed decisions about behavior and lifestyle that affect their health.

Just as many scientists are reluctant to deal with media representatives because of past negative experiences, media representatives also often complain—with justification—that scientists do not care about or respond to the constraints and demands under which the mass media operate: extremely short turnaround times, changing priorities, pressure to compete for market share with a station (or newspaper) that may be less particular than it should be about following expected ethical standards.

Most media representatives are ethical, conscientious, hardworking people dedicated to the notion that they serve as representatives for the public in its ongoing quest for well-being. The mistakes they make—the misquotations, the incorrect interpretations—result from the fact that, despite their best efforts, they do not really understand what the scientists are saying because scientists use scientific language rather than plain language. Scientists overwhelm media representatives with too much information or present information in vague, general terms and couched in risks and probabilities that do not make clear the message (SOCO) they intend to convey.

Guidelines for Dealing with a Health Crisis

A health crisis is an unplanned event that triggers a real, perceived, or possible threat to the well-being of the public (or some segment of it), the environment, or the affected health agency. Many times, organizations do not handle crisis situations such as following an earthquake disaster as effectively as they might. Two major problems related to such failures can be solved by foresight and planning:

1. The failure to react quickly enough. In a crisis situation, the first 24 hours are critical. If you do not provide the facts and the implications of those facts, the media and the public will speculate and form opinions on their own.
2. The failure to name a primary person (and one who is experienced in media matters) to be "the voice" for your organization. If a reporter states that "Dr. Jones *said* everything was fine, but he *looked* worried and seemed to be in a big

hurry,'' Dr. Jones may have done more harm than good by serving as agency spokesperson. (Of course, in this case one might also accuse the reporter of being irresponsible for speculating on the mood behind the scientist's words.) Furthermore, it is almost impossible for different people to convey *exactly* the same message—even if they read from the same prepared script. Even when delivering the same information, multiple spokespersons may be perceived as conveying different messages.

Regarding the first problem noted above, it is important for the agency spokesperson to define the problem accurately from the start. If there are delays in response on the part of the appropriate agency, the media and the public will define the problem for themselves—probably inaccurately. On the premise that "bad news is always news," it is important to remember that a shift from "safety violation" to "a history of cover-ups" can occur easily and rapidly. It is important to anticipate (or determine) how (and when) the media will report the problem so the agency can react calmly and responsibly or make an appropriate announcement before the media version of the story is reported.

Regarding the second problem noted above, it is important that the primary agency or organization spokesperson for a crisis such as a disaster have the following attributes:

- be in a key position (administration or public affairs)
- experience in dealing with media

Table 7-1 Most Frequently Asked Questions by the Media and the Public

- What happened?
- When and where?
- Who was involved?
- What caused the situation?
- How was this allowed to happen?
- What are you doing (going to do) about it?
- How much (what kind) of damage is there?
- What safety measures are being (will be) taken?
- Who (what) is to blame?
- Do you (your agency) accept responsibility?
- Has this ever happened before? With what result?
- What do you have to say to those who were injured (endangered, inconvenienced, etc.)?
- How does (will) this problem affect your operations?

Table 7-2 Guidelines for the Agency Spokesperson

- Do not give names of injured or dead until next of kin have been officially notified.

- Acknowledge responsibility, but avoid prematurely assigning blame. Assure the media that results of the investigation will be given to them.

- Avoid conjecture, speculation, and personal opinions.

- Always tell the truth. Admit it when you do not know the answer to a question.

- Prepare a brief written statement, and make it available to the media representatives (include background information and accompany photos, audiotapes, and videotapes, as appropriate).

- Do not give exclusive interviews. Schedule a press conference for all media representatives, and give them all the same information at the same time. If you are only going to read a prepared statement (and not answer questions until later), say so at the beginning.

- Be as accessible as possible to take follow-up inquiries from the media so that it does not appear that you are hiding from them.

- Stay calm.

- responsible, calm, and confident manner
- ability to speak clearly (accent, quality of voice) and convincingly.

Finally, an agency or organization can actually enlist the aid of the media. Since the media are going to be involved following all disasters, acknowledge the role they can play in assisting the agency to deal with the problem. The media's interest and efforts can provide valuable assistance in the following areas:

- Assist in precrisis education.
- Convey warnings.
- Convey instructions or other information to target audiences.
- Reassure the public.
- Defuse inaccurate rumors.
- Assist in the response effort.
- Provide the agency with updated information.
- Solicit and obtain help from the outside as needed.

Tables 7-1 to 7-8 provide other practical guidelines for dealing with reporters and other representatives of the mass media during a crisis.

Table 7-3 Checklist for Public Health Practitioners to Use in Dealing with Media Representatives

1. Prepare fact sheets (statements about problem to be discussed) for reporters about all problems to be covered. Keep reporters updated.

2. Avoid jargon (that means all jargon).

3. Respect reporters' deadlines (which you determine by asking).

4. Always be polite and straightforward. Humor, sarcasm, irony, and other linguistic devices that are appropriate in some settings need to be avoided when dealing with reporters; it is too easy to be misunderstood—with respect to both your information and your attitude.

5. Always tell the truth. If information is not available or unreliable, say so.

6. Always have your own agenda set the SOCO, or message you need to convey, and stick to it. Answer the reporters' questions as completely as possible, but return to your own agenda.

7. If you are not sure about a question (whether you do not know what it means or simply do not hear it), ask the reporters to repeat it.

8. If you do not know an answer, and it is within your area of responsibility, try to find it. If it is outside your area of expertise, do not try to answer it. Admit that you do not know.

9. Stick to facts; do not offer your own opinions.

10. Explain the context and relevance of your message (e.g., the public health significance).

11. Make notes (or a tape) of the meeting (interview).

12. Provide feedback to the reporter and his/her editor on the results of your interaction.

Table 7-4 A Proactive Approach to Media Relations for the Public Health Practitioner

1. Do not wait for the media representatives to contact you. Study the patterns and type of reporting in your area and determine which media representatives appear to be most knowledgeable, most responsible, and most effective. Then contact them. You may want to begin with one representative and branch out after you have gained some experience.

2. Be able to write and state clearly and concisely not just your facts but your messages as well.

3. Explain at each meeting the relative importance of the issues you have discussed and how they fit into the overall context of public health practice.

4. Do your part in maintaining an image (and the integrity to back it up) of truthfulness, expertise, and candor.

5. Be responsive when media representatives contact you for information—regardless of whether it is about your pet problem. They remember who helps them and who does not.

Table 7-5 Guidelines for News Releases

News releases are intended to take the place of a person-to-person interview. The subject must be current and of sufficient interest.

1. Make sure the item is of sufficient interest and scope to make it worthwhile for media representatives to use it.

2. Distribute only to a list of media representatives who are preselected on the basis of (1) their documented interest in public health issues, (2) the appropriateness of their target audiences for your purposes, and (3) their past responsiveness and responsibility. However, do not bar any official media representative from obtaining a copy of a news release. The perception that you are refusing to deal with a particular media representative may generate damaging ill will.

3. Use the inverted pyramid style of writing: Put most important items first, and taper down to detail.

4. Open the press release with a summary lead, a paragraph in which you answer "Who?" "What?" "When?" "Where?" "Who cares?" and "How?" Depending on the subject matter, you may or may not need or be able to answer "Why."

5. Make the news release no longer than two pages.

6. Use short, straightforward sentences. Define any specialized terms you *must* use, but generally avoid using jargon or specialized vocabulary.

7. Provide direct quotations, with the source and credentials of that source provided.

8. Consider providing audio or video segments to accompany the news release, if appropriate. If not feasible, supply appropriate still photographs and useful graphic material to illustrate or dramatize the message in the press release.

Summary

All of these problems described by the media representative and the scientist are serious, but they are not insoluble. What is necessary is the triad of truth, trust, and time.

- Truth means just that—on the part of all participants in the process. Period. No compromise.
- Trust must be developed among scientists and media representatives, who all are out to achieve the same objective: good information provided in a responsible manner to the targeted audience in an appropriate time frame. The motivations may differ (e.g., profit for the media and public health for the scientist), but that is not a problem if mutual trust is established, earned, and maintained.
- Time is needed to allow the scientist to be comfortable with the quality of the information provided, but not so much that the media's deadlines are missed. Compromises are required on all sides.

Table 7-6 Sample News Release

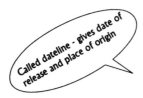

May 20, 1994   Atlanta, Georgia

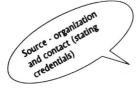

Centers for Disease Control and Prevention
Contact: Dr. S.A. Jones
Investigative Epid.
Center for Inf. Dis.
Telephone: (404) 633-2121

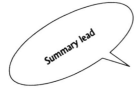

Infectious disease investigators at CDC announced today that an outbreak of meningitis at the U. of Ga. Athens campus is now under control.

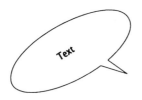

More than 100 students and staff at the University has had a laboratory-confirmed diagnosis of meningitis in the past week. Meningitis, a potentially serious infection, is caused by a bacterium. More than 50% of all known cases of this disease have led to complications, and 10% of patients have died.

"This outbreak at (U of) Georgia is certainly serious," acknowledges investigative epidemiologist, Dr. S.A. Jones, "but we are now confident that it is under control."

Ill students and staff have been hospitalized and placed in strict isolation for their protection and the protection of other patients and hospital staff.

In addition, all known contacts of students and staff with meningitis have been vaccinated against meningitis. This means that even if they do become infected and have the illness, they should only have mild cases.

- More -

Table 7-6 (Continued)

"Each year," says Dr. Jones, "we see outbreaks of meningitis on college campuses. Group settings and the age of the university population make the risk of this infection higher for these people than it is for the population in general."

CDC does not recommend that all school and college-age young people be vaccinated at this time.

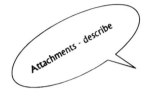

Attachments--photograph of Dr. Jones in his office, photograph of group of students being examined, CDC report on meningitis (1994)

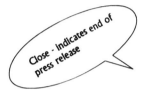

- 30 -

Table 7-7 Guidelines for Fact Sheets

The public health fact sheet is a brief (no more than two pages) report that describes background and context for a particular health problem. For example, a fact sheet on hurricanes, intended for general audiences in the United States, would do the following:

- Describe the mechanisms that cause hurricanes.
- Tell when and where hurricanes usually occur.
- Give some examples of detailed (unusual, particularly hazardous) problems associated with hurricanes.
- Provide recommendations for actions to be taken by target audiences if a hurricane occurs.

Fact sheets are often used by journalists and other media representatives as reference material when they prepare their reports. Fact sheets ("backgrounders") may be kept and used several times before they need to be replaced with more current information. They are also useful to the public health staff who prepare them, because fact sheets in reporters' files can obviate the need for public health staff to answer the same questions repeatedly as different reporters (and members of target audiences) call with inquiries.

Table 7-8 Important "Pearls" in Dealing With a Health Crisis Such as a Disaster

- Silence kills. It is equated by the media and the public alike with guilt.

- Do not delay. The first 24 hours are critical.

- Permit controlled access to the site (or the agency premises) as soon as possible.

- Never speculate or give your own opinions. Only state the facts as you know them.

- If you cannot answer a question (because you do not know the answer or because the answer is confidential information), admit it. Follow up on promises to get answers to questions.

- Monitor what the media report after your initial conference with them. Correct any incorrect information and clarify points of confusion as needed.

Recommended Reading

Ambron A, Hooper K (eds). *Interactive multimedia*. Redmond, Washington: Microsoft Press, 1988.

Bourque LB, Russell LA, Goltz JD. Human behavior during and immediately after the Loma Prieta earthquake. In: Bolton P, editor. *The Loma Prieta, California, earthquake of October 17, 1989: Public response. USGS Professional Paper 1553-B*. Washington, DC: U.S. Government Printing Office, 1993:B3–B22.

Burkett W. *News reporting: science, medicine, and high technology*. Ames: The University of Iowa Press, 1986.

Churchill RE. *MOD:Comm—a communications module*. Atlanta: Centers for Disease Control and Prevention, 1996.

Committee on Disasters and the Mass Media. *Disasters and the media. Proceedings of the Committee on Disasters and the Mass Media Workshop, February 1979*. Washington, DC: National Academy of Sciences, 1980.

Imperato PJ. Dealing with the press and the media. In: *The administration of a public health agency: a case study of the New York City Department of Health*. New York: Human Sciences Press, 1983.

Kotler P, Roberto EL. *Social marketing*. New York: The Free Press, 1989.

Lipson GL, Kroloff GK. *Understanding the news media and public relations in Washington (a reference manual)*. Washington, DC: The Washington Monitor, 1977.

Wurman RS. *Information anxiety*. New York: Bantam Books, 1990.

II

GEOPHYSICAL EVENTS

8

Earthquakes

ERIC K. NOJI

Background and Nature of Earthquakes

A major earthquake affecting a large city has the potential to be the most catastrophic natural disaster for the United States. Earthquakes of sufficient size threaten lives and damage property by setting off a chain of effects that disrupts the natural and human-built environments. Widespread strong ground shaking is a geological effect that can severely damage buildings or cause them to collapse completely. Vibratory earthquake motion, in turn, can induce secondary geological effects such as soil liquefaction, land-slides, and related ground failure hazardous to the built environment or can trigger seismic sea waves (tsunamis) that may wreak coastal destruction thousands of miles from the earthquake source. Earthquakes may also result in major nongeological effects (e.g., widespread fires, flooding of populated areas caused by failure of large dams, or release of toxic or radioactive materials) that could be more catastrophic than the initial effects of the earthquake.

Worldwide, more than a million earthquakes occur each year, an average of about 2 each minute (1). Research indicates a 60% probability that an earthquake of Richter magnitude 7.5 or greater will occur on the San Andreas Fault in southern California within the next 30 years, and a 50% probability that an earthquake of 7.0 or greater magnitude will occur on the San Andreas or Hayward faults in the San Francisco Bay region within the same time period (2). A recent study estimates a 40% to 63% prob-ability of a Richter magnitude 6.0 earthquake occurring in the New Madrid seismic of the central United States zone before the year 2000 (3). As previewed by the significant damages resulting from the 1989 Loma Prieta earthquake in northern California (magnitude 7.1) and the 1994 Northridge earthquake in southern California (magnitude 6.8), the impact of the predicted higher-magnitude earthquakes in California and the central United States could potentially kill and injure thousands of people, result in billions of dollars in property loss, and cause severe disruptions to the economy (*4*).

Despite the remarkable scientific progress in seismology and earthquake engineering during the past several years, the aim of achieving high standards of life safety against earthquakes globally has yet to be achieved.

Scope/Relative Importance of Earthquake Disasters

During the past 20 years, earthquakes alone have caused more than a million deaths worldwide (*5*). Nine countries account for more than 80% of all fatalities this century, and almost half of the total number of earthquake deaths in the world during this period have occurred in just one country—China (Fig. 8-1). On July 28, 1976, at 3:42 A.M., an earthquake of magnitude 7.8 occurred in Tangshan in the northeastern part of China. In a matter of seconds, an industrial city of a million people was reduced to rubble, with more than 240,000 people killed (*6*). Recent accelerated urbanization in other seismically active parts of the world whose population densities reach 20,000 to 60,000 inhabitants per square kilometer underscores the vulnerability of such areas to similar

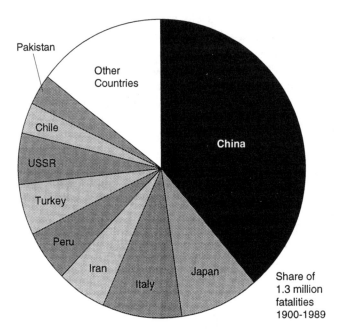

Figure 8-1. Location of earthquake deaths across the world. Figure adapted from: Coburn AW, Pomonis A, Sakai S. Assessing strategies to reduce fatalities in earthquakes. In: *Proceedings of the International Workshop on Earthquake Injury Epidemiology for Mitigation and Response, 10–12 July, 1989, Baltimore, Maryland.* Baltimore, Johns Hopkins University, 1989:112. (*96*)

catastrophic numbers of earthquake-related deaths and injuries. In just the past 10 years, the world has witnessed four catastrophic earthquakes resulting in great loss of life: in Mexico City in 1985 (10,000 deaths); in Armenia in 1988 (25,000 deaths); in Iran in 1990 (40,000 deaths); and in India in 1993 (10,000 deaths) (Table 8-1).

The United States has been relatively fortunate in terms of earthquake-related casualties so far (7). Only an estimated 1,600 deaths have been attributed to earthquakes since colonial times, with over 60% of these having been recorded in California. The most serious earthquake in terms of loss of life was the 1906 San Francisco earthquake and fire that killed an estimated 700 people. Only four other earthquakes in United States territory have killed more than 100 people: 173 people died in Unimake Island, Alaska, in 1946; 131 died in Prince William Sound, Alaska, in 1964; 120 died in Long Beach, California, in 1933; and 116 died in Mona Passage, Puerto Rico, in 1918. More recent earthquakes continue to exact smaller but significant tolls: 64 died in the 1971 San Fernando earthquake; 67 died in the 1989 Loma Prieta earthquake; and most recently, 60 died in the 1994 Northridge, California, earthquake (8–10) (Table 8-2).

Table 8-1 Earthquakes in the Twentieth Century that Caused More than 10,000 Deaths

Year	Location (Magnitude)	No. Killed
1985	Mexico City, Mexico (M 8.1 and 7.3)	10,000
1993	India (M 6.4)	10,000
1960	Agadir, Morocco (M 5.9)	12,000
1968	Dasht-i-Biyaz, Iran (M 7.3)	12,000
1962	Buyin Zhara, Iran (M 7.3)	12,225
1917	Indonesia (M 7.0+)	15,000
1978	Tabas, Iran (M 7.7)	18,200
1905	Kangra, India (M 8.6)	19,000
1948	Ashkabad, USSR (M 7.3)	19.800
1974	China (M 6.8)	20,000
1976	Guatemala City (M 7.5)	23,000
1988	Armenia, USSR (M 6.9)	25,000
1935	Quetta, Pakistan (M 7.5)	25,000
1923	Concepcion, Chile (M 8.3)	25,000
1939	Chillán, Chile (M 8.3)	28,000
1915	Avezzano, Italy (M 7.5)	32,610
1939	Erzincan, Turkey (M 8.0)	32,700
1990	Iran (M 7.7)	40,000
1927	Tsinghai, China (M 8.0)	40,912
1908	Messina, Italy (M 7.5)	58,000
1970	Ankash, Peru (M 8.3)	66,794
1923	Kanto, Japan (M 8.3)	142,807
1920	Kansu, China (M 8.5)	200,000
1976	Tangshan, China (M 7.8)	242,000
Total		Approximately 1,500,000

Table 8-2 The Eight Most Fatal Earthquakes in the United States Since 1900

No. Killed	Location	Year
700	San Francisco (earthquake and fire)	1906
173	Alaska (earthquake/tsunami hitting Hawaii and California)	1946
120	Long Beach, California	1933
117	Alaska (earthquake/tsunami)	1964
116	Puerto Rico	1918
64	San Fernando Valley, California	1971
62	Loma Prieta, northern California	1989
60	Northridge, southern California	1994

As mentioned above, population growth in areas of high seismic risk in the United States has greatly increased the number of people at risk since the last earthquake of great magnitude struck (1906 in San Francisco). Researchers estimate that a repetition of the 1906 San Francisco earthquake, which measured 8.3 on the Richter scale, could cause 2,000 to 6,000 deaths, 6,000 to 20,000 serious injuries, and total economic losses exceeding $120 billion (*11, 12*). Approximately 90% of the seismic activity in the contiguous United States occurs in California and western Nevada (Fig. 8-2). Although the risk of catastrophic earthquakes in the western part of the United States is widely recognized, few people realize the high probability that a major earthquake will hit the eastern United States in the next several decades. For example, a series of three great earthquakes (estimated magnitudes 8.6, 8.4, and 8.7), all of intensity XII, occurred during a 3-month period in the winter of 1811–1812 near the town of New Madrid, Missouri. Although little loss of life occurred in the then sparsely populated area, the earthquakes were felt over most of the United States east of the Rocky Mountains and caused destruction for hundreds of miles. The New Madrid fault system is less well studied than the San Andreas system, but New Madrid–size earthquakes may recur at 600- to 700-year intervals. Seismologists now feel that enough strain may have developed in the New Madrid seismic zone to produce a magnitude 7.6 earthquake, which would be damaging over 200,000 square miles.

Earthquakes have even occurred on the East Coast. For example, Charleston, South Carolina, experienced a magnitude 6.8 (Intensity X) earthquake in 1886 that killed 83 people and was felt over most of the United States east of the Mississippi River (*13*). Although the eastern United States has considerably less seismic activity than the area west of the Rocky Mountains, the lower probability of major earthquakes in the East needs to be balanced against the greater population densities, less stringent seismic codes, less well-developed earthquake-preparedness programs, and lower public awareness of the earthquake problem in the eastern states, as well as the fact that earthquakes in the East exert damaging effects over a much wider area for an event of a given magnitude. Other vulnerable regions in the United States include the Puget Sound

U. S. Seismicity: 1960-1988

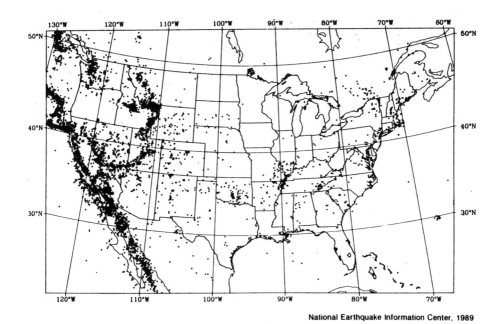

National Earthquake Information Center, 1989

Figure 8-2. United States seismic activity. This U.S. Geological Survey map depicts earthquake risk in the continental United States. The dots represent active seismic areas from 1960 to 1988. *Source*: National Earthquake Information Center, 1989.

region in Washington State and the Salt Lake City region in Utah. Only a few Gulf states, such as Florida, are considered at very low risk.

Factors that Contribute to Earthquake Disasters

Depending on its magnitude, its proximity to an urban center, and the degree of earthquake disaster preparedness and mitigation measures implemented in the urban center, an earthquake can cause large numbers of casualties. At 5:04 P.M. on Tuesday, October 17, 1989, a magnitude 7.1 earthquake centered near Loma Prieta Peak in the Santa Cruz mountains of northern California caused 62 deaths and 3,000 injuries (*14*). The Loma Prieta earthquake was this country's most damaging earthquake since the 1971 San Fernando Valley earthquake in southern California. The Loma Prieta earthquake brought to memory the December 7, 1988, earthquake in Armenia, which, although about one-half its size in terms of energy release (magnitude 6.9), caused an estimated 25,000 deaths and 18,000 injuries. The differences in impacts between these two earthquakes is directly related to differences in the degree of disaster-mitigation and disaster-preparedness measures taken in northern California and in the former Soviet Union (*15–17*). Strict adherence to building codes during the past two decades in the San Francisco Bay region undoubtedly saved many lives and kept thousands of buildings from collapsing in the Loma Prieta earthquake (*18–20*).

With population increases and rapid urbanization in seismic-risk zones, earthquakes producing high numbers of casualties are expected to continue to occur in the future. Other factors affecting earthquake-related morbidity and mortality will be discussed in more detail in the next sections of this chapter.

Factors Affecting Earthquake Occurrence and Severity

Natural Factors

As shown in Figure 8-3, earthquakes tend to be concentrated in particular zones on the earth's surface that coincide with the boundaries of the tectonic plates into which the

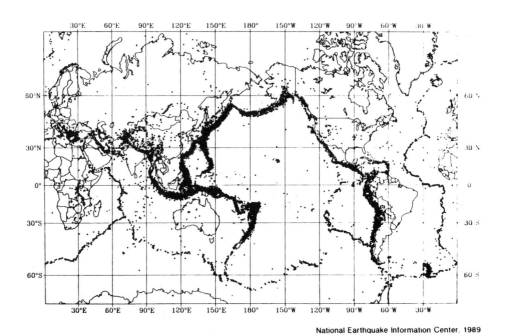

Earthquakes with Magnitudes ≥ 5.0: 1963-1988

National Earthquake Information Center, 1989

Figure 8-3. This U.S. Geological Survey map depicts earthquakes in the world with magnitude ≥5.0: 1963–1988. *Source*: National Earthquake Information Center, 1989.

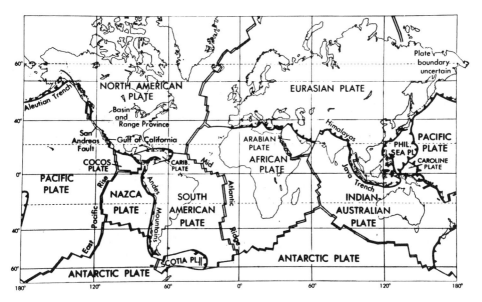

Figure 8-4. This U.S. Geological Survey map depicts the major tectonic plates of the world. Most earthquakes occur in the areas of plate boundaries.

earth's crust is divided (Fig. 8-4). As the plates move relative to each other along the plate boundaries, they tend not to slide smoothly but to become interlocked. This interlocking causes deformations to occur in the rocks on either side of the plate boundaries, with the result that stresses build up. As the rocks deform on either side of the plate boundary, they store energy—and the amounts of such energy that can be stored in the large volumes of rock involved can be truly massive. When the fault ruptures, the energy stored in the rocks is released in a few seconds—partly as heat and partly as shock waves. These waves constitute the earthquake (*21*). The resultant vibrational energy is then transmitted through the earth's surface, and when it reaches the surface, it may cause damage and collapse of structures, which in turn may kill and injure the occupants of these structures (Fig. 8-5). These large and inexorable forces are responsible for the band of seismic activity that extends along the Pacific rim to South America and to Japan (Fig. 8-3).

Earthquake Strength

Magnitude and intensity are two measures of the strength of an earthquake and are frequently confused by laypeople (*22*). The magnitude of an earthquake is a measure of actual physical energy release at its source as estimated from instrumental observations. A number of magnitude scales are in use. The oldest and most widely used is the

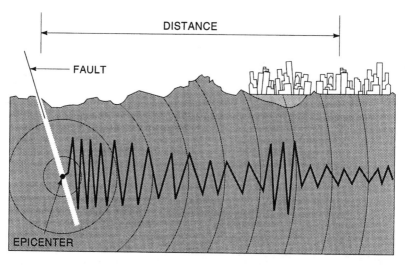

Figure 8-5. Motion of the earth's plates causes increased pressure at faults where the plates meet. Eventually the rock structure collapses and movement occurs along the fault. Energy is propagated to the surface above and radiates outward. These waves of motion in the earth's crust shake landforms and buildings, causing damage.

Richter magnitude scale, developed by Charles Richter in 1936. Although the scale is open-ended, the strongest earthquake recorded to date has been of Richter magnitude 8.9.

On the other hand, intensity is a measure of the felt or perceived effects of an earthquake rather than the strength of the earthquake itself. It is a measure of how severe the shaking was at a particular location. Thus, whereas magnitude refers to the force of the earthquake as a whole (i.e., an earthquake can have just one magnitude), intensity refers to the effects of an earthquake at a particular site. The intensity is usually strongest close to the epicenter and is weaker the farther a site is from the epicenter. Intensity is determined by classifying the degree of shaking severity as measured by an intensity scale. The intensity is assigned for a particular location on the basis of the visible consequences left by the earthquake and from subjective reports by people who experience the shaking. There are many intensity scales in use today around the world. The most commonly used scale for intensity in the United States is the Modified Mercalli (MM) scale, a 12-point scale that ranges from barely perceptible earthquakes at MM I to near total destruction at MM XII (Table 8-3).

The intensity of an earthquake is more germane to its public health consequences than its magnitude. Intensity scales also allow comparisons with earthquakes that occurred before the development of seismic monitoring instruments. The destruction that an earthquake causes is a function of its intensity and the resistance of structures to seismic damage.

Table 8-3 Modified Mercalli (MM) Scale Categories

I. Felt only by a very few people under especially favorable circumstances

II. Felt only by a few people at rest, especially on the upper floors of buildings. Suspended objects may swing.

III. Felt quite noticeably indoors. Standing motor vehicles may rock slightly. Vibration like the passing of a truck.

IV. Felt indoors by many, outdoors by a few. At night, some awakened. Crockery, glassware, windows, doors rattle.

V. Felt by nearly everyone; damage to contents and structures uncommon but possible.

VI. Felt by all; many frightened and run outdoors; damage slight.

VII. Everybody runs outdoors; damage negligible to buildings seismically well-designed and constructed; slight to moderate to ordinary structures; considerable damage to poorly built or badly designed structures.

VIII. Damage slight in well-designed, considerable in ordinary, and great in poorly built structures; chimneys, monuments, walls, etc., fall.

IX. Damage considerable to well-designed structures, and great (including partial or complete collapse) in other buildings; buildings shifted off foundations; underground pipelines disrupted.

X. Some well-built wooden structures destroyed; most masonry and ordinary structures destroyed; railroad tracks bent; landslides common; water spills over banks of streams, lakes, etc.

XI. Few, if any, masonry structures remain standing; bridges are destroyed; broad fissures open in the ground; underground pipelines are completely out of service; earth subsides.

XII. Damage is total; waves are seen propagating along surface of the ground; nearly impossible to stand; objects thrown up into the air.

Topographic Factors

Topographic factors substantially affect the impact of earthquakes. Violent ground shaking in areas constructed on alluvial soils or landfill, both of which tend to liquify and exacerbate seismic oscillations, can produce significant damage and injuries at a given location far from the actual earthquake epicenter (*23*). Both the impact of the 1985 earthquake on Mexico City, where an estimated 10,000 people died, and that of the 1989 Loma Prieta earthquake are good examples of how local soil conditions can play important roles in producing building damage of greater severity than what may occur in areas closer to the earthquake's epicenter.

Meteorological Factors

Meteorology plays only a minor direct role in the events that initiate earthquakes. However, it can substantially affect the secondary effects of earthquakes. High tides and high water levels from storm runoff exacerbate the impact of seismic sea waves.

Water saturation of soils increases the likelihood of landslides, avalanches, and earthen dam failures, as well as the probability of soil liquefaction during seismic shaking. Earthquake-induced failure of dams when streams are near flood stage would be catastrophic. If housing is substantially damaged, rain or subfreezing temperatures would be, at the least, a nuisance and could contribute substantially to morbidity and mortality, as such conditions did following the December earthquake in mountainous Armenia in 1988.

Volcanic Activity

Earthquakes often occur in association with active volcanoes, sometimes triggered by magmatic flow and sometimes releasing pressure that allows magmatic intrusion. The so-called harmonic tremors associated with actual magmatic flow are generally not damaging; however, relatively severe earthquakes can immediately precede or accompany actual volcanic eruptions and can contribute to devastating mudslides.

Human-Generated Factors (Artificial Causes of Earthquakes)

Four human activities or consequences of human activities have been known to induce earthquakes: (1) the filling of large water impoundments; (2) deep well injection; (3) underground explosions of nuclear devices, and (4) the collapse of underground mine-workings. Some observers have speculated that nuclear detonations along a fault may release strain in a controlled fashion and prevent a major earthquake, but the potential liability of such an experiment gone awry has proved daunting for even the most intrepid seismic investigators (*24*).

Public Health Impacts of Earthquakes: Historical Perspective

In most earthquakes, people are killed by mechanical energy as a direct result of being crushed by falling building materials. Deaths resulting from major earthquakes can be instantaneous, rapid, or delayed (*25*). Instantaneous death can be due to severe crushing injuries to the head or chest, external or internal hemorrhage, or drowning from earthquake-induced tidal waves (tsunamis). Rapid death occurs within minutes or hours and can be due to asphyxia from dust inhalation or chest compression, hypovolemic shock, or environmental exposure (e.g., hypothermia). Delayed death occurs within days and can be due to dehydration, hypothermia, hyperthermia, crush syndrome, wound infections, or postoperative sepsis (*26, 27*).

As with most natural disasters, the majority of people requiring medical assistance following earthquakes have minor lacerations and contusions caused by falling elements like pieces of masonry, roof tiles, and timber beams (*28*). The next most frequent reason for seeking medical attention is simple fractures not requiring operative intervention (*29*). Such light injuries usually require only outpatient-level treatment and tend to be much more common than severe injuries requiring hospitalization. For example, after the 1968 earthquake south of Khorasan, Iran, only 368 (3.3%) of 11,254 people injured required inpatient care (*30*). A similar pattern of injuries is discussed in reports by Durkin, Thiel, *et al.*, which indicated that following the 1989 Loma Prieta earthquake as many as 60% of those with earthquake-related injuries either treated themselves or received treatment in nonhospital settings (*31*). These findings suggest that a substantial number of earthquake-related injuries are treated outside the formal health care system.

Major injuries requiring hospitalization include skull fractures with intracranial hemorrhage (e.g., subdural hematoma); cervical spine injuries with neurologic impairment; and damage to intrathoracic, intraabdominal, and intrapelvic organs such as pneumothorax, liver lacerations, and ruptured spleen (*32*). Most seriously injured people will sustain combination injuries, such as pneumothorax in addition to an extremity fracture. More detailed inpatient information is available from data collected on 4,832 patients admitted to hospitals following the 1988 earthquake in Armenia (*33*). Consistent with findings from other major earthquakes, these data show that combination injuries constituted 39.7% of the cases. Superficial trauma such as lacerations and contusions were the most frequently observed (24.9%), followed by head injuries (22%), lower-extremity injuries (19%), crush syndrome (11%), and upper-extremity trauma (10%).

Hypothermia, secondary wound infections, gangrene requiring amputation, sepsis, adult respiratory distress syndrome (ARDS), multiple organ failure, and crush syndrome have been identified as major medical complications in past earthquakes. Crush syndrome results from prolonged pressure on limbs, causing disintegration of muscle tissue (rhabdomyolysis) and release of myoglobin, potassium, and phosphate into the circulation (*34*). Systemic effects include hypovolemic shock, hyperkalemia, renal failure, and fatal cardiac arrhythmias. Patients with crush syndrome may develop kidney failure and require dialysis (*35*). Following the 1988 earthquake in Armenia, more than 1,000 victims trapped in collapsed buildings developed crush syndrome as a result of limb compression; 323 developed secondary acute renal failure requiring renal dialysis (*36*). Amputations and chronic sequelae of orthopedic and neurologic injuries, especially spinal cord injuries, can be expected (*37*). For example, a rate of 1.5 cases of paraplegia/ 1,000 injured was observed after the Guatemalan earthquake (*38*), and more than 2,200 people became paraplegics as a result of injuries sustained in the 1976 Tangshan quake (*6*). Following the Tangshan earthquake, all these chronically disabled people required extensive treatment and rehabilitation in long-term-care facilities. This care significantly taxed the health care system in the region for years to come.

As noted above, trauma caused by the collapse of buildings is the cause of most deaths and injuries in most earthquake (*5*). However, a surprisingly large number of patients require acute care for nonsurgical problems such as acute myocardial infarction, exacerbation of chronic diseases such as diabetes or hypertension, anxiety and other mental health problems such as depression (*39, 40*), respiratory disease caused by exposure to dust and asbestos fibers from rubble, and near drowning caused by flooding from broken dams. An example of the adverse effects of an earthquake on medical conditions was observed in 1981 after a magnitude 6.7 earthquake in Athens, Greece. A 50% increase in deaths due to myocardial infarction was documented during the first 3 days after the earthquake, with the death rate peaking on the third day (*41, 42*). There may be a plausible biological mechanism for increased risk of cardiac problems after a natural disaster: emotional stress and physical activity cause increased levels of catecholamines, vasoconstriction, and increased coagulability (*43*). If stress has such an acute physiological effect, then the proportion of sudden deaths might be expected to increase. On the day of the 1985 Mexico City earthquake, the number of abortions, premature births, and normal deliveries in chronic care facilities rose and together constituted the primary cause of all admissions seen on that day (*44, 45*). Even more admissions for these causes occurred 4 days later, again probably because of the effects of stress related to the disaster (*44*).

Huge amounts of dust are generated when a building is damaged or collapses, and dust clogging the air passages and filling the lungs is a major cause of death for many building-collapse victims (*6, 33, 46*). Fulminant pulmonary edema from dust inhalation may also be a delayed cause of death (*47*). Dust has hampered rescue and cleanup operations by causing eye and respiratory-tract irritation. Anecdotal accounts from the 1985 Mexico City earthquake indicate that rescue workers finally resorted to full-face respirators, equipment that will probably be in short supply after most major earthquakes (*45*). Many commercial and school buildings in the United States are heavily laden with asbestos, which will likely pulverize if the buildings collapse. Asbestos and other particulate matter in the dust could pose both subacute and chronic respiratory hazards to entrapped victims as well as to rescue and cleanup personnel, depending on the characteristics and toxicity of the dust (*48*).

Burns and smoke inhalation from fires used to be major hazards after an earthquake. For example, following the 1923 earthquake in Tokyo, more than 140,000 people perished, principally because of fires that broke out in a city where most buildings were constructed from highly flammable paper (shoji) and wood material. Since 1950, however, the incidence of burns in the aftermath of earthquakes has decreased considerably (*5*).

There is a growing body of evidence that nonstructural elements (e.g., facade cladding, partition walls, roof parapets, external architectural ornaments) and building contents (e.g., glass, furniture, fixtures, appliances, chemical substances) can cause substantial morbidity following earthquakes (*49*). In a study from the 1987 Whittier Narrows earthquake in southern California (magnitude 5.9), Bourque and others reported that injuries occurred "primarily because objects fell from shelves or walls, because parts of buildings fell, because of how the injured person behaved during or immediately after the earthquake, or because the person fell during the earthquake" (*50*). In another study, fall-related injuries were those most frequently reported in the absence of structural collapse (*31*). This type of injury accounted for almost 30% of those occurring during and after shaking. Most people who incurred fall-related injuries after the shaking stopped were attempting to evacuate down darkened exit stairs. Although most injuries from falls or from being struck by nonstructural elements are minor compared with those sustained as a result of building collapse, some physical objects (e.g., tall metal lockers, wine barrels, heavy filing cabinets) and some settings (e.g., stairwells) are particularly hazardous and can cause serious injuries.

Although many structures may be at risk of damage in highly seismic areas, most deaths or serious injuries from earthquakes tend to occur in a relatively small number of damaged facilities widely scattered throughout the earthquake-affected area (*5, 51*). For example, 50 of 62 deaths in the Loma Prieta earthquake occurred at the Cypress freeway structure in Oakland, and 40 of 64 deaths in the 1971 San Fernando earthquake occurred as a result of a collapse of a Veterans Hospital. Data on earthquakes in other countries also suggest that a relatively small number of damaged structures are the source of the vast majority of the serious casualties (*5*).

Factors Influencing Earthquake Morbidity and Mortality

Natural Factors

Landslides

Landslides and mudflows triggered by earthquakes accounted for most of the fatalities and serious injuries in several recent earthquakes, including those in Tajikstan (1989), the Philippines (1990), and Colombia (1994) (*52*). Earlier this century, landslides were clearly the dominant feature in earthquakes in China that killed 100,000 in 1920 and one that killed more than 66, 000 in Peru in 1970 (*53*). Landslides can bury villages and hillside houses and sweep vehicles off roads into ravines, especially in mountainous areas. Debris flows caused by earthquakes may also dam rivers. Such blocking of rivers may cause land upstream to flood and, if the dam is suddenly breached, may cause waves of water to be sent suddenly downstream. Both of these occurrences may pose additional hazards to human settlements.

Tsunamis ("Seismic Sea Waves")

Submarine earthquakes can generate damaging tsunamis (also known as seismic sea waves), which can travel thousands of miles undiminished before bringing destruction to low-lying coastal areas and around bays and harbors. A tsunami can be created directly by underwater ground motion during earthquakes or by landslides, including underwater landslides. Tsunamis can travel thousands of miles at 300–600 mph with very little loss of energy. Wave heights in deep ocean water may be only a few feet and pass under ships with little disturbance, but in shallow coastal waters wave heights can reach 100 feet with devastating impact on local shipping and shoreline communities. Successive crests may arrive at intervals of every 10–45 minutes and wreak destruction for several hours.

The Pacific coast of the United States is at greatest risk from tsunamis, primarily from earthquakes in South America and the Alaska/Aleutian Island region. For example, the 1964 Alaska earthquake generated tsunamis up to 20 feet in height along the coasts of Washington, Oregon, and California and caused extensive damage in Alaska and Hawaii. The death toll from these tsunamis was 122 compared with only 9 nearer the epicenter of the earthquake itself. Tsunamis are clearly the leading earthquake-related threat to the inhabitants of Hawaii. More recently, tsunamis triggered by earthquakes accounted for the majority of the deaths and serious injuries in Nicaragua (1992), northern Japan (1993), and Indonesia (1992 and 1994) (*54–56*).

Aftershocks

Most earthquakes are followed by many aftershocks, some of which may be as strong as the main shock itself. Many fatalities and serious injuries occurred from a strong aftershock 2 days after the September 19, 1985, Mexico City earthquake that killed an estimated 10,000 people (*45*). In some cases landslides may be triggered by an aftershock, after having been primed by the main shock. Some major debris flows start slowly with a minor trickle and then are triggered in waves. In these cases there may be sufficient warning that allows a community that is aware of this hazard to evacuate in time.

Local Weather Conditions

Local weather conditions, which are known to affect survival time among people trapped in collapsed buildings after an earthquake, have a major influence on the percentage of those injured who subsequently die before they can be rescued. For example, the harsh winter conditions that were present during the 1988 earthquake in Armenia, which killed an estimated 25,000 people, decreased the ability of those trapped to survive even if their original injuries were minor. Some of the people who could otherwise have been rescued may have perished because of the intense cold in the mountainous region.

Time of Day

Time of day is an important determinant of a population's risk for death or injury, primarily because it affects people's likelihood of being caught in a collapsing building. For example, the 1988 Armenia earthquake occurred at 11:41 A.M., and thus many people were trapped in schools, office buildings, or factories. If the earthquake had occurred at another time of day, very different patterns of injury and places of injury would have occurred. The 1933 earthquake in Long Beach, California, caused significant damage to school buildings but no deaths, because it occurred at a time when school was not in session (*57*). In Guatemala, the 1976 quake, which killed 24,000 people, occurred at 3:05 A.M. while most people were asleep. If the same quake had occurred later in the day, many more people would have been outside and thus would not have been injured (*58*). On the other hand, the 1994 Northridge earthquake in southern California killed about 60 people (*9, 59*), yet the number of injuries and deaths among the 700,000 schoolchildren and 6 million commuters likely would have been much worse if the earthquake had occurred at 9:31 A.M. on a school and work day instead of 4:31 A.M. on a holiday. Thus, the time of day that an earthquake occurs is a crucial factor in the number of casualties.

Human-Generated Factors

Fires and dam bursts following an earthquake are examples of major human-caused complications that aggravate the destructive effects of the earthquake itself. In industrialized countries, an earthquake may also be the cause of a major technological disaster by damaging or destroying nuclear power stations, research centers, hydrocarbon-storage areas, and complexes making chemical and toxic products. In some cases, such "follow-on" disasters can lead to many more deaths than those caused directly by the earthquake (*60*).

Hazardous Materials

Our modern industrial cities are laden with chemical and petroleum products that could contribute substantially to the generation of toxic products following an earthquake (*61*). Industrial storage facilities for hazardous materials might explode or leak, and damage at a nuclear power plant could lead to widespread contamination by radioactive materials. In a major earthquake, pipelines carrying natural gas, water, and sewage can be expected to be disrupted. Following the Loma Prieta earthquake, about 20% of after-earthquake injuries were caused by toxic materials (*31*).

Efforts to remove trapped occupants from a collapsed building may also expose rescuers to a variety of hazards, such as those from damaged utilities (*48*). For example, the destruction of buildings and industrial facilities by any catastrophe will invariably result in ruptured electrical, water, gas, and sewer lines. Other hazards will be escaping gases and chemicals used in refrigeration units and in certain industrial operations. Thus, rescue personnel must constantly observe all safety precautions to protect themselves from injury.

Fire Risks

One of the most severe follow-on or secondary disasters that can follow earthquakes is fire (*62*). Severe shaking may cause overturning of stoves, heating appliances, lights, and other items that can ignite materials into flame. Historically, earthquakes in Japan that trigger urban fires cause 10 times as many deaths as those that do not (*62*). The Tokyo earthquake of 1923, which killed more than 140,000 people, is a classic example of the potential that fires have to produce enormous numbers of casualties following earthquakes. Similarly, the large fire that occurred after the 1906 San Francisco earthquake was responsible for much of the death toll following that event. More recently, the 1994 Northridge earthquake in southern California showed that strong vibrations may sever underground fuel lines or gas connection points, causing spills of volatile or explosive mixtures and resultant fires (*10, 59*). Similarly, during the first 7 hours following the 1989 Loma Prieta earthquake in northern California, San Francisco had 27 structural fires and more than 500 reported incidents of fire (*18*). Furthermore, the city water supply was disrupted, significantly impairing the city's ability to fight these fires (*63*).

Perhaps the most vulnerable areas of all are the informal housing sectors on the periphery of many rapidly growing cities in developing countries (so-called "squatter housing" or "shantytown" settlements). Many of these have the potential for catastrophic conflagrations following an earthquake.

Dams

Dams may also fail, threatening communities downstream. A standard procedure after any sizable earthquake should be an immediate damage inspection of all dams in the vicinity and a rapid reduction of water levels in reservoirs behind any dam suspected of having incurred structural damage.

Structural Factors

Trauma caused by partial or complete collapse of human-made structures is overwhelmingly the most common cause of death and injury in most earthquakes (*5*). About 75% of fatalities attributed to earthquakes this century were caused by the collapse of buildings that were not adequately designed for earthquake resistance, were built with inadequate materials, or were poorly constructed (*64*). Results of field surveys following earthquakes have demonstrated that different building types and structural systems deteriorate in different ways when subjected to strong earthquake ground-motion vibration. There is also evidence that different types of buildings inflict injuries in different ways and to different degrees of severity when they collapse (*33, 65, 66*).

Glass (1976) was one of the first to apply epidemiology to the study of building collapse (*67*). He identified the type of housing construction as a major risk factor for injuries. Those living in the newer-style adobe houses were at highest risk for injury or death, while those living in the traditional mud-and-stick houses were at the least risk. Figure 8-6 shows the breakdown of earthquake fatalities by cause for each half of this century. By far the greatest proportion of victims have died in the collapse of

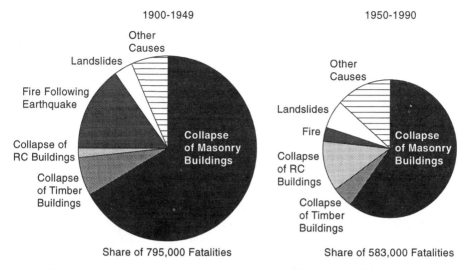

Figure 8-6. Fatalities attributed to earthquake, by cause. Figure from: Coburn A, Spence R. *Earthquake protection.* Chichester: John Wiley & Sons Ltd., 1992:6. (5)

unreinforced masonry (URM) buildings (e.g., adobe, rubble stone, or rammed earth) or unreinforced fired-brick and concrete-block masonry buildings that can collapse even at low intensities of ground shaking and will collapse very rapidly at high intensities. Adobe structures in many highly seismic parts of the world (e.g., eastern Turkey, Iran, Pakistan, Latin America) not only have collapse-prone walls but also very heavy roofs (*68, 69*). When collapsing, these heavy walls and roofs tend to kill many of the people in the homes (*70, 71*). In the United States, unreinforced masonry buildings abound throughout earthquake-prone regions of the central United States (e.g., the New Madrid seismic zone). Most of these unreinforced masonry buildings also remain without any degree of earthquake retrofit for seismic safety.

Concrete-frame houses are generally safer (i.e., less likely to collapse), but they are also vulnerable, and when they do collapse, they are considerably more lethal and kill a higher percentage of their occupants than do masonry buildings. In the second half of this century, most of the earthquakes striking urban centers have involved collapses of reinforced concrete buildings, and the proportion of deaths due to the collapse of concrete buildings is significantly greater than it was earlier in the century (Fig. 8-6). Reinforced concrete requires sophisticated construction techniques; however, it is often used in communities around the world where either technical competence is inadequate or inspection and control are lacking. Catastrophic failures of modern reinforced, con-crete-slab buildings caused by the collapse of their supports have recently been de-scribed in Mexico City (1985), El Salvador (1986), and Armenia (1988) (*72–74*). Whereas the debris of buildings of adobe, rubble masonry, and brick can be removed with primitive tools, reinforced concrete poses grave problems for rescuers, particularly if not enough special and heavy equipment is available (*48*).

Time and again, wood-frame buildings such as suburban houses in California have been pronounced among the safest structures one could be in during an earthquake. Indeed, these buildings are constructed of light wood elements—wood studs for walls, wood beams and joists for floors, and wood beams and rafters for roofs (*75*). Even if they did collapse, their potential to cause injury is much less than that of unresistant old stone buildings, like those often used for businesses, offices, or schools. The relative safety of wood-frame buildings was shown quantitatively following the 1990 Philippine earthquake. People inside buildings constructed of concrete or mixed materials were three times more likely to sustain injuries (odds ratio [OR] = 3.4; 95% confidence interval [CI], 1.1–13.5) than were those inside wooden buildings (*76*).

Another structural risk factor for death and severe injury in earthquakes is the building height. In the 1988 Armenian earthquake, people inside buildings with five or more floors were 3.65 times more likely to be injured compared to those inside buildings less than five floors in height (95% CI, 2.12–6.33) (*65*), and in the 1990 Philippine earthquake, people inside buildings with seven or more floors were 34.7 times more likely to be injured (95% CI, 8.1–306.9) (*66*). In a high-rise building, escape from upper floors is unlikely before the building collapses, and if it collapses completely, as many as 70% of the building's occupants are likely to be trapped inside (*64*). On the other hand, in a low-rise building that takes perhaps 20 or 30 seconds to collapse, more than three-quarters of the building's occupants may be able to escape before the collapse (*64*).

Damage to other human-engineered structures, such as transportation networks (e.g., bridges, roads, and railways), can also pose serious threats to life in earthquakes. For example, in the 1989 Loma Prieta earthquake, 42 of the 62 total deaths resulted from the collapse of the upper section of the Cypress Viaduct of Interstate 880 in Oakland, which trapped motorists driving on the lower section (*77*).

Nonstructural Factors

Nonstructural elements and building contents have been known to fail and cause significant damage in past earthquakes. Facade cladding, partition walls, roof parapets, external architectural ornaments, unreinforced masonry chimneys, ceiling tiles, elevator shafts, roof water tanks, suspended ceilings and light fixtures, raised computer floors, and building contents such as heavy fixtures in hospitals are among the numerous nonstructural elements that can fall in an earthquake, sometimes causing injury or death (*78*). The frequent collapse of stairways makes escape particularly difficult, since many buildings have only one stairway (*79*). Furthermore, heavy furniture, appliances, bookshelves, equipment, and objects placed high can fall and cause injury unless secured (*49*). Although recent research indicates that nonstructural elements such as ceiling tiles and building contents such as office equipment and household furnishings have a low likelihood of causing fatal injuries, such elements are responsible for numerous minor and moderate injuries that can tax emergency health services (*80*).

Individual Risk Factors

Demographic Characteristics

In earthquakes, people over 60 years of age are at increased risk for death and injury and have a death rate that can be five times higher than that of the rest of the population (*67*). Children between 5 and 9 years of age, women, and the chronically ill also seem to be at an elevated risk for injury and death (*67*). Lack of mobility to flee collapsing structures, inability to withstand trauma, and exacerbation of underlying disease are factors that may contribute to the vulnerability of these groups. Mortality distribution by age will also be affected to a certain degree by the social attitudes and habits of different communities. For example, in some societies young children sleep close to their mothers and may be more easily protected by them.

Entrapment

As might be expected, entrapment appears to be the single most significant factor associated with death or injury (*81*). In the 1988 Armenia earthquake, death rates were 67 times higher and injury rates more than 11 times higher for people who were trapped than for those who were not (*33*). In the 1980 southern Italian earthquake, entrapment requiring assistance to escape was the most important risk factor: the death rate was 35.0% for trapped people versus 0.3% for untrapped people (*82*). In the Philippine earthquake of 1990, people who died were 30 times more likely to have been trapped than were injured survivors (OR = 29.74; 95% CI, 12.35–74.96) (*66*).

Occupant's Location Within a Building

In several past earthquakes in the United States and in other countries, the location of people at the time of the earthquake's impact has been shown to be an important determinant of morbidity. For example, the morbidity and mortality rate was significantly greater for people who were indoors than for those who were outdoors when earthquake shaking began (*33, 65, 76, 83*).

Furthermore, occupants of upper floors of multistory buildings have been observed to fare less well than ground-floor occupants. For example, in Armenia, there was a significant "dose-response" increase in risk for injury associated with the building floor people were on at the moment of the earthquake. People on the second to the fourth floor at the time of the earthquake were 3.84 times more likely to be injured than those on the first floor, and those on the fifth floor and higher were 11.20 times more likely to be injured (*65*).

Four out of five deaths in the Loma Prieta earthquake occurred in motor vehicles on public roadways (*14*). As in nonearthquake situations, where motor vehicles account for more than half of unintentional injury deaths (*84*), occupants of motor vehicles appear to have a special risk of fatal injury in an earthquake. As mentioned above, in the Loma Prieta earthquake, a single circumstance, the collapse of the Cypress Viaduct of Interstate 880 in Oakland, accounted for 40 of 62 total earthquake-related deaths.

Occupants' Behavior

The behavior of people during an earthquake is an important predictor of their survival (*85*). In several recent earthquakes (e.g., 1990 Philippines and 1992 Egypt earthquakes), there were widespread reports of deaths and injuries due to stampedes, as panicked building occupants and students rushed for the nearest exits (*76, 86*). On the other hand, a review of the first reaction of people following an initial earthquake shock revealed that those who immediately ran out of buildings had a lower incidence of injury than did those who stayed inside (*65, 66*). Other reports, however, suggest that running outside may actually increase the risk of injury. For example, during the 1976 Tangshan earthquake, many were struck by the collapse of outer walls after running out of their houses. Such victims actually accounted for 16% of the total number of deaths (*6*). Other anecdotal reports suggest the efficacy of moving to a protected area such as a doorway or under a desk. Clearly, the behavior of occupants during and immediately after an earthquake has been inadequately studied (*87, 88*).

From the 1985 Mexico City earthquake, anecdotal reports of little islands of concrete slab perched on the tops of children's school desks while the rest of the ceiling had collapsed to the floor suggest that earthquake drills might be worthwhile (*89*). The real question, of course, is whether the children would have been able to get under the desks in time to prevent injury if the school had been occupied. In the best-documented study of occupant behavior during earthquakes, the behavior of 118 employees of a county office building in Imperial County, California, was studied after a magnitude 6.5 earthquake damaged their building (*90*). Of interest here is the finding that 30% of the desks under which people in this building sought refuge moved away during the shaking, thus exposing the person to possible injury from falling objects. Following the 1989 Loma Prieta earthquake, Durkin et al. examined the value of taking protective actions commonly suggested in citizen safety advisories (e.g., standing in a doorway or crawling under a desk) (*31, 79*). They found that at least 60% of those injured during the period of shaking were engaged in some form of protective action at the time of their injury, but those injuries tended to be minor. Durkin's results suggest that while commonly recommended self-protective actions may enhance people's safety in total-building-collapse situations, people who rush to protect themselves in less hazardous settings may actually be increasing their risk of minor injury.

Time Until Rescue

Although the probability of finding live victims diminishes very rapidly with time, entrapped people have survived for many days. People have been rescued alive 5, 10, and even 14 days after an earthquake (*91*); these "miracle rescues" are often the result of exceptional circumstances—for example, someone with very light injuries is trapped in a void deep in the rubble with air and possibly water available. In the 1988 Armenia earthquake, 89% of those rescued alive from collapsed buildings were extricated during the first 24 hours (*33*). The probability of being extricated alive from the debris declined sharply over time, with no rescues after day 6. In the 1990 Philippine earthquake, survival among the trapped also fell off rapidly with time, from 88% on Day 1, to 35% on Day 2, to 9% on Day 3, to 0% from Day 4 onward (*66*). Of all the trapped who were extricated alive, 333 (94%) were rescued during the first 24 hours following the earthquake.

Prevention and Control Measures

Until earthquake prevention and control measures are adopted and mitigation actions implemented throughout the United States, a single severe earthquake could cause tens of thousands of deaths and serious injuries and economic losses exceeding $100 billion (*5*). Prevention and control efforts need to be multidisciplinary, and should include public education programs as well as better building design and improved quality of construction in those areas most likely to suffer an earthquake (*92*). The problem of ''earthquake casualties'' involves questions of seismology, the engineering of the built environment, the nature of both the physical and the sociological environments, aspects of personal and group psychology and behavior, short- and long-term economic issues, and many planning and preparedness aspects. Public health and disaster-response officials need to work together in the effort to develop and maintain effective seismic safety-planning and earthquake mitigation programs (*79*).

Primary Prevention of Earthquakes

Although we can neither prevent earthquakes nor set off small ones to prevent big ones, we should take earthquakes into consideration before undertaking activities known to precipitate earthquakes, such as making deep well injections, filling water impoundments, and discharging nuclear explosives underground.

Avoidance of Construction in Areas of High Seismic Risk

Avoiding unnecessary residential and commercial construction on or near active faults and in areas subject to tsunamis or landslide slope failures, soil liquefaction, and rockfalls is technically a secondary prevention measure for earthquakes, but it is a primary prevention measure for earthquake-related injuries (*93*). Areas of high seismic risk have been fairly well delineated, and information about such areas should be available to local planners and developers. It is also well known that certain types of ground (e.g., landfill areas) vibrate more severely during earthquakes and so cause more damage to the buildings built on them. By avoiding building on areas of potentially higher hazard, builders can help reduce future earthquake damage.

Safer Construction

Recent research findings support the view that preventing structural collapse is the most effective approach to reducing earthquake-related fatalities and serious injuries (5). Engineering interventions have largely been directed to increasing the ability of new buildings to withstand ground shaking or to retrofitting existing hazardous buildings. The most stringent level of seismic security will allow buildings to withstand earthquakes with little or no damage (94). At a minimum, buildings should be designed so that they will remain functional even though damaged (an important design criterion for hospitals). In developing countries, there may be rules of thumb or standard construction practices that could be established and learned even by village builders so that gross errors in construction are avoided in the future.

A building may still fail in an earthquake, but injuries may be prevented or reduced if those parts of the building likely to be occupied by large numbers of people can be designed in such a way that there is less risk of injury to the occupants (95). It may be possible to design buildings so that if they do "fail," they collapse in such a manner that occupants have the best possible chance of being rescued (96). For example, almost all types of damaged buildings will contain voids or spaces in which trapped people may remain alive for comparatively long periods of time. The design of new buildings could incorporate features such as a structural core or deep-beam structure that is believed to produce more potential safe spaces or voids for entrapped victims following complete or partial collapse.

Anecdotal evidence from earthquakes in Guatemala (1976), Mexico City (1985), and Armenia (1988) suggests that suffocation from dust inhalation may be a significant factor in the deaths of many people who die without apparent severe external trauma (15, 46, 97). However, the use of certain building materials and finishes may reduce dust production—for example, plasterboard may produce less dust on collapse than wet applied plaster. Developing and using methods of reducing dust release during a building collapse could perhaps prevent many deaths.

Retrofitting existing buildings (e.g., anchoring houses, bracing walls) can be expensive, and many owners do not have the funds for compliance even with minor strengthening requirements. Thus, a policy of selectively retrofitting buildings on the basis of relative risk may be appropriate. For example, in the case of unreinforced masonry buildings, Durkin and Thiel's research shows that many injuries in recent California earthquakes have occurred outside the buildings, often to occupants attempting to evacuate (31, 79, 98). This finding suggests that protecting the evacuation route out of URM buildings and along the buildings' perimeters may yield substantial reductions in the number of injuries and deaths at a modest cost (99). Other relatively simple modifications that may increase the probability that severe damage will cause fewer injuries include strengthening stairwells or bathrooms and creating "safe" corridors (*95*).

Finally, many of the 22,000 highway bridges in California are at risk of severe damage or collapse in a major earthquake (*77*). Any plan for earthquake hazard mitigation in a seismically active area such as California should also give high priority to the systematic retrofitting of transportation structures.

Development and Enforcement of Seismic Safety Codes

Because of improved building construction codes, land use planning, and preparedness, the losses in the San Francisco Bay area from the 1989 Loma Prieta earthquake and in the Los Angeles area from the 1994 Northridge earthquake were kept much lower than would have occurred in a less-well-prepared region. Aseismic design is an evolving science, and codes need to be updated periodically to reflect what has been learned from building performance during actual earthquakes. Particular attention should be paid to areas in the eastern part of the United States and in the upper Mississippi River Valley, where actual risk may be higher than perceived and where, consequently, local codes may not be adequate. How and when and at what expense older buildings should be brought up to code is a major public health issue, since these buildings are likely to be the most vulnerable.

However, the good design required by seismic codes can be negated if builders cut corners on materials and construction techniques. Rigorous enforcement of building codes can prevent shoddy and below-code-level work.

Nonstructural Measures

Many injuries and much of the cost and disruption from earthquakes are caused by the contents of buildings, including equipment, machinery, and other nonstructural elements. Therefore, the structural stability and robustness to violent shaking of all of these elements should be reviewed. A room-by-room review is likely to reveal many items that could cause injury to the room's occupants in the event of violent shaking. Although often beyond the purview of building codes (or any reasonable hope of enforcement, for that matter), heavy furniture, glass cabinets, appliances, and objects placed where they could fall or be thrown about should be firmly secured to prevent them from striking people in the event of an earthquake. Special precautions must be taken with sources of flame or electric filaments in boilers, heaters, space heaters, pilot lights, cookers, etc., because violent shaking could cause fires.

Prediction of Earthquakes

The science of predicting the time, place, and magnitude of an earthquake is still in its infancy (*100*). Although some major earthquakes have been presaged by foreshocks, changes in groundwater and geothermal activity, and even animal behavior, most major earthquakes have occurred suddenly and without warning. Nevertheless, the theoretical possibility of routine earthquake prediction remains, and if everybody was warned in time and evacuated their buildings, then very few people would be killed by building collapse. Thus, earthquake prediction certainly holds out the possibility of highly effective casualty prevention in the future (*101*).

Drills for Evasive Actions During Earthquakes

Earthquake drills are important. Earthquakes, although sudden, are usually not instantaneous. Building occupants usually have a few seconds to react before the shaking reaches maximum intensity, raising the possibility of taking evasive action to escape injury (*50, 87, 102*). Despite the relative lack of data on the efficacy of various evasive actions, it seems worthwhile for people to practice taking some evasive actions, particularly since they will have just a few seconds to act when an earthquake strikes.

Foreshocks may provide valuable warnings that can lead to lifesaving actions. For example, the Montenegro earthquake of 1979 came in two shocks with enough time between them for people to get outside their houses (*103*). Studies of the 1980 Italian earthquakes suggest that those who immediately ran outside were less likely to be injured or killed (*82*). However, while running outside may be good advice in rural areas, it may not necessarily be the best thing to do in densely populated urban areas. Narrow streets provide no protection and can rapidly fill with debris falling from collapsing side walls or roofs of buildings, whereas the central portion of the same buildings may be left standing and provide protection. Reports from the 1985 Chilean earthquakes suggest that a number of people were killed by building overhangs that fell on them as they tried to escape (*104, 105*). The most popular preparedness action recommended in this country is "duck and cover," which is based on anecdotal stories of people surviving under desks or beds.

However, anecdotal stories should not be the basis for responding to an earthquake: there is a distinct need to reassess all such widely accepted citizen safety actions to ensure that they are indeed the best responses (*31, 79, 106*). Only by conducting epidemiologic studies of the location of injured and noninjured people can we determine which behaviors are truly most likely to reduce the risk for injury. Determining the safest behaviors is likely to depend on the quality of construction and collapse potential of individual building types, and will be different for densely populated urban areas than for rural areas. If one is in a building with good antiseismic construction that is not likely to suffer total collapse, probably the best approach is to crawl under a desk and cover one's nose and mouth with a piece of cloth to protect the respiratory system against excessive dust. On the other hand, if one is in a building that is highly prone to total collapse (because of poor design, poor building materials, or poor construction practices), the only hope may be to run outside quickly.

Deaths and injuries caused by stampedes in public facilities such as schools underline the need for earthquake drills. People should therefore be encouraged to practice those actions that they would take during an earthquake. Earthquake-preparedness programs and educational materials, ranging from regular reminders or "earthquake tips" disseminated through the media to earthquake drills for occupants of specific institutions, such as hospitals and schools, should prove useful (Table 8-4).

Planning Scenarios for Earthquakes

Relative chaos is likely to prevail immediately after a major earthquake. Area residents, cut off from the outside, will initially have to help themselves and their neighbors (*16, 17*). They can best do this if they have already planned their responses to the most likely earthquake scenarios and practiced the necessary skills (*107*). Medical preparedness plans can be built around similar earthquake scenario calculations based on the building types likely to be affected, the population densities and settlement patterns, the size and characteristic of earthquakes expected in the region, and the medical facilities available in any study area (*108*). Such a regional hazard assessment, including "casualty scenarios," would permit the development of specific training programs for medical and rescue personnel as well as the appropriate deployment of medical and rescue equipment in advance of an earthquake disaster (*109*).

On the basis of the earthquake scenario that they develop, public health officials should devise a response plan. This plan should include the following:

- recommended actions for individuals to take during earthquake shaking
- instructions for evacuating buildings after the shaking has ceased (or during the earthquake itself if easy and safe to do so)
- a list of safe sites where people living in areas threatened by landslides during secondary tremors could be relocated
- means of caring for young, elderly, sick, or infirm people
- procedures for the safe shutdown of any machinery or processes
- procedures for extinguishing any potential fire sources and making hazardous situations safer
- a protocol for checking personnel and accounting for any missing persons
- a plan for dispensing first aid and dealing with distressed people
- procedures for checking and reporting damage
- damage limitation measures
- procedures for informing the workforce of whether and when it is safe to return to work or go home

Because there never are enough rescuers or medical providers in major disasters, communities vulnerable to earthquakes should establish ongoing programs to teach the

Table 8-4 Earthquake Safety Measures

Before an earthquake:

- Hold family earthquake drills so that each member of the family knows what to do in the event of an earthquake.
- Bolt down water heaters and gas appliances.
- Know where and how to shut off water, gas, and electricity at main valves and switches.
- Place large and heavy objects on lower shelves.
- Fasten bookcases and modular wall units to walls.
- Secure hanging plants in heavy pots.
- Secure large picture frames, mirrors, and heavy objects on open shelves.
- Have on hand emergency supplies, such as flashlights, extra batteries, and a portable battery-operated radio.

During an earthquake:

- Stay calm. Think through any action you might take for the consequences it may cause.
- Stay where you are. Do not go inside if you are outside. Do not go outside if you are inside. Most injuries occur as people are entering or leaving buildings. Never use elevators.
- If you are indoors, take cover under a heavy desk, table, bench, supported doorway, or alongside an inside wall. Cover your head and face to protect them from falling debris. If you are under a table, desk, etc., hold on to it.
- Pull a cloth, sheet, or piece of clothing over your head to protect yourself from breathing the thick dust that may be thrown up if the building suffers any damage.
- Stay away from glass, fireplaces, or anything that could fall on you. Do not use candles or open flames because of possible gas leaks.
- If you are cooking, working with machinery, or standing near a fire or naked flame, shut down the machinery, switch off your cooker, and extinguish any flames. If you cannot do so quickly, stay away from the machinery or flame and shut it down as soon as the shaking has stopped.
- If you are outdoors, move away from buildings, poles, and electrical wires. Stay away from doorways. Once in the open, stay there until the shaking stops.
- If you are driving, pull to the side of the road, away from bridges, overpasses, power lines, tall buildings, or any other structures that could fall onto the car. Stay inside the car until the shaking has finished. Watch for hazards in the road after an earthquake. Once the shaking has stopped, proceed with caution. Avoid bridges or ramps that might have been damaged by the quake.

After an earthquake:

- Be prepared for aftershocks. Some may be large enough to cause additional damage.
- Check for injuries. Do not attempt to move seriously injured people. Do not stay to collect belongings or valuables. As you go outdoors, put your arms over your head to protect yourself against objects possibly falling from above and move as far away from nearby buildings as possible. Do not look up until you are well clear of the buildings.
- If your building has been damaged, do not reenter it. Another earthquake can come at any time. Even if your building has not been damaged, stay outdoors for an hour or so.
- Do not use the telephone unless somebody has been injured or a building is damaged or burning. The emergency services may need all available lines.

Table 8-4 (*Continued*)

- Get your news from a portable radio or television.
- Check for gas leaks. If you smell gas, shut off your gas at the meter, or have someone else do it. Check for fallen or loose wires; disconnect damaged appliances.
- Check your home for damage and evacuate it if it appears dangerous. Check your chimney for cracks. Approach chimneys with caution. If you find severe damage, leave immediately; aftershocks could bring the structure down.
- Assume that tap water is contaminated; don't use plumbing until you are told sewer lines are safe. Plug drains to prevent sewage backup. You can use water from the water heater or toilet tank (not the bowl) for uses other than drinking; purify it by bringing to a rolling boil for one minute, or use purification tablets.
- Clean up hazardous materials. Be careful of falling objects when you open cabinets or closets.
- Cover broken windows with plywood or plastic sheeting.
- Listen to the radio for advisories.
- Wear protective shoes and clothing. After a large quake, there will be a lot of broken glass around.
- Do not use your vehicle unless there is an emergency. Do not go sight-seeing; you will only hamper relief efforts.

public what to do when an earthquake occurs, such as first-aid education, basic rescue training, and fire drills (*15*). Simulation exercises can be carried out jointly by volunteer groups, local fire brigades, and hospitals. This training also might help to improve bystanders' responses during everyday emergencies.

Disaster Response to Earthquakes

Disaster response to earthquakes is more akin to medical treatment than to prevention, but some aspects of the response may be likened to tertiary prevention in that those responding seek to limit further injury and to control the secondary effects of the earthquake (*92*). Prompt rescue should improve the outcome of victims, and early medical treatment should lessen the sequelae of the primary injuries (e.g., wound complications, chronic neurological disabilities). Provision of adequate food, water, and shelter should especially help people in vulnerable age groups and those with preexisting diseases. Effective environmental control measures should prevent secondary environmental health problems. Identification and control of long-term hazards (e.g., asbestos in rubble) should reduce chronic health effects.

Early Rapid Assessment of the Earthquake's Impact

Because rapid rescue of trapped victims and prompt treatment of those with life-threatening injuries can improve their outcome, early rapid assessment of the extent of damage and injuries is needed to help mobilize resources and direct them to where they are most needed (*110*). Unfortunately, the very factors likely to cause large numbers of injuries are also likely to disrupt communications and transportation and to damage medical-care facilities. Public health officials need to establish in advance how the affected areas will be surveyed (see Chapter 3, "Surveillance and Epidemiology").

Search and Rescue

People trapped in the rubble will die if they are not rescued and given medical treatment. To maximize trapped victims' chances of survival, search-and-rescue teams must respond rapidly after a building collapses. Studies of the 1980 earthquake in Campania-Irpinia, Italy (*111*), the 1976 earthquake in Tangshan, China (*112*), the 1988 earthquake in Armenia (*33*), and the 1990 earthquake in the Philippines (*66*) show that the proportion of trapped people found alive declined as the duration of entrapment increased. In the Italian study, a survey of 3,619 survivors showed (1) that 93% of those who were trapped and survived were extricated within the first 24 hours and (2) that 95% of the deaths recorded occurred while the victims were still trapped in rubble (*111*). Estimates of the survivability of victims buried under collapsed earthen buildings in Turkey and China indicate that within 2 to 6 hours fewer than 50% of those buried are still alive (*82*). Although we cannot determine whether a trapped person died immediately or survived for some time under the debris, we can safely assume that more people would be saved if they were extricated sooner. As suggested by these data, teams with specialized expertise in areas such as search and rescue and on-site resuscitation and medical first aid arriving more than a couple of days after an earthquake's impact are unlikely to make much difference in the overall death toll of a large earthquake (*91*).

With the exception of personnel from countries in close geographical proximity, foreign assistance usually arrives after the local community has already engaged in much of the rescue activity. For example, in southern Italy in 1980, 90% of the survivors of an earthquake were extricated by untrained, uninjured survivors who used their bare hands and simple tools such as shovels and axes (*111*). Following the 1976 Tangshan earthquake, about 200,000 to 300,000 entrapped people crawled out of the debris on their own and went on to rescue others (*6*). They became the backbone of the rescue teams, and it was to their credit that more than 80% of those buried under the debris were rescued. Thus, lifesaving efforts in a stricken community rely heavily on the capabilities of relatively uninjured survivors, including untrained volunteers, as well as those of local firefighters and other relevant professionals (*113*). This does not mean that people who were dead when they were extricated could not have been saved by a skilled team with sophisticated resources. However, people from the community clearly play the most important role in rescue efforts, if they are appropriately prepared.

Surveillance of Search-and-Rescue Activities

The conduct of future rescue operations can be enhanced by lessons learned from the position and circumstances of trapped victims and from specific details about the extrication process itself. Knowledge of collapse conditions helps set rescue priorities. For example, almost all types of damaged buildings will contain voids or spaces in which trapped people may remain alive for long periods of time. To know where these safe places may be, one needs to know the characteristics of various types of construction. Buildings of the same class and type of construction collapse in much the same way, and common factors are present. It is important that rescuers study these factors, since this knowledge will prove helpful when extricating casualties.

Ideally, search-and-rescue teams should have surveillance forms to record important information, including the building type, the collapse-site address, the nature of the collapse, the amount of dust present, the presence of fire or toxic hazards, the location of victims, and the nature and severity of injuries. Victims pronounced dead at the scene should be tagged with an identification number so that the medical examiner's data can later be linked to the search-and-rescue surveillance form. Surveillance of search-and-rescue activities should be used to direct resources to sites where the most good can be done in the first 24 to 48 hours—the most critical time.

Medical Treatment

Just as speed is required for effective search and extrication, it is also essential for effective emergency medical services: the greatest demand occurs within the first 24 hours (*33*). Ideally, "disaster medicine" (medical care for victims of disaster) would include immediate life-supporting first aid (LSFA), advanced trauma life support (ATLS), resuscitative surgery, field analgesia and anesthesia, resuscitative engineering (search-and-rescue technology), and intensive care (*26*). Unconscious patients with either upper-airway obstruction or inhalation injury or any patients with correctable hypovolemia resulting from hemorrhage or burns would be especially likely to benefit from early medical intervention. Safar, studying the 1980 earthquake in Italy, concluded that 25% to 50% of victims who were injured and died slowly could have been saved if lifesaving first aid had been rendered immediately (*114*).

Data from the 1976 earthquake in Guatemala (*115, 116*), the 1985 Mexico City earthquake (*29*), the 1988 Armenia earthquake (*33*), and the 1992 earthquake in Egypt (*86*) showed that injured people usually seek emergency medical attention only during the first 3 to 5 days following the earthquake, after which hospital case-mix patterns return almost to normal. From Day 6 onward, the need for emergency medical attention declined rapidly and the majority of the wounded required only ambulatory medical attention—indicating that specialized field hospitals that arrive 1 week or more after an earthquake are generally too late to help during the emergency phase. Following the

1992 earthquake in Egypt, nearly 70% of all patients with earthquake-related injuries were admitted within the first 36 hours after this earthquake (*86*).

The medical and public health impact of a severe earthquake may well be compounded by significant damage to medical facilities, hospitals, clinics, and supply stores within the affected area (*117*). In the worst-case scenario, a hospital building may itself be damaged by the earthquake, and the hospital staff may have to continue emergency treatment without using the buildings (*118*). For example, on January 17, 1994, at 4:31 A.M. Pacific Standard Time, an earthquake registering 6.8 on the Richter scale occurred in a previously unrecognized fault in Los Angeles County's San Fernando Valley, killing at least 60 people. The earthquake caused considerable damage to health facilities and significant health service disruption. Immediately after the shaking stopped, structural and nonstructural damage forced several hospitals to evacuate patients and move operations outside (*9, 10*). Structural damage forced several older hospitals and medical buildings to cease or reduce operations. During the 1985 Mexico City earthquake, which killed an estimated 7,000 people, a total of 4,397 hospital beds were lost—about one in four of those available in the metropolitan Mexico City area (*119*). Hospital emergency plans in earthquake areas should provide for the contingency of evacuating patients from the wards; safely removing critical equipment from operating theaters, radiology departments, and other parts of the hospital; and reestablishing routine patient-care services (*120*).

Surveillance of Injuries at Medical Treatment Sites

Treatment sites, whether at hospitals or in temporary field clinics, should designate someone to organize surveillance of injuries, collect data, and see that the data are tabulated and reported to disaster-response health officials. In addition to collecting adequate information on the location and severity of the injury and disposition of each patient, the surveillance team should attempt to record, for each patient, a permanent point of contact outside the disaster impact area so that epidemiologists conducting follow-up studies and/or surveillance efforts can find them, even if they are not able to return to their previous addresses because of earthquake damage. Depending on the urgency of the situation, some information can be collected on the spot about how an injury was sustained. Good basic data collected at the outset will both provide decision-makers with accurate data on injuries and form the basis for lessons applicable to the next earthquake.

Dissemination of Public Health Information

Public health organizations should work out scenarios for various information-dissemination contingencies before an earthquake occurs. This will be difficult. Telephone service is likely to be disrupted in the impact area of an earthquake. However, police, fire, and many emergency service organizations maintain radio networks, which public health officials may be able to use. Furthermore, radio and television news crews often arrive at the scene of a disaster with sophisticated communications equipment. The electronic news media can be another effective vehicle for disseminating health advisories and updates on casualties and relief efforts. For example, during the emergency phase, warnings of possible landslides disseminated by the media may help populations maintain a vigilance and possibly evacuate areas if minor rockfalls, slope failures, or debris flows suggest that a more severe failure is imminent. Prompt evacuation of low-lying areas near the coast should also be a priority whenever the National Oceanic and Atmospheric Administration's tsunami warning network (headquartered in Hawaii) issues a warning.

In a survey conducted after the 1989 Loma Prieta earthquake, Bourque et al. found that while the majority of deaths and injuries happened at the time of earthquake shaking, a rather high proportion—about 40%—of deaths and injuries occurred during the 72-hour period after the earthquake, some of which might have been prevented had advisory warnings been issued to the public (*87*). Ideally, public officials should work out media guidelines for information dissemination so that all parties will know what to expect when an earthquake strikes (see chapter on Effective Media Relations [Chapter 5]).

Environmental Health

In the day or so immediately following an earthquake, the priorities are undoubtedly rescuing and treating victims. Saving the lives of those injured or trapped far outweighs most other needs. However, the other needs of a population suddenly deprived of homes, possessions, urban services, and other essentials cannot be ignored and will assume greater significance as soon as the life-threatening situation stabilizes. If large areas of buildings are destroyed, the population made homeless will have an urgent need for shelter and food (*121*). They will also need drinking water, clothing, sanitation, hygiene education, and basic comfort provision. Effective environmental control measures should prevent secondary environmental health problems.

Surveillance for Communicable Diseases

Rumors and fears of epidemics generally circulate in the aftermath of disasters, and earthquakes are no exception. Outbreaks of infectious disease generally have not followed earthquakes in other countries and are unlikely to occur in the United States. Health officials, however, should be prepared to recommend appropriate sanitary precautions and to dispel unfounded rumors and inaccurate information. They should set up a disease surveillance mechanism appropriate to the circumstances and provide regular reports to disaster-response officials. Any unusually high incidence of disease should be investigated and control measures implemented. Mass vaccination campaigns not based on results of public health surveillance are inappropriate following earthquakes (see Chapter 3, "Surveillance and Epidemiology," and Chapter 5, "Communicable Diseases and Disease Control").

Detailed Follow-up Epidemiology

Few earthquakes have been adequately studied epidemiologically, with the exceptions previously noted (122). It is vital that plans for follow-up epidemiology be developed before an earthquake occurs so that the initial surveillance data collected will allow proper follow-up (123). Disaster-response officials must be convinced to invest time and resources in the initial surveillance effort, even though their attention is likely to be focused on emergency medical services and disaster relief (124). Without this investment, the opportunity to learn many lessons useful for future earthquakes may be lost (125). Again, it is important to recognize that earthquakes will recur and that lessons learned during the surveillance effort following a particular earthquake can help save lives during later earthquakes.

Critical Knowledge Gaps

Because we do not know enough about the precise causes of deaths and nature of injuries that occur during earthquakes, relief services are often misdirected and community medical/health planning for earthquakes is often inadequate (126). The more we know about the manner in which injuries and deaths occur, the better we can prepare for and respond to earthquakes. The following are steps researchers can take to help health officials and individuals better prepare for earthquakes:

- Classify the earthquake-related risks of populations around the world by the construction class of buildings in which they live and by the seismic intensity possible in the area. Such classifications will help improve the accuracy of loss prediction studies before disasters (127).
- Determine the role of physical elements (e.g., type of building, nonstructural elements) in producing specific types and severities of earthquake-related injuries. Currently, data on deaths and injuries and other related data are usually gathered without being correlated with building design information, the dynamic characteristics of soil around each building, or the characteristics of the population at risk in individual buildings. Furthermore, few studies have looked at exactly what components of a building cause the injuries, particularly in those situations in which some people are killed and others are only injured or escape without injury (79).

- Evaluate the role of occupant behavior in earthquake injury susceptibility.
- Collect more extensive data concerning the circumstances of entrapment (e.g., location of victims in the collapsed structure). Lack of such data has made planning search-and-rescue actions, providing proper medical care, and requesting the appropriate outside aid more difficult.
- Formally evaluate the effectiveness and appropriateness of the different methods and strategies of search and rescue (*128*).
- Integrate knowledge obtained from different disciplines. Most earthquake casualty studies have addressed the problem from the point of view of a single discipline, either that of engineers or that of health researchers. This lack of active collaboration between workers from different disciplines has been a major shortcoming of past research into the health effects of disasters. Successful epidemiologic studies will require close interdisciplinary collaboration among structural engineers, physicians, and epidemiologists.
- Incorporate postearthquake research findings into specific emergency-preparedness and response-guidance protocols. The gap between what researchers have learned and the knowledge base underlying the protocols of the "user community" (e.g., response and recovery organizations) can be lessened considerably if researchers and members of the user community interface more effectively. Results of research should be communicated to key decision-makers and citizens at national, state, and local levels so that they can incorporate such findings into community earthquake-preparedness and earthquake-response programs.
- Develop valid earthquake casualty estimation models for planning and response (e.g., predisaster models of the medical impact of earthquakes for simulation of disaster impacts) (*129, 130*).
- Determine whether and to what extent prior citizen safety training changes people's behavior under stress. Few studies have evaluated the extent to which people know about or follow earthquake safety recommendations or the effectiveness of recommended procedures (e.g., "duck and cover"). More research clearly needs to be done in these areas, and more effective teaching and training tools need to be developed.

Methodologic Problems

The data needed for comparative earthquake studies is often lacking. These data include such basic information as the magnitude or intensity of the earthquake, the number of deaths, the number of people injured (using standard definitions) and the size of the affected population (*131*).

The study of earthquake injuries is difficult to approach from any narrow background, as it requires the active collaboration of workers having a number of areas of expertise

(*122*). First, one must understand the mechanisms of physical failure in earthquakes. This requires structural engineering and architectural competence. Second, one must understand the process of human injury in earthquake-induced building failure. Third, one must develop the analytical framework for the analysis of injury patterns and for the analysis of the relationship between specific causative agents and negative consequences (*129*).

Furthermore, the causal mechanisms and nature of earthquake-related injuries are difficult to determine precisely, as are the appropriate variables and indicators describing such injuries. One must consider hazard exposure; construction types and their performance during earthquakes; the influence of nonstructural components, building components, and building contents; building occupancy and the behavior of occupants; emergency and rescue response; and medical treatment provided. Not surprisingly, one is soon faced with the problem that such information is very difficult to collect because it must be collected immediately after the impact, when conditions are most chaotic and all qualified personnel are directed to the primary lifesaving effort (*132*). This use of personnel is, in most cases, justifiable; however, without the active assistance of search-and-rescue personnel, "backtracking" injuries from hospitals to specific building-collapse sites may be impossible.

The difficulty of collecting information on entrapped people is compounded by the fact that traditional, institutionalized sources of injury data (e.g., hospital medical records) do not usually document information such as where in a building the injury occurred, which attributes of the building contributed to the injury, the injured person's initial behavior when ground shaking began, and the circumstances of entrapment. Unfortunately, this lack of data on the circumstances of entrapment tends to hinder the development of effective search-and-rescue techniques and effective injury-prevention strategies.

General earthquake injury statistics based only on statistics from hospital emergency departments tend to overestimate the number of people seeking hospital treatment for earthquake-related problems, since they also include individuals who seek treatment for medical complaints that are not earthquake-related. On the other hand, looking only at hospitals and the problems they treat will likely underestimate the total health impact of an earthquake, since such information does not take into account other settings in which people seek and receive treatment. These settings include (but are not limited to) community clinics, urgent-care centers, and Red Cross and Salvation Army shelters. Of course, it is also difficult to obtain documentation on those patients whose injuries are self-treated. According to Durkin, injury statistics based solely on data collected from hospitals may account for only 40% of the number of injuries that actually occurred (e.g., the actual number of injuries in the 1989 Loma Prieta earthquake may have been as high as 9,500 instead of the officially reported 3,800) (*31*).

Analytic studies that establish and quantify the magnitude of the relationship between significant risk factors and injuries are also very difficult to organize and conduct in an earthquake-devastated region where most dwellings have been destroyed and populations relocated—factors that make locating injured people extremely difficult. Furthermore, in most areas of the world where major earthquakes have occurred, official census records are poor. Even when good census data are available, as in California, other factors, such as the proportion of people commuting to and from the affected area, may greatly affect the size of the population present at the actual time of the earthquake. Thus, even estimating the population at risk may be difficult, let alone selecting appropriate control subjects (*133*). As a result, almost all of the published epidemiologic studies on earthquake-related injuries are descriptive; they are not the analytic studies necessary to test hypotheses that particular types of exposures or hazards (e.g., collapsing buildings) are associated with injuries.

(See Chapter 2, "The Use of Epidemiologic Methods in Disasters", for a more in-depth discussion of the problems of conducting studies following disasters [e.g., collecting reliable data on injuries under difficult field conditions, collecting "perishable" data, dealing with a lack of definition of disaster-related injury, working with poor documentation in medical records, and selecting appropriate control subjects]).

Research Recommendations

- Seek to understand the mechanism by which people are killed or injured in earthquakes (e.g., what components of the building have directly caused trauma). Such knowledge is essential to developing effective prevention strategies (*134*).
- Attempt to identify factors related to the survival of those rescued following a building collapse. For example, study the relationship between the incidence of injuries and a building's structural design, the construction materials used, non-structural components in the building, demographic factors of the community, and the physical circumstances of entrapment. Determining where people are located when they are injured or killed can provide valuable information to assist both in locating potential survivors and in making recommendations to building occupants as to what to do during an earthquake.
- Establish the cause and approximate time of death of a body removed from a collapsed structure in concert with experts in forensic medicine. Then correlate time-of-death estimates with duration of entrapment. Understanding when people die following a building collapse can provide important information for planning rescue efforts and evaluating needed resources.
- Establish detailed autopsy data on a sample of earthquake victims to determine the exact cause of death. Such information could provide the basis upon which to suggest modifications to buildings to prevent death. Similar autopsy information has been valuable in analyzing automobile crashes and making appropriate modifications to automobile interiors.

- Evaluate the efficacy of search-and-rescue efforts and of medical care rendered following earthquakes. A careful investigation of the organizational barriers to rapid response is required to improve the ability of rescue and field medical teams to respond rapidly enough to save the lives of the most seriously injured disaster victims. Studies of the epidemiology of injured survivors may also help to identify the best way to dismantle a collapsed building (*135*) and to conduct rescue without doing more damage to those trapped.
- Study immediate medical needs of people entrapped in buildings following earthquakes. Such studies could help identify effective interventions to prevent or to manage casualties (e.g. treatment of crush syndrome) as well as to minimize disability (e.g., by reducing the incidence of wound infections and postoperative complications in the field).
- Determine whether knowledge of injury patterns following an earthquake can be used to suggest design changes in the structural and nonstructural components of a building.
- Analyze previous building failures in the context of injury studies. The results could lead to the development of simple but effective retrofit prevention strategies designed to mitigate injury or death.
- Study behavioral factors related to death and injury in earthquakes. Only by developing reliable data on the location of injured and noninjured people can disaster officials offer building occupants sound advice as to the best actions to take in order to reduce the likelihood of death or injury.
- Gather data that will allow us to predict what types of injuries to expect when an earthquake occurs given a knowledge of building design, local soil conditions, earthquake intensity, population density, etc. (*95*). This information is essential both for rapidly assessing the magnitude of the problem and for anticipating rescue and health and medical service demands following a major earthquake (e.g., predicting the amount of supplies and number of personnel needed) (*136*).
- Examine the manner in which buildings collapse during other kinds of disasters. For example, structural collapses caused by tornadoes, hurricanes, single-building construction failures, mine disasters, terrorist bombings, aircraft or train crashes, wartime experiences, and so on could provide valuable insights into the manner in which buildings collapse during earthquakes.
- Determine the risk of toxic releases and other nontraditional hazards following earthquakes.
- Identify the cultural and socioeconomic determinants of earthquake injury. For example, despite the potential hazards associated with unreinforced masonry buildings, such buildings frequently offer the only affordable shelter for economically and socially disadvantaged residents and marginal minority businesses. Therefore, we should direct research at developing architectural, administrative, and managerial hazard-reduction techniques that are tailored to reduce the risks of different ethnic minorities in earthquake-prone areas of the country.

- Attempt to determine worldwide and by country or disaster-prone area (1) the proportion of people who are effectively protected at that moment by aseismic buildings, both at home and in the workplace, and (2) the cost of providing complete protection for the population in question (*137*).

Summary

A major earthquake in one of our urban areas ranks as the largest potential natural disaster for the United States. Most of what can be done to mitigate injuries must be done before an earthquake occurs. Researchers have identified a number of potentially important risk factors for injuries associated (either directly or indirectly) with earthquakes. Because structural collapse is the single greatest risk factor, priority should be given to seismic safety in land-use planning and in the design and construction of safer buildings.

The integration of epidemiologic studies with those of other disciplines such as engineering, architecture, the social sciences and other medical sciences is essential for improved understanding of injuries following earthquakes (*138*). Better epidemiologic knowledge of risk factors for death and the type of injuries and illnesses caused by earthquakes is clearly an essential element for determining what relief supplies, equipment, and personnel are needed to respond effectively to earthquakes.

Strengthening communities' self-reliance in disaster preparedness is the most fruitful way to improve the effectiveness of relief operations. In disaster-prone areas, training and education in basic first aid and rescue methods should be an integral part of any community preparedness program.Unfortunately, because of the relatively long time periods between major earthquakes, the public health community faces a special challenge in effectively communicating the hazards posed by potential earthquakes and the necessity to plan and take action before an earthquake occurs.

References

1. Hays WW. Perspectives on the International Decade for Natural Disaster Reduction. *Earthquake Spectra* 1990;6:125–143.
2. Perez E, Thompson P. Natural hazards: causes and effects. Earthquakes. *Prehospital and Disaster Med* 1994;9:260–271.
3. Hamilton RM, Johnston AC. *Tecumseh's prophecy: preparing for the next New Madrid earthquake*. US Geological Survey Circular 1066. Denver: USGS, 1990.
4. U.S. Geological Survey. *Scenarios of possible earthquakes affecting major California population centers, with estimates of intensity and ground shaking*. Open-File Report 81–115. Menlo Park, CA: USGS, 1981.
5. Coburn A, Spence R. *Earthquake protection*. Chichester: John Wiley & Sons Ltd., 1992:2–12, 74–80, 277–284.

6. Chen Y, Tsoi KL, Chen F, *et al. The Great Tangshan Earthquake of 1976: An anatomy of disaster.* Oxford: Pergamon Press, 1988.

7. U.S. Department of Commerce, National Oceanic and Atmospheric Administration, and U.S. Department of Interior, Geological Survey. *Earthquake history of the United States,* rev. ed. with supplement for 197140. Boulder, CO: 1982. Pub. no. 41–1.

8. Haynes BE, Freeman C, Rubin JL, *et al.* Medical response to catastrophic events: California's planning and the Loma Prieta earthquake. *Ann Emerg Med* 1992;21:368–74.

9. Tierney K. Social impacts and emergency response. In: Hall JF, editor. *Northridge earthquake, January 17, 1994: Preliminary reconnaissance report.* Oakland: Earthquake Engineering Research Institute, 1994:86–93.

10. Goltz JD. *The Northridge, California, earthquake of January 17, 1994: general reconnaissance report.* Technical Report NCEER 94–0005. Buffalo, NY: National Center for Earthquake Engineering Research, 1994.

11. Davis JF, Bennett JH, Borchardt GA, *et al. Earthquake planning scenario for a magnitude 8.3 earthquake on the San Andreas fault in Southern California.* Special Publication No 60. Sacramento (CA): California Department of Commerce, Division of Mines and Geology. 1982.

12. National Oceanic and Atmospheric Administration. *A study of earthquake losses in the San Francisco Bay Region.* Washington, D.C.: Office of Emergency Preparedness, 1972.

13. Fitzgerald RH. Medical consequences of the earthquake of 1886 in Charleston, South Carolina. *South Med J* 1985;78:458–462.

14. Centers for Disease Control. Earthquake-associated deaths: California. *MMWR* 1989; 38:767–770.

15. Noji EK. The 1988 earthquake in Soviet Armenia: implications for earthquake preparedness. *Disasters: The International Journal of Disaster Studies and Practice* 1989;13:255–262.

16. Pointer JE. The 1989 Loma Prieta earthquake: impact on hospital care. *Ann Emerg Med* 1992;21:1228–1233.

17. Palafox J, Pointer JE, Martchenke J, *et al.* The 1989 Loma Prieta earthquake: issues in medical control. *Prehospital and Disaster Medicine* 1993;8:291–297.

18. Benuska L, editor. Loma Prieta earthquake reconnaissance report. *Earthquake Spectra* 1990;6(Suppl.):1–448.

19. Fratessa PF. Buildings. In: *Practical lessons from the Loma Prieta earthquake.* Washington, (DC): National Academy Press, 1994:1–274.

20. Noji EK, Armenian HK, Oganessian AP. Mass casualties and major injuries: Medical management in the Armenian earthquake. In: *Proceedings of the International Symposium on "Medical Aspects of Earthquake Consequences" in Yerevan, Armenia 9–11 October 1990.* Yerevan (Armenia): Armenian Ministry of Health, 1990.

21. Perez E, Thompson P. Natural hazards: causes and effects. Earthquakes. *Prehospital and Disaster Medicine* 1994;9:260–271.

22. California Department of Commerce, Division of Mines and Geology. *How earthquakes are measured.* California Geology February 1979:35–37.

23. U.S. Atomic Energy Commission. *Report on structural damage in Anchorage, Alaska caused by the earthquake of March 27, 1964.* Nevada Operations Office. NV0–9949. (Contract AT [2S1] 99), Jan. 1966.

24. Stratton JW. Earthquakes. In: Gregg MB, editor. *The public health consequences of disasters.* Atlanta: Centers for Disease Control, 1989:13–24.

25. Pretto E, Safar P. Disaster reanimatology potentials revealed by interviews of survivors of five major earthquakes. *Prehospital and Disaster Medicine* 1993;8:S139.

26. Pretto EA, Angus DC, Abrams JI, *et al.* An analysis of prehospital mortality in an earthquake. *Prehospital and Disaster Medicine* 1994;9:107–124.

27. Mikaelyan AL, Belorusov O, Lebedeva RN, *et al.* The experience of the All-Union Surgery Scientific Center of the USSR Academy of Medical Scientific Center of the USSR Academy of Medical Sciences and its branch in the treatment of the Armenian earthquake victims. In: *Proceedings of the International Conference on Disaster Medicine Moscow 22–23 May 1990.* Moscow: Ministry of Health, 1990:1;467.

28. Jones NP, Noji EK, Smith GS, Krimgold F. Preliminary earthquake injury epidemiology report. In: Bolin R, editor. *The Loma Prieta earthquake: studies of short-term impacts.* A Natural Hazards Center monograph. Boulder: University of Colorado, 1990:33–43.

29. Malilay JM. *Comparison of morbidity patterns in two hospitals following the September 19, 1985 earthquake in Mexico City.* Washington, D.C.: Pan American Health Organization, 1986.

30. Memarzadeh P. The earthquake of August 31, 1968, in the south of Khorasan, Iran. In: *Proceedings of the Joint IHF/IUA/UNDRO/WHO Seminar.* Manila: World Health Organization Regional Office, 1978:13.

31. Durkin ME, Thiel CC, Schneider JE, *et al.* Injuries and emergency medical response in the Loma Prieta earthquake. *Bull Seismological Society of America* 1991;81:2143–2166.

32. Noji EK. Medical and Health Care Aspects of the Spitak-88 Earthquake. In: *Proceedings of the International Seminar on the Spitak-88 Earthquake,* 23–26 May, 1989, Yerevan, S.S.R. of Armenia. Paris: UN Educational, Scientific and Cultural Organization, 1992:241–246.

33. Noji EK, Kelen GD, Armenian HK, *et al.* The 1988 earthquake in Soviet Armenia: a case study. *Ann Emerg Med* 1990;19:891–897.

34. Noji EK. Acute renal failure in natural disasters. *Ren Fail* 1992;14:245–249.

35. Eknoyan G. Acute renal failure in the Armenian earthquake. *Kidney Int* 1993;44:241–244.

36. Aznaurian AV, Haroutunian GM, Atabekian AL, *et al.* Medical aspects of the consequences of earthquake in Armenia. In: *Proceedings of the International Symposium on ''Medical Aspects of Earthquake Consequences'' in Yerevan, Armenia 9–11 October 1990.* Yerevan (Armenia): Armenian Ministry of Health, 1990:9–10.

37. Frechette CN. Rescuing earthquake victims in Armenia. *Plast Reconstr Surg* 1989;84:838–840.

38. de Ville de Goyet C, Jeannee E. Epidemiological data on morbidity and mortality following the Guatemala earthquake *IRCS Medical Sciences: Social and Med* 1976;4:212.

39. Alexander DE. Disease epidemiology and earthquake disaster: the example of Southern Italy after the Nov. 23rd, 1980 Earthquake. *Soc Sci Med* 1982;16:1959–1969.

40. Arvidson RM. On some mental effects of earthquake [letter]. *Am Psychol* 1969;24:605–606.

41. Katsouyanni K, Kogevinas M, Trichopoulos D. Earthquake-related stress and cardiac mortality. *Int J Epidemiol* 1986;15:326–330.

42. Trichopoulos D, Katsouyanni K, Zavitsanos X. Psychological stress and fatal heart attack: the Athens 1981 earthquake natural experiment. *Lancet* 1983;1:441–443.

43. Dobson AJ, Alexander HM, Malcolm JA, *et al.* Heart attacks and the Newcastle earthquake. *Med J Aust* 1991;155:757–761.

44. Malilay JM. *Comparison of morbidity patterns in two hospitals following the September 19, 1985 earthquake in Mexico City.* Washington, D.C.: Pan American Health Organization, 1986.

45. Diaz de la Garza JA. *Earthquake in Mexico, Sept. 19 and 20 of 1985. Disaster Chronicles. No. 3.* Washington, D.C.: Pan American Health Organization, 1987.

46. Hingston RA, Hingston L. Respiratory injuries in earthquakes in Latin America in the 1970s: a personal experience in Peru, 1970; Nicaragua, 1972–73; and Guatemala, 1976. *Disaster Med* 1983:1:425–426.

47. Noji EK. Natural disasters. *Crit Care Clin* 1991;7:271–292.

48. Noji EK. Training of search and rescue teams for structural collapse events: a multidisciplinary approach. In: Ohta M, Ukai T, Yamamoto Y, editors. *New aspects of disaster medicine.* Tokyo, Japan: Herusu Publishing Co., Inc., 1989:150–155.

49. Rahimi M, Azevedo G. Building content hazards and behavior of mobility-restricted residents. In: Bolton P, editor. *The Loma Prieta, California, earthquake of October 17, 1989—public response.* USGS Professional Paper 1553-B. Washington, D.C.: US Government Printing Office, 1993:B51–B62.

50. Goltz JD, Russell LA, Bourque LB. Initial behavioral response to a rapid onset disaster: a case study of the October 1, 1987 Whittier Narrows earthquake. *Int J Mass Emergencies* 1992;10:43–69.

51. Haynes BE, Freeman C, Rubin JL, *et al.* Medical response to catastrophic events: California's planning and the Loma Prieta earthquake. *Ann Emerg Med* 1992;21:368–474.

52. Garcia LE. The Paez, Colombia earthquake of June 6, 1994. *Earthquake Engineering Research Institute Newsletter* 1994;8:7.

53. Blake P. *Peru earthquake, May 31, 1970. Report of the CDC epidemiologic team.* Atlanta: Center for Disease Control, 1970.

54. UN Economic Commission for Latin America (ECLAC). *The tsunami of September 1992 in Nicaragua.* Santiago, Chile: ECLAC, 1992.

55. Yanev P. Hokkaido Nansei-Oki earthquake of July 12, 1993. *EQE Review*, Fall 1993;1–6.

56. Synolakis C. The June 3, 1994 East Java Earthquake—Tsunami takes it toll on local villages. *Earthquake Engineering Research Institute Newsletter* 1994;28:6–7.

57. Jones NP, Noji EK, Krimgold F, Smith GS, editors. *Proceedings of the International Workshop on Earthquake Injury Epidemiology for Mitigation and Response, 10–12 July, 1989.* Baltimore: Johns Hopkins University, 1989.

58. US Agency for International Development (USAID). *Case report: Guatemala earthquake 1976.* Washington, D.C.: USAID, 1978.

59. Hall JF. *The January 17, 1994 Northridge, California earthquake: an EQE summary report.* San Francisco: EQE International, 1994.

60. Alexander DE. Death and injury in earthquakes. *Disasters* 1985;9:57–60.

61. Showalter PS, Myers MF. Natural disasters in the United States as release agents of oil, chemicals, or radiological materials between 1980–1989: analysis and recommendations. *Risk Anal* 1994;14:169–182.

62. Coburn AW, Murakami HO, Ohta Y. *Factors affecting fatalities and injury in earthquakes.* Internal Report, Engineering Seismology and Earthquake Disaster Prevention Planning. Hokkaido, Japan: Hokkaido University, 1987.

63. EQE Engineering. *The October 17, 1989 Loma Prieta earthquake: a quick look report.* San Francisco: EQE Engineering, 1989.

64. Coburn AW, Spence RJS, Pomonis A. Factors determining human casualty levels in earthquakes: mortality prediction in building collapse. In: *Proceedings of the First International Forum on Earthquake-Related Casualties. Madrid Spain, July 1992.* Reston, VA: U.S. Geological Survey, 1992.

65. Armenian HK, Noji EK, Oganessian AP. Case control study of injuries due to the earthquake in Soviet Armenia. *Bull World Health Organ* 1992;70:251–257.

66. Roces MC, White ME, Dayrit MM, Durkin ME. Risk factors for injuries due to the 1990 earthquake in Luzon, Philippines. *Bull World Health Organ* 1992;70;509–514.

67. Glass RI, Urrutia JJ, Sibony S, *et al*. Earthquake injuries related to housing in a Guatemalan village. *Science* 1977;197:638–643.

68. Mitchell WA, Wolniewicz R, Kolars JF. *Predicting casualties and damages caused by earthquakes in Turkey. A preliminary report*. Colorado Springs (CO): U.S. Air Force Academy, 1983.

69. Mehrain M. A reconnaissance report on the Iran Earthquake. *National Center for Earthquake Engineering Research Bulletin* 1991;5:1–4.

70. Coburn AW, Petrovski J, Ristic D, *et al*. *Mission report and technical review of the impact of the earthquake of 21 June 1990 in the provinces of Gilan and Zanjan. Earthquake reconstruction program formulation mission to the Islamic Republic of Iran*. Geneva: UN Disaster Relief Office, 1990.

71. Ceciliano N, Pretto E, Watoh Y, *et al*. The earthquake in Turkey in 1992: a mortality study. *Prehospital and Disaster Medicine* 1993;8:S139.

72. Bertero VV. *Lessons learned from the 1985 Mexico City earthquake*. El Cerrito, CA: Earthquake Engineering Research Institute, 1989.

73. Bommer J, Ledbetter S. The San Salvador earthquake of 10th October 1986. *Disasters* 1987;11:83–95.

74. Wyllie LA, Lew HS. Performance of engineered structures. *Earthquake Spectra* 1989(Special Supplement):70–92.

75. Mochizuki T, Hayasaka S, Kosaka S. Human behavior and casualties in wooden houses with little ductility. In: *Proceedings of Ninth World Conference on Earthquake Engineering*. Tokyo: Japan Association for Earthquake Disaster Prevention 1988;8:983–988.

76. Centers for Disease Control: Earthquake Disaster—Luzon, Philippines. *MMWR* 1990; 39:573–577.

77. Governors Board of Inquiry on the 1989 Loma Prieta Earthquake. *Competing against time: report to Governor George Deukmejian*. North Highlands (CA): California Department of General Services, 1990.

78. Ohashi T. Importance of indoor and environmental performance against an earthquake for mitigating casualties. In: *Proceedings of the Eighth World Conference on Earthquake Engineering*, Vol. VII. Englewood Cliffs, NJ: Prentice-Hall, 1984;7:655–662.

79. Durkin ME, Thiel CC. Improving measures to reduce earthquake casualties. *Earthquake Spectra* 1992;8:95–113.

80. Wagner RM, Jones NP, Smith GS, Krimgold F. Study methods and progress report: a case-control study of physical injuries associated with the earthquake in the County of Santa Cruz. In: Tubbesing SK, editor. *The Loma Prieta, California, earthquake of October 17, 1989—Loss estimation and procedures*. USGS Professional Paper 1553-A. Washington, DC: U.S. Government Printing Office, 1993:A39–A61.

81. Durkin ME, Murakami HO. Casualties, survival and entrapment in heavy damaged buildings. In: *Proceedings of the 9th World Conference on Earthquake Engineering*. Tokyo: Japan Association for Earthquake Disaster Prevention, 1988;8:977–982.

82. de Bruycker M, Greco D, Lechat MF. The 1980 earthquake in Southern Italy: morbidity and mortality. *Int J Epidemiol* 1985;14:113–117.

83. Jones NP, Wagner RM, Smith GS. Injuries and building data pertinent to the Loma Prieta earthquake: County of Santa Cruz. In: *Proceedings of the 1993 National Earthquake Conference, 2–5 May, 1993, Memphis, Tennessee*. Monograph #5. Memphis: Central U.S. Earthquake Consortium, 1993:531–540.

84. National Safety Council (NSC): *Accident facts*. Chicago: National Safety Council, 1989.

85. Aroni S, Durkin M. Injuries and occupant behavior in earthquakes. In: *Proceedings of the Joint US-Romanian Seminar on Earthquakes and Energy*. Washington, D.C.: Architectural Research Centers Consortium, 1985:3–40.

86. Malilay J. Medical and healthcare aspects of the 1992 earthquake in Egypt. *Report of the Earthquake Engineering Research Institute reconnaissance team.* Oakland: Earthquake Engineering Research Institute, 1992.

87. Bourque LB, Russell LA, Goltz JD. Human behavior during and immediately after the Loma Prieta earthquake. In: Bolton P, editor. *The Loma Prieta, California earthquake of October 17, 1989—public response.* USGS Professional Paper 1553-B. Washington, D.C.: U.S. Government Printing Office, 1993: B3–B22.

88. Archea J. Immediate reactions of people in houses. In: Bolin R, editor. *The Loma Prieta earthquake: studies of short-term impacts.* Monograph #50. Boulder: Univ. of Colorado, 1990:56–64.

89. Durkin ME. Behavior of building occupants in earthquakes. *Earthquake Spectra* 1985; 1(2):271–83.

90. Arnold C, Durkin M, Eisner R, Whittaker D. *Imperial County Services Building: occupant behavior and operational consequences as a result of the 1979 Imperial Valley earthquake* [grant monograph]. San Mateo, CA: Building Systems Development, Inc., 1982.

91. Noji EK. Medical consequences of earthquakes: coordinating medical and rescue response. *Disaster Management* 1991;4:32–40.

92. Noji EK, Sivertson KT. Injury prevention in natural disasters: a theoretical framework. *Disasters* 1987;11(4):290–296.

93. National working group in Japan: *Tsunami protective measures in Japan.* Tokyo: Tokyo University, 1961.

94. Special Subcommittee of the Joint Committee on Seismic Safety. *The San Fernando earthquake of February 9, 1971 and public policy.* San Jose, CA: California Legislature, 1972.

95. Smith GS. Research issues in the epidemiology of injuries following earthquakes. In: *Proceedings of the International Workshop on Earthquake Injury Epidemiology for Mitigation and Response, 10–12 July, 1989, Baltimore, Maryland.* Baltimore: Johns Hopkins University, 1989:61–81.

96. Coburn AW, Pomonis A, Sakai S. Assessing strategies to reduce fatalities in earthquakes. In: *Proceedings of the International Workshop on Earthquake Injury Epidemiology for Mitigation and Response, 10–12 July, 1989, Baltimore, Maryland.* Baltimore: Johns Hopkins University, 1989:107–132.

97. Sanchez-Carrillo CI: Morbidity following Mexico City's 1985 earthquakes: clinical and epidemiologic findings from hospitals and emergency units. *Public Health Rep* 1989; 104(5):483–488.

98. Durkin M, Aroni S, Coulson A. Injuries in the Coalinga earthquake. In: *The Coalinga earthquake of May 2, 1983.* Berkeley (CA): Earthquake Engineering Research Institute, 1983.

99. Durkin ME, Thiel CC, Schneider JE. Casualties and emergency medical response. In: Tubbesing SK, editor. *The Loma Prieta, California, earthquake of October 17, 1989—loss estimation and procedures.* USGS Professional Paper 1553-A. Washington, D.C.: US Government Printing Office, 1993:A9–A38.

100. Disaster trends. Real-time earthquake monitoring. *Disaster Trends Summary* 1992;5:2.

101. Chengye T. A criterion for calling an earthquake alert: forecasting mortality for various kinds of earthquakes. *Earthquake Research in China* 1991;5:83–93.

102. Lomnitz C. Casualties and the behavior of populations during earthquakes. *Bulletin of the Seismological Society of America* 1970;60(4):1309–1313.

103. Tiedemann H. Casualties as a function of building quality and earthquake intensity. In: *Proceedings of the International Workshop on Earthquake Injury Epidemiology for Mitigation and Response, 10–12 July, 1989, Baltimore, Maryland.* Baltimore: Johns Hopkins University, 1989:420–434.

104. Durkin ME. The Chile earthquake of March 3, 1985: casualties and effects on the health care system. *Earthquake Spectra* 1986;2(2):487–497.
105. Reyes Ortiz M, Reyes Roman M, Vial Latorre A, *et al*. Brief description of the effects of the earthquake of 3rd March 1985—Chile. *Disasters* 1986;10:125–140.
106. Archea J. The behavior of people in dwellings during the Loma Prieta California earthquake of October 17, 1989. *National Center for Earthquake Engineering Research Bulletin* 1990;4:8–9.
107. Ohta Y, Ohashi H, Kagami H. A semi-empirical equation for estimating occupant casualty in an earthquake. In: *Proceedings of the 8th European Conference on Earthquake Engineering*. Lisbon: European Association for Earthquake Engineering, 1986;2(3): 81–88.
108. Spence RJ, Coburn AW, Sakai S, *et al: Reducing human casualties in building collapse: methods of optimizing disaster plans to reduce injury levels*. Cambridge: Martin Center for Architectural and Urban Studies, Cambridge University, 1990.
109. Noji EK. Health impact of earthquakes: implications for hazard assessment and vulnerability analysis. In: *Proceedings of the First International Forum on Earthquake-Related Casualties, Madrid Spain, July 1992*. Reston, VA: U.S. Geological Survey, 1992.
110. Schneider E. *Northridge earthquake rapid health needs assessment of households—Los Angeles County, California. January 20, 1994*. Atlanta: Centers for Disease Control and Prevention, 1994.
111. de Bruycker M, Greco D, Annino I, *et al*. The 1980 earthquake in Southern Italy: rescue of trapped victims and mortality. *Bull World Health Organ* 1983;61:1021–1025.
112. Sheng ZY. Medical support in the Tangshan earthquake: a review of the management of mass casualties and certain major injuries. *J Trauma* 1987;27:1130–1135.
113. Noji EK, Armenian HK, Oganessian A. Issues of rescue and medical care following the 1988 Armenian earthquake. *Int J Epidemiol* 1993;22:1070–1076.
114. Safar P. Resuscitation potentials in earthquakes. An international panel. *Prehospital and Disaster Medicine*. 1987;3(2):77.
115. de Ville de Goyet C, del Cid E, Romero A, *et al*. Earthquake in Guatemala: epidemiologic evaluation of the relief effort. *Bull Pan Am Health Organ* 1976;10:95–109.
116. Chatterson J. Guatemala after the earthquake. *Can J Public Health* 1976;67:192–195.
117. Degler RR, Hicks SM. The destruction of a medical center by earthquake: initial effects on patients and staff. *Calif Med* (now *West J Med*) 1972;116:63–67.
118. Arnold C, Durkin M. *Hospitals and the San Fernando earthquake of 1971: the operational experience*. San Mateo, CA: Building Systems Development, Inc., 1983.
119. Zeballos JL. Health effects of the Mexico earthquake—19th Sept. 1985. *Disasters* 1986; 10:141–149.
120. Noji EK, Jones NP. Hospital preparedness for earthquakes. In: Tomasik KM, editor. *Emergency preparedness: when the disaster strikes. Plant, Technology & Safety Management Series*. Oakbrook Terrace, IL: Joint Commission on the Accreditation of Health Care Organizations, 1990:13–20.
121. Malilay J. *The damnificados of Mexico City: morbidity, health care utilization, and population movement following the September 1985 earthquakes* [dissertation]. New Orleans, LA: Tulane University, 1987.
122. Jones NP, Noji EK, Krimgold FR, Smith GS. Considerations in the epidemiology of earthquake injuries. *Earthquake Spectra* 1990;6:507–528.
123. Centers for Disease Control, US Geological Survey, Office of US Foreign Disaster Assistance, National Science Foundation and Federal Emergency Management Agency. *Proceedings of the First International Forum on Earthquake-Related Casualties, Madrid Spain, July 1992*. Reston, VA: U.S. Geological Survey, 1992.

124. Moorhead GV, Freeman C, Van Ness C. *Injury patterns in a major earthquake.* Sacramento, CA: Emergency Medical Services Authority, California, 1984.

125. Noji EK. Need for a sound research program on earthquake epidemiology. In: Hays WW, editor. *Proceedings of a meeting of the U.S. working group on earthquake-related casualties.* Open-file Report 90–244. Reston, VA: U.S. Geological Survey, 1990:71–80.

126. Lechat MF. An epidemiologist's view of earthquakes. In: Solnes J, editor. *Engineering seismology and earthquake engineering.* Leiden, Holland: Noordhoff, 1974;3:285–306.

127. Centers for Disease Control, US Geological Survey, Office of US Foreign Disaster Assistance, National Science Foundation and Federal Emergency Management Agency. *Proceedings of the meeting of the U.S. ad hoc working group on earthquake-related casualties, Washington, D.C., May 1992.* Reston, VA: U.S. Geological Survey, 1992.

128. Krimgold F. Search and rescue in collapsed buildings. In: Bertero VV, *Lessons learned from the 1985 Mexico City earthquake.* El Cerrito, CA: Earthquake Engineering Research Institute, 1989:217–219.

129. Olsen R. *Proceedings of the workshop on modelling earthquake casualties for planning and response.* Sacramento: California Emergency Medical Services Authority, 1990.

130. Shiono K, Krimgold F, Ohta Y. Postevent rapid estimation of earthquake fatalities for the management of rescue activity. *Comprehensive Urban Studies* 1991;44:61–105.

131. Pollander GS, Rund DA. Analysis of medical needs in disasters caused by earthquakes: the need for a uniform injury reporting scheme. *Disasters* 1989;13(4):365–369.

132. Comfort LK. Suggested problems for field research in earthquake disaster operation. In: *Proceedings of the International Workshop on Earthquake Injury Epidemiology for Mitigation and Response, 10–12 July 1989, Baltimore, Maryland.* Baltimore: Johns Hopkins University, 1989:458–461.

133. Armenian HK, Oganessian AP, Noji EK. The case control method for the investigation of the risk of morbidity in earthquakes. In: *Proceedings of the International Symposium on "Medical Aspects of Earthquake Consequences" in Yerevan, Armenia 9–11 October 1990.* Yerevan (Armenia): Armenian Ministry of Health, 1990.

134. Jones NP, Noji EK, Smith GS, Wagner RM. Casualty in earthquakes. In: *Proceedings of the 1993 National Earthquake Conference, 2–5 May 1993, Memphis, Tennessee. Monograph #5.* Memphis: Central U.S. Earthquake Consortium, 1993:19–68.

135. Applied Technology Council. *Earthquake damaged buildings: an overview of heavy debris and victim extrication.* Earthquake Hazards Reduction Series 43 (ATC 21–2). Washington, D.C.: Federal Emergency Management Agency, 1988.

136. Durkin ME, Thiel CC. Toward a comprehensive regional earthquake casualty modeling process. In: *Proceedings of the 1993 National Earthquake Conference, 2–5 May 1993, Memphis, Tennessee. Monograph #5.* Memphis: Central U.S. Earthquake Consortium, 1993:557.

137. Lechat MF. Corporal damage as related to building structure and design: the need for an international survey. In: *Proceedings of the International Workshop on Earthquake Injury Epidemiology for Mitigation and Response, 10–12 July 1989, Baltimore, Maryland.* Baltimore: Johns Hopkins University, 1989:1–16.

138. Wagner RM, Jones NP, Smith GS. Risk factors for casualty in earthquakes: the application of epidemiologic principles to structural engineering. *Structural Safety* 1994;13:177–200.

9

Volcanoes

PETER J. BAXTER, M.D.

Human and economic losses from volcanic eruptions have been dwarfed by those from floods, earthquakes, and hurricanes, but the potential for devastating events from volcanic eruptions is so great that volcanic hazards now warrant close attention. The main factors that contribute to volcanic disasters include the lack of accurate volcanic-hazard mapping, the few resources devoted exclusively to monitoring the most dangerous volcanoes, and the continuing growth and spread of populations with the result that about 500 million people will live in areas of volcanic activity by the end of this century. Hundreds of dangerous and explosive volcanoes exist, yet few of them have been subjected to any detailed hazard analysis. To advance hazard-zonation studies around volcanoes, the United Nations' International Decade for Natural Disaster Reduction (IDNDR) has designated some of the most hazardous volcanoes in developing and developed countries as Decade Volcanoes for special study (*1*) (Table 9-1).

Factors Affecting the Occurrence and Severity of Volcanic Disasters

Historically, some 600 volcanoes have been active worldwide, and 100 or more of these have been notorious for the frequency or severity of their eruptions in populated areas (*2, 3*). On average, about 50 volcanoes erupt each year. Most volcanoes, including those in the United States, are in a belt bordering the Pacific Ocean that is referred to as the "Ring of Fire"; historically, most deaths from volcanic eruptions have occurred in Indonesia. Another important belt stretches from southeastern Europe through the Med-

Table 9-1 Volcanoes Designated as Decade Volcanoes by the United Nations International Decade for Natural Disaster Reduction (IDNDR)

Colima (Mexico)	Mount Rainier (USA)	Teide (Spain)
Etna (Italy)	Nyiragongo (Zaire)	Ulawun (Papua New Guinea)
Galeras (Colombia)	Sakurajima (Japan)	Unzen (Japan)
Mauna Loa (United States)	Santa Maria (Guatemala)	Vesuvius (Italy)
Merapi (Indonesia)	Taal (Philippines)	

iterranean. In addition, volcanic islands are found in the Pacific, Atlantic, and Indian oceans. Interestingly, most volcanoes lie within 300 km of the sea in areas that are frequently also at high risk for earthquakes.

About 400 to 500 volcanoes lie in areas known as subduction zones, where tectonic plates undergo compression (e.g., the "Ring of Fire"), and these volcanoes tend to be explosive. Explosive volcanoes can erupt violently and release large quantities of ash. Conversely, some volcanoes, such as those in Hawaii, are characterized by large lava flows and copious gas emissions but little ash. Other volcanoes, such as the Icelandic volcanoes, can erupt with large lava flows (e.g., the mid-Atlantic rift volcano Krafla), or can erupt explosively and emit highly toxic ash, as does the volcano Hekla. Volcanoes having both explosive and effusive characteristics are classified as "mixed." Geologists now believe that there are at least 35 volcanoes with explosive potential located in the eastern United States and Alaska, with about two dozen in the Cascade range; six of these volcanoes have erupted in the last 200 years. Another dangerous area contains the Mono-Inya craters of California. The Hawaiian volcanoes of Mauna Loa and Kilauea have major lava eruptions every few years and have been intensively studied by geologists, but these volcanoes pose little risk to human life compared with their explosive cousins, such as Mount St. Helens, on the U.S. mainland.

Until the eruption of Mount St. Helens, and excluding volcanic activity in Hawaii, the most recent previous eruptions in the United States had been a minor one at Mount Lassen, California, in 1914 and the massive eruption of Mount Katmai in Alaska in 1912. The eruption of Mount St. Helens in Washington State on May 18, 1980, provided an important stimulus to volcanic disaster mitigation in the United States and elsewhere. Although Mount St. Helens is the most active volcano in the Cascade range, erupting approximately every 100 years, authorities were unprepared for the scale and destructiveness of its explosive eruption. Since then further disastrous eruptions around the world (e.g., of Mount Galungung, Indonesia, in 1984; of Nevado del Ruiz, Colombia, in 1985; of El Chichón, Mexico, in 1982; of Mount Pinatubo, the Philippines, in 1991; and of Mount Unzen, Japan, in 1991) (Table 9-2) have highlighted the dangers of inadequate preparedness.

Scientific work in recent years has confirmed the critical effect volcanoes may have on world climate. For example, an eruption on the scale of that which occurred at

Table 9-2 Volcanic Eruptions Since A.D. 1600 That Have Caused More Than 8,000 Deaths

Volcano	Date of Eruption	No. Killed	Lethal Agent
Laki, Iceland	1783	9,350	Ashfalls destroyed crops and animals, causing starvation
Unzen, Japan	1792	14,300	70% killed by cone collapse; 30% by tsunami
Tambora, Indonesia	1815	92,000	Most deaths from starvation
Krakatoa, Indonesia	1883	36,147	90% killed by tsunami
Mont Pelée, Martinique	1902	29,025	Pyroclastic flows
Nevado del Ruiz, Colombia	1985	23,000	Lahar

Source: Modified from Blong RJ. *Volcanic hazards: a source book on the effects of eruptions.* Sydney: Academic Press, 1984. (6)

Tambora, Indonesia, in 1815, and which is regarded as the deadliest eruption in historic times, would, if repeated today, likely lead to major loss of life from famine in many parts of the world because of the eruption's impact on climate. Plumes from certain eruptions, such as that of El Chichón in Mexico in 1982 and Mount Pinatubo in the Philippines in 1991, produced abundant sulphate aerosols in the stratosphere that prevented sunlight from penetrating completely through the aerosols and thus affected global surface temperatures (*4*). Massive caldera eruptions are hugely destructive and capable of global disruption on a grand scale; the last occurred in prehistoric times. Currently we possess no way to predict or plan for them.

Predicting Eruptions and Issuing Warnings

Volcanologists predict the general behavior of a volcano from available evidence of its geological characteristics and past activity (*5*). Assessing hazards associated with volcanoes can be an expensive and costly scientific activity, but it is an essential first step before undertaking a risk assessment or developing disaster plans. Using statistical information on the timing of previous eruptive events to predict future eruptions is difficult because such information is often sparse. For the few volcanoes on which data exist, random eruption patterns (e.g., at Mauna Loa), clustering (e.g., at Kilauea), and the increasing probability of a violent eruption as time passes since the last eruption (e.g., in Vesuvius, Italy) have all been identified.

If the timing, size, and nature of a volcanic eruption could be accurately foretold, then loss of life could be prevented through the enactment of timely evacuation measures. In practice, however, achieving this goal is remote. Warning of a reawakening of volcanic activity may be given by certain premonitory events, such as small earthquakes or minor emissions of gas and ash over weeks or months. Specific monitoring techniques, including seismography and ground deformation and the monitoring of gas emissions, microgravity, and thermal activity, may all be used (5). Even with close surveillance, however, it is impossible to infer from precursor activity whether there will be an eruption or to determine the size or character of the eruption. A hazard evaluation made by the U.S. Geological Survey in 1978 successfully predicted the scale of the eruption of Mount St. Helens on May 18, 1980, but the eruption could be foretold only as a likely occurrence, "possibly within this century"; even when premonitory activity began, there was no scientific consensus on whether a major eruption would occur. For subsequent minor eruptions, however, monitoring techniques were able to predict these eruptions a day or less beforehand and thus provided important information for emergency services personnel and people who continued to work in the volcano's vicinity.

As a further drawback, we know that disastrous eruptions can occur at places where volcanoes were not known to be located—for example, at Mount Lamington, Papua New Guinea, where 2,942 people were killed in 1951. In 1991, Philippine authorities were surprised when Mount Pinatubo first showed signs of eruptive activity because it had last erupted more than 600 years before and was not even considered to be a volcano warranting serious study. Not until volcanologists conducted an urgent assessment of Mount Pinatubo's stratigraphy did they recognize the extensive pyroclastic flow deposits and hazards. The volcano's explosive eruption on June 14, 1991, was one of the largest of the century.

Unfortunately, this inability to accurately predict when a volcano will erupt and with what force creates serious problems in heavily populated areas where long lead times may be required to successfully evacuate the population. For the foreseeable future, catastrophes such as the eruption at Nevado del Ruiz (Table 9-2) seem inevitable. One of the most dangerous volcanoes today is Mount Vesuvius in Italy. Now overdue for an eruption, the volcano threatens at least 800,000 people residing in houses and buildings that have spread relentlessly up the volcano's flanks. The examples illustrate the importance of placing the highest priority on efforts in disaster mitigation that are directed toward community preparedness and emergency response measures as long as such predictive uncertainties remain.

Hazards Associated with Eruptions and Factors Influencing Morbidity and Mortality

Volcanoes have been revered for their awesome power and feared for their ability to cause death and destruction. The range of eruptive phenomena and the secondary consequences is wide, and this diversity makes the study of volcanoes a particularly complex undertaking for scientists and health care workers (6). The most hazardous of these phenomena are pyroclastic flows and lahars (mudflows containing volcanic debris), which move like gravity currents. The risks for injury or death associated with these phenomena depend on (1) the size and nature of an eruption, (2) local topographic factors, and (3) the proximity of a population to the volcano. In addition, asphyxiant gases that form during an eruption are most dangerous near craters or fissures that are on or close to a volcano's flanks. Because gravity is crucial in determining the flow of volcanic solids and these dense gases, people living in low-lying areas and valleys near the volcano are at greatest risk for injury or death. Volcanologists studying critically active volcanoes know well the importance of ensuring that people avoid living in these areas as much as possible and of paying special attention to the risks faced by communities in low-lying areas surrounding volcanoes.

Hazards from Blasts and Projectiles

A blast is an explosive force, and if it occurs during an eruption, it is likely to be confined close to the vent or to arise locally from explosions, such as occur when hot material falls into lakes. Producing noise audible over long distances, sound waves will shatter windows and can lead to lacerations from broken glass. Rock fragments of varying sizes can be explosively ejected at any time, causing injury or death, and in massive eruptions can be released over a wide area around the volcano. Large projectiles may damage houses and, if hot, can set the houses afire.

Small explosive eruptions may occur in craters with little warning. For example, at Mount Etna in Sicily in 1979, nine tourists visiting the volcano were killed after a small eruption occurred, and at Galeras, Colombia, in 1993, six scientists who were working inside the crater were killed without warning. Such small-scale releases of energy caused by pent-up gases or similar mechanisms are a serious occupational hazard to volcanologists working close to volcanic vents (1).

Hazards from Pyroclastic Flows and Surges

Pyroclastic flows and surges are mixtures of hot gases, ash, fine pumice, and rocks that are propelled primarily by gravity and may be formed by the collapse of a vertical eruption column or may erupt directly over the crater rim (3). It is important to visualize these flows and surges as gravity currents that move like clouds of dense gas and that are capable of spreading out from a point source over a wide area and causing massive destruction. These flows may travel at speeds of 50–150 km per hour, a speed that, together with the flows content of solids, creates a powerful destructive momentum much like that of a hurricane-force wind. The dynamic pressure of the flow is responsible for flattening trees and buildings. Many flows and surges start at high temperatures (e.g., 600–900°C), and some may cool rapidly if they are turbulent and mix with air during their travel. In some places at the periphery of the flow, the temperature peak and dense particle concentration may be so short-lived that people can survive even out-of-doors: often sturdy housing can protect people who remain indoors. Pyroclastic surges are dilute flows that may leave deposits only a few centimeters deep; nevertheless, they can be highly destructive when they erupt from the volcano at high temperatures and energy levels. Many pyroclastic flows come to rest with a surge that extends several kilometers farther and which can still be hot enough to cause severe burns and that to vegetation. Gases such as steam, carbon dioxide, and sulfur dioxide are also likely to be present, at least in small concentrations.

The first opportunity to investigate the causes of death from pyroclastic flows was in the aftermath of the lateral pyroclastic flow from the May 18, 1980, eruption of Mount St. Helens. Despite official warnings and the establishment of restricted zones by local officials, more than 160 people, including a few loggers going about their work, were within close range of the volcano at the time it erupted. Lines of downed trees marked an abrupt cutoff of the maximal dynamic forces in an area of destruction that was as far as 27 km from the crater. Autopsies conducted on the 25 retrieved bodies (7) showed that 17 deaths had been caused by asphyxia due to inhalation of ash and that 5 deaths were the result of thermal injuries. Three people who died were loggers located at a spot 19 km from the crater; two survived the flow but suffered second- and third-degree burns affecting 33% and 47% of their body surfaces, respectively. However, these two loggers later died from adult respiratory distress syndrome induced by inhaling of hot, fine ash particles (8). Three people were killed by trauma to the head from fallen trees (2) or rocks (1).

The mortality rate associated with this eruption was about 50% after everyone, including those located in the periphery of the flow, was accounted for. This figure is surprisingly low, considering that all the victims and survivors were caught by the eruption out-of-doors (9). The best available evidence for the protection afforded by housing was obtained after the eruption of the St. Vincent volcano in 1902 (10). People who protected themselves from the eruption inside sturdy houses with shuttered windows survived, whereas those who were outside were killed, as were unprotected animals. In an eruption of Mount Unzen in Japan in 1991, two volcanologists and 39 journalists were killed by a high-temperature surge, but 8 people who were in nearby houses and 1 inside a car survived. Findings from these different eruptions have important implications for emergency planning in built-up areas around volcanoes. Nonetheless, evacuation must be the key preventive measure, because the magnitude and energy of flows are unpredictable. For example, in another eruption in 1902, at Mont Pelée in Martinique, only 2 of the 28,000 people inside the town of Saint Pierre survived the pyroclastic flow that devastated that town.

Lahars and Floods

Lahars (mudflows is another, but not necessarily accurate, designation for this slurry of water and volcanic debris) are frequent concomitants of eruptions and are at least as deadly as pyroclastic flows. The heat from pyroclastic flows, lava, and steam blasts may melt glaciers and snow, or heavy rain may accompany ash eruptions when the water mixes with ash and rock debris to form a huge volume of material that has a consistency that varies from that of a dilute slurry to that of a thick paste or wet concrete. Crater lakes, if present, can also be a major source of water, and lahars can greatly expand their volume as they flow by the lakes and incorporate loose soil that has eroded from river valleys. A large lahar is capable of flattening everything in its path, including houses, roads, and bridges. After the May 18, 1980, eruption of Mount St. Helens, lahars traveled down the Cowlitz and Toutle rivers into the Columbia River as far as the city of Portland. The average speed of these flows along the valley was only about 32 km/hr (20 mph), so that people living in their path downriver had time to escape (*11*). Conversely, in 1985 lack of preparedness resulted in the vast lahar from Nevado del Ruiz volcano, in Colombia, overwhelming the town of Armero located 48 km (30 miles) away and killing at least 23,000 people (*12*). Because river valleys are natural courses for lahars, flooding may be an immediate consequence as the debris fills in rivers and lakes. In addition, the deposited material alters the levels and courses of existing rivers, thereby posing a serious risk for future flooding in the event of heavy rain. Floods may also be caused by avalanches into lakes or by melting ice and snow.

Huge eruptions, such as the eruption of Mount Pinatubo in the Philippines in 1991, will fill deep valleys with pyroclastic and other eruptive material, and then heavy rains may mobilize the material for years afterward. Water overfilling rivers and channels rapidly erodes banks, and nearby housing is undermined or readily flooded. This problem has been particularly serious in flat areas around Mount Pinatubo and has resulted in the continued displacement of tens of thousands of people.

Tephra Fallout

Ashfalls from large eruptions can cause destruction and environmental damage across wide areas, as far as hundreds of kilometers downwind from the volcano. Heavy ashfalls (more than 25 cm deep) can be a major risk to life from their loads on the roofs of buildings. In the past, the hazards of ashfalls have not been emphasized enough, as two recent eruptions illustrate. At the eruptions of Mount St. Helens in 1980, the impact and size of the ashfall in central Washington State had not been anticipated (*13*). Even though the maximum depth of ash was only slightly more than 4 cm in places (Fig. 9-1), when the May 18 plume arrived, all economic activity, especially road, rail, and air transport, ceased for 5 days because of the drastically reduced visibility and as a result of the interference caused by the ash being suspended in the air. The paralysis continued until an unexpectedly heavy rainfall made the ash compact and adhere to the ground. The three large 1980 eruptions were of only average size for Mount St. Helens, which in a past eruption has left a deposit of ash over 30 cm deep for a distance of 80 km (50 miles). Depending on the prevailing wind direction, if such an ashfall were to

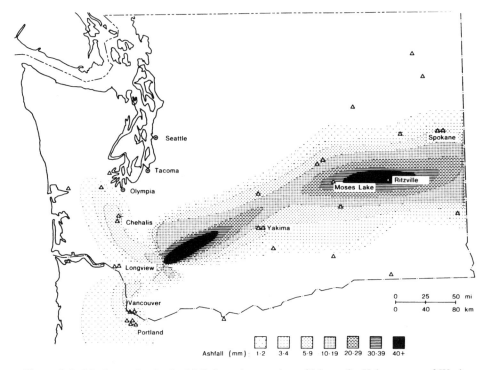

Figure 9-1. Maximum depth of ashfall from the eruption of Mount St. Helens, state of Washington, 1980.

occur today, it would cause massive disruption in the large cities, such as Portland, Oregon, that are west of the volcano. In 1991, at Mount Pinatubo, at least 300 people died and a similar number were seriously injured in buildings whose roofs collapsed under the weight of the ash; although the depth of ash in some of the affected cities was only 10 cm, its density had been augmented by heavy rains during the eruption (*14*).

A volcanic plume contains ash and gases and will be driven in the direction of prevailing winds, with the finer and lighter ash particles carried the farthest. Gases and other volatile materials are adsorbed onto the ash particles and, being readily soluble, will be washed off by rain into watercourses or onto crops. Depending on the type of volcano, fluoride from hydrogen fluoride can be a toxic hazard during ashfalls. Farmers in Iceland are well aware of the dangers posed by eruptions of the Hekla volcano, as only a 1 mm deposit of ash on grass killed thousands of grazing sheep. Fluoride poisoning was also believed to be the cause of death of livestock after the Lonquimay eruption in Chile in 1988. Many sheep also died after the eruption of Mount Hudson in Chile in 1991, but these deaths were probably due to starvation rather than to toxic causes (*15*). During major eruptions, a deep layer of ash can cause great hardship to foraging animals that may be unable to find food or adequate supplies of water.

Volcanic ash can be produced from the explosion and shattering of old rock (lithics) as well as from the release of pressure on the magma (fresh liquid rock) inside the volcano. The size of ash particles and their mineral composition varies between volcanoes and even between eruptions of the same volcano. Freshly emitted ash may impart a sulfurous or pungent smell to the air, and the adherent volatile material will add to the irritant effects that fine ash may have on the lungs. The ash particles produced in explosive eruptions are often small enough to be readily inhaled deep into the lungs, and coarser particles may lodge in the nose or eyes and irritate the skin. In the ashfall from the Mount St. Helens eruption on May 18, 1980, more than 90% of the particles by count were within the respirable range (<10 micrometers).

Respiratory and Ocular Effects

The Mount St. Helens eruptions of 1980 remain the only well-documented examples in which epidemiological surveillance was undertaken after a volcanic eruption (*16*). Trends in emergency department visits and hospital admissions after each eruption revealed increases in the number of patients seeking treatment for asthma and bronchitis (Fig. 9-2) (*16*). In addition, a household survey in Yakima, Washington, showed that about a third of patients with chronic lung disease who did not become ill enough to visit a hospital at the time of the eruption nevertheless experienced a marked exacerbation of their respiratory symptoms during the period when the raised levels of respirable ash were elevated and continued to persist in the ambient air for more than 3 months after the eruption (*17*). These patients would undoubtedly have been more seriously affected if they had not heeded the advice of public health authorities and their own common sense by staying indoors during the worst conditions. No deaths were attributable to the respiratory effects of the ash. Despite the absence of epidemiologic data, there is little doubt that the impact of similar eruptions would be greater in less-privileged countries where the housing is less resistant to particle infiltration. Thus, in 1992, after the eruption of Cerro Negro in Nicaragua, a substantial increase in asthma cases was reported, but the underutilization of health services by the population made a complete epidemiologic assessment of the size of the impact impossible. In contrast, an epidemiologic surveillance system established by the Philippine Department of Health after the massive Mount Pinatubo ashfall failed to find any increases in acute respiratory problems in the affected communities, an unexpected finding that may have been attributable to the compaction and settling of the ash by the heavy rainfall that accompanied the eruption.

In the eruptions of Mount Pinatubo and Mount St. Helens (*18*), the ash contained 3%–7% crystalline silica, a mineral that causes silicosis; most of the particles were

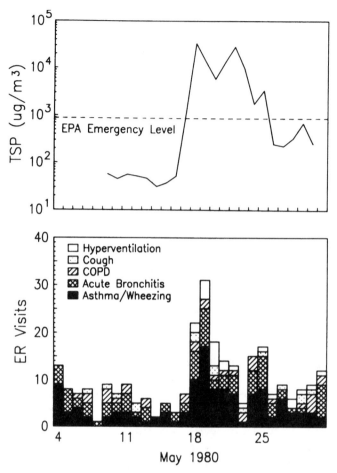

Figure 9-2. *Above*: Total suspended particulate concentrations (TSP) from the huge numbers of ash particles produced in explosive eruptions of Mount St. Helens, state of Washington, 1980. *Below*: Trends in emergency department visits after the eruption of Mount St. Helens, state of Washington, 1980, revealed increases in the number of patients seeking treatment for asthma and bronchitis.

within the respirable range. Outdoor occupational exposure to resuspended ash for groups such as loggers and farmworkers could be potentially high enough to cause silicosis if the exposure were maintained, for example, as a result of the volcano erupting ash repeatedly over a period of years. So much ash erupted at Mount Pinatubo in 1991 that resuspension of this material occurred during the dry seasons of subsequent years.

Eye irritation and minor corneal abrasions can result from ash particles entering the eye. These effects are not normally serious, but people who work outdoors and those who wear contact lenses should wear protective eye shields or goggles when working outdoors.

Collapse of Buildings

Many buildings are vulnerable to the heavy loading that a large depth of accumulated ash can produce, particularly if the ash is wet. In the Mount Pinatubo eruption, wide-span buildings, such as churches and halls, were at 5 times greater risk for collapse than was residential housing (*14*). The susceptibility of large buildings to collapse is especially important because they may be used for shelter by displaced groups of people. Flimsy dwellings are especially prone to collapse under the weight of ash. Accumulations of ash may be rapid (e.g., as much as 25 cm may accumulate in an hour) in certain eruptions. Advice to keep roofs swept of ash may be impossible to follow under such circumstances, and special advice may be needed on temporarily strengthening roofs with supports or on taking shelter in the most resistant part of a house until an ashfall is over.

Toxic Effects

Ash should be routinely tested for chemical toxicity after eruptions, because people are usually anxious about real and imagined health risks of the ash to their families and to livestock. As well as being directly poisoned by ingesting ash, grazing animals can also be exposed from contaminated surface waters. Furthermore, the pH of rivers can be lowered by acidic ash and thus endanger fish. Lakes and rivers used for drinking water for both humans and animals need to be tested if the ash is known to have or is suspected of having a high fluoride content. Elevated fluoride levels (as high as 9 ppm) were measured in streams after the Hekla eruptions of 1947 and 1970 in Iceland. Susceptible people also could have adverse reactions from drinking contaminated water, and thus it is best to advise that people use alternative water sources until the levels fall, as should occur within a few days, especially after heavy rains.

Ionizing Radiation Risks

Radon may be emitted in large quantities in eruption columns where it is unlikely to pose a health risk, but radon "daughters" may adhere to ash particles and thus expose the population to radiation risks. Ash itself may have a high uranium content, and its radioactivity needs to be checked if it is from a volcano with a well-differentiated magma. In the past, using certain volcanic materials to build homes has resulted in elevated indoor air radon levels in contemporary housing in some parts of Italy.

Adverse Mental Health Effects

As with other types of natural disasters or chaotic situations, the threat of an impending eruption from a volcano previously assumed to be inactive, or having to cope with the aftermath of a major eruption, may cause people to become anxious or depressed or to experience post-traumatic stress disorders. The upheavals and disruption to normal living caused by phenomena such as repeated ashfalls, air pollution from degassing volcanoes, or the continuing threats from lahars can be disturbing, particularly if families have to be relocated or if houses, businesses, or farmland have been destroyed or severely damaged. For example, although there was no evidence of severe acute mental health disturbances in the immediate aftermath of the Mount St. Helens eruption on May 18, 1980, adverse mental health reactions were subsequently experienced by people in local communities (*19*) (see Chapter 6, "Mental Health Consequences of Disasters").

Transportation Hazards

Virtually all transportation will come to a halt in a heavy ashfall because of the impenetrable darkness and the damaging effect ash may have on automobile, train, and plane engines. In the worst but most likely scenarios in the future, cities could come to a virtual standstill for days in the event of a massive ashfall, with all the obvious implications for emergency services and supply lines. Automobile breakdowns and accidents due to slippery roads or poor visibility may greatly add to the chaos, and an important task for the police is traffic control with roadblocks to permit only essential vehicles to pass.

Problems with Communications

Not only will transportation services be severely affected by ashfall, but radio and television transmission may suffer serious interference while the ash is falling, and antennae can be damaged by heavy fallout. Telephone systems will become rapidly overloaded with anxious callers and should not be relied upon in emergencies. Telephone and electronic switch gear and computers are easily damaged by fine, infiltrating ash particles. Satellite communications have a valuable role if they are available.

Problems with Public Utilities

Moist ash is a good conductor of electricity, and a layer of ash on an unprotected insulator can cause short-circuiting of outdoor power equipment and, consequently, power outages. In addition, engineers may be hampered in their repair tasks if visibility is so restricted that vehicles cannot move. Many of the consequences of power outages are well known, but less obvious is the failure of water supplies dependent on electrical pumping.

Water supplies can also be restricted because of ashfall into reservoirs and rivers that causes clogging of inlets and filtration plants. In addition, water quality may be impaired through increased turbidity as well as through changes in pH. Sewage disposal machinery is rapidly overloaded and put out of action by abrasive ash.

Lightning

Heavy lightning frequently accompanies ash plumes for many kilometers from the volcano and can add to the general sense of alarm and fear. Ground strikes can cause fatalities and fires in a volcano's vicinity.

Infectious Hazards

Debris and tephra that fall around volcanoes may obstruct rivers and fill in lakes, and unusual flooding and pooling of water can lead to conditions conducive to the spread of endemic infectious diseases such as leptospirosis and malaria. (For a thorough discussion of such problems, see Chapter 5, "Communicable Diseases and Disease Control".)

Gases

Tall volcanoes exert a "stack" effect that, together with the heat and force of an eruption, results in the dispersal of gases into the atmosphere. However, there are occasions when gases may concentrate, or be released, at ground level. Some volcanoes quietly release gases ("degas") during quiescent periods between major eruptive phases. Recent research has shown that even volcanoes with minimal evidence of activity may be actively releasing carbon dioxide and radon from deep magma through ground soil diffusion (20), and the flux of these gases could rise rapidly before or during an eruption. Deaths caused by gases are uncommon compared with other volcano-associated fatalities, although it must be admitted that the effects of gases on humans during eruptions have not been well documented.

The chief volatile emissions are water vapor, carbon dioxide (CO_2), hydrogen sulfide (H_2S), and sulphur dioxide (SO_2), followed by hydrogen chloride (HCl), hydrogen fluoride (HF), carbon monoxide (CO), hydrogen (H), helium (He), and radon (Rn). Inorganic volatile emissions such as mercury may also be important in certain volcanoes (e.g., in Kilauea, with the potential for environmental contamination). Volatile organic materials (e.g., polynuclear aromatic and halogenated hydrocarbons) may also be detected in small quantities in eruptive plumes, particularly if the heat of the eruption has incinerated trees and other vegetation. Plumes from the Mount St. Helens eruptions were also found to contain appreciable quantities of carbonyl sulfide, carbon disulfide, and nitrogen dioxide (21).

From the health effects viewpoint, volcanic gases can be classified as asphyxiants (e.g., carbon dioxide [CO_2]) or as respiratory irritants (e.g., sulfur dioxide [SO_2]). Buildup of asphyxiant gases to lethal concentrations is most likely on the slopes of a volcano, inside a crater, or close to a fissure, whereas irritant gases may exert their effects in much lower concentrations for many kilometers downwind of the volcano.

Quiescent Volcanoes

Animals grazing in enclosed or low-lying regions on the slopes of certain hazardous volcanoes have been asphyxiated, probably by CO_2, which is denser than air. Hydrogen sulfide has also been reported to kill birds and to cause blindness in sheep. People roaming volcanic areas are also at risk from asphyxiant gases. Near fumaroles the presence of the highly irritant acid gases makes breathing difficult when high concentrations are reached, and this intolerance helps protect against overexposure to the less irritant but more poisonous gas H_2S (20). However, deaths have occurred during still weather on the Kusatsu-Shirane volcano in Japan, where the emissions have been mainly H_2S and CO_2 only, so that skiers had no warning that H_2S was present (the rotten-egg smell of H_2S cannot be detected in elevated concentrations). Volcanologists working in crater areas can also be deceived over the presence of H_2S and should always carry meters for detecting this gas (20).

Soil gas emissions on the flanks of volcanoes or in quiescent calderas may be sufficiently high to pose a hazard inside houses. For example, in the town of Furnas in the Azores, a town of 2,000 people that was built inside a volcanic caldera, elevated levels of CO_2 and radon can be measured in houses built.

Degassing Volcanoes

Several examples of volcanoes that release gases (i.e., degassing volcanoes) and that thus can pose an air pollution hazard for people living downwind of the volcano are to be found in Central America, where strong prevailing winds and local topography combine to direct plumes into inhabited areas on the volcanoes' flanks. In 1986, in Nicaragua, people had·to evacuate the area around the Concepción volcano. The last gas-emission crisis at the Masaya volcano in Nicaragua ceased in the early 1980s, but this volcano undergoes a cyclical phase of degassing every 25 years, with severe consequences to agriculture, particularly coffee plants, downwind (22). The effects of the San Cristobal volcano, also in Nicaragua, have not been studied, but plumes of gas can travel down the slope to populated areas on some days, depending on weather conditions. In 1983, during eruptions of the Kilauea volcano in Hawaii, gas sampling was undertaken to exclude a threat of high SO_2 exposure in local populations (23).

One of the most intriguing examples of a degassing volcano occurs at the Poas volcano in Costa Rica, which releases gases through a crater lake. Since 1986 the lake has cyclically evaporated to a low level during successive dry seasons and refilled again during the rainy seasons. Principal gases in the plume are carbon dioxide, sulfur dioxide, hydrogen sulfide, hydrogen chloride, and hydrogen fluoride, but outbreaks of respiratory complaints in the communities downwind of the volcano and damage to crops have probably been due to the concentrated acid aerosols that are generated as the lake level falls. Other fine particulate matter is formed by rock dissolving in the acid lake waters, and this matter may also be entrained in the plume. Over several months in 1994, the volcano's activity and gas emissions peaked, and equipment was used to monitor levels of SO_2 in the nearby populated area on the volcanos flanks.

Sulfur dioxide and fine sulfuric acid aerosols are likely to be the most important constituents of the plume as far as human respiratory health is concerned. Acute irritation of the airways by SO_2 may lead to effects ranging from constriction of small airways among healthy adults (concentrations in inspired air of 1–5 ppm for a few minutes) to frank asthma among susceptible people (levels as low as 200 ppb) (24). Acid aerosols can be generated through gaseous bubble formation at the surface of crater lakes or possibly inside craters, and these aerosols can evaporate to form fine submicrometer-size particles capable of traveling long distances in a plume. The levels at which acid aerosols can cause adverse health effects are controversial. Sulfur dioxide is a good marker constituent of plumes, and it has been well studied as an air pollutant in industrial countries. Health effects may also be caused by the mixture of constituents in the plume, and too much reliance should not be placed solely on SO_2 concentrations as an indicator of health risk. All degassing volcanoes should be actively monitored, since sudden increases in gas flux may be a warning of new violent eruptive activity. In addition, if air concentrations in inhabited areas readily exceed the World Health Organization's air-quality standard for SO_2 (25), affected communities may need advice about respiratory protection measures or about the desirability of evacuation.

Gas Emissions in Eruptions

The potential for catastrophic releases of gases from erupting volcanoes was demonstrated on the Dieng Plateau, Java, in 1979, when 142 people died while attempting to flee from a mild eruption. Apparently, they were overwhelmed by a powerful emission of CO_2 from a source less than 2 km above them on the volcano's flanks (26). The insidious risk gases may pose was illustrated in 1973 at Vestmannaeyjar on the island of Heimaey, Iceland, when a fissure eruption began without warning and the town had to be rapidly evacuated. Workers saved homes from copious ashfalls, but they were hampered by accumulations of gas, particularly by CO_2, and also by carbon monoxide and methane that seeped through the ground into buildings (27). The possibility of fissures and vents suddenly opening and releasing gases on erupting volcanoes is an important hazard that needs to be considered in disaster planning. For CO_2 to flow down into valleys, it will almost certainly have to be released at temperatures not much higher than those of the ambient air. Therefore, the source is likely a reservoir beneath the ground or within the volcano.

A dramatic example of a massive release of CO_2 carbon from a reservoir, on this occasion from the bottom layers of a crater lake, occurred at Lake Nyos, Cameroon, on August 21, 1986, and resulted in the deaths of 1,700 people (28). About a quarter of a million tons of CO_2 flowed as far as 20 km away along the valleys below the lake. The area was a mountainous, remote part of northern Cameroon; in a densely populated region the death toll would have been enormous. In 1984, a similar event, killing 37 people, occurred at Lake Monoun, which is situated only 95 km (59 miles) to the southeast of Lake Nyos. The cause of both events was thought to be an overturning of the deep layers of well-stratified water in which CO_2 had slowly accumulated from soda springs at the bottom of the lakes. Suggestions have been made to degas Lake Nyos and Lake Monoun; meanwhile, both lakes are slowly recharging with carbon dioxide and remain serious potential threats. Fortunately, it seems that there are few other such lakes in the world, but in volcanic fields any deep lake with a depth of 200 m or greater should be regarded as a potential hazard.

Other Hazardous or Eruptive Phenomena

Acid Rain

Acid rain is not a direct health hazard to humans, although it causes damage to vegetation and crops and has other adverse environmental effects. Rain falling through a plume from a degassing volcano will readily dissolve hydrogen chloride, which is the main component of volcanic acid rain. Rainwater at the Poas volcano in Costa Rica or at the Masaya volcano in Nicaragua during their degassing cycles may have a pH as acidic as 2.5–3.5 when people complain that the rain causes eye and skin irritation (22). In developing countries, rainwater is often collected from the sheet-metal roofs of houses and used for drinking. Health problems may arise if the acid rain dissolves metals or has a high fluoride content; the latter situation would occur only if the plume contained a high concentration of hydrogen fluoride. Acid aerosols and acid rain will corrode materials such as machinery or metal fences (e.g., barbed wire) and attack galvanized roofs and painted surfaces. Interestingly, the flower of the coffee plant seems particularly sensitive to air pollution at levels at which human respiratory symptoms also occur.

Lava Flows

Lava flows from effusive volcanoes are destructive, but their slow speed usually permits inhabitants to evacuate the affected area in plenty of time. Unfortunately, people do not always have a chance to escape. In 1977, a fluid lake of lava at Nyiragongo, Zaire, drained suddenly, killing 300 people (29); in 1994, a potential recurrence of this deadly phenomenon threatened Rwandan refugee camps at Goma in Zaire. Diversion barriers and other methods of influencing the direction of the lava flow may be attempted to mitigate lava flows from large effusive eruptions. One of the most interesting recent examples of such mitigation measures taken occurred during the fissure eruption of Mount Etna in 1991–1993, its most extensive eruption in three centuries. The lava threatened the village of Zefferana, but engineers were able to divert the lava flow into an artificial channel and to limit the flow's advance. The possibility of a sudden release of fluid lava from a fissure close to another settlement also required close monitoring during the main lava eruption (*30*).

Earthquakes

The onset of an explosive eruption may be heralded by localized earthquakes of magnitude 4–5, but because these can be quite shallow, their intensity may be sufficient to bring down structures and to endanger life. The limited lava eruption of Mount Etna on December 25, 1985, was accompanied by several earth tremors, one of which destroyed a hotel in the vicinity and killed one person. Special consideration needs to be given not only to housing but to the possibility of bridge collapse and landslips onto roads that would thereby block evacuation routes.

Tsunamis

Tsunamis are giant sea waves that are produced by subterranean shocks and explosions and are capable of devastating coastlines. The greatest loss of life from an eruption in recent times was caused by tsunamis after the 1883 eruption of Krakatoa when 36,000 people were drowned on the coasts of nearby Java and Sumatra (*2*). A tsunami's occurrence is unpredictable, but technological innovations are now making it possible to warn coastal communities at risk for an incoming tsunami (e.g., one that will occur as a result of an earthquake at sea). Another important cause of tsunamis is a slope collapse on a volcano that runs into the sea.

Slope Collapse

The importance of the stability of volcanic slopes was made clear to volcanologists during the eruption of Mount St. Helens in 1980. The eruption was triggered by an earthquake that caused the unstable northern slope to give way, and a major eruption followed the release of pressure on the magma. Fieldwork around volcanoes in recent years has confirmed that slope collapse is not the rare phenomenon it was once thought to be, and many volcanoes may show some degree of instability as they increase their mass with eruptive activity over time. Massive edifice failure has occurred about four times every century during the past 500 years (*31*). When the Unzen volcano erupted in Japan in 1792, it triggered the collapse of the Mount Mauyama complex and led to one of the worst natural disasters in Japan (Table 9-2); the slope slid into the sea, and the resultant tsunami swept across settlements on the opposite side of the bay. Two hundred years later, anxiety developed over a possible recurrence of this fearsome phenomenon when the volcano's activity resumed. Unfortunately, it is impossible to accurately predict such events at the present time, but certain unstable-looking active volcanoes (e.g., Colima in Mexico and Mount St. Augustine in Alaska) are being closely monitored for premonitory signs.

Public Health Implications and Preventive Measures

In most volcanic areas, the time between one major eruption and another is so long that communities do not remember the disaster (poor "disaster memory") or do not establish a set of traditional coping strategies for warding off disaster. Even in those areas where eruptions involving loss of life are frequent within each generation (e.g., in Merapi, Indonesia), communities still tend to resettle in the same hazardous places.

Since the reawakening of a volcano will usually be a new experience for a generation or several generations of inhabitants, there is commonly an initial acceptance of volcanic risk along with other life risks. When an eruption actually starts to threaten, or disaster workers attempt to encourage planning as part of a disaster-mitigation project, citizens and officials alike usually have little concept of what an eruption can do, and the volcanologists' description of eruptive phenomena may make remarkably little impression. Above all, the threat of economic disruption by volcanic activity strongly influences risk perceptions in a community. Consequently, people, or at least their political leaders, may have little appetite for dealing with criteria for warning and evacuation or for other potentially alarming aspects of community preparedness. The evacuation of whole cities raises fundamental questions of community viability and is unlikely to be successful unless volcanologists can almost guarantee that a major eruption will occur. As long as volcanic prediction remains an inexact science, local decision-makers will continue to find volcanic hazards a most difficult political issue. However, there have been two successful responses that resulted in the saving of tens of thousands of lives in eruptions at Mount Pinatubo in 1991 and at Rabaul in New Guinea in 1994. Fifty thousand people were evacuated from the area around Mount Pinatubo, and 30,000 were evacuated from the Rabaul area; in both instances, the buildup to the eruptions was obvious and people needed little persuading to leave. At Rabaul, extensive planning for more than a decade had prepared citizens to leave the area rapidly—within the 24 hours that elapsed between the time when the first earthquakes were felt and the cataclysmic eruption occurred. These successes need to be highlighted in developing strategies for future mitigation work.

Disaster Preparedness

Although one of the main goals of the U.N.'s IDNDR is to ensure that volcanic hazard-mapping is rapidly extended to as many dangerous volcanoes as possible, the response to date has been slow. Consequently, the main challenge facing volcanologists in the near future will be the conducting of rapid hazard assessments for understudied volcanoes that have begun to threaten populations with renewed activity. A brief description of the main aspects of disaster preparedness follows.

Hazard Assessment

Hazard assessment involves the study and mapping of the geology and stratigraphy of the volcano, including its previous eruptive products. This task, which for a large volcano may take several years to complete, requires a team of volcanologists and requires considerable resources if it is to be comprehensive. In difficult or inhospitable terrain, hazard assessment can be logistically difficult. Its purpose is to characterize the frequency and extent of previous activity and to use the findings to predict the probabilities of different types of future eruptions and their consequences (*32, 33*).

In a particularly threatening situation, there may only be time for a rapid hazard assessment over a few days or weeks. This may be enough to characterize the degree of danger (e.g., at Mount Pinatubo even a brief field survey was sufficient to recognize the magnitude of past pyroclastic flows and to appreciate the extreme danger another explosive eruption could pose).

Risk Assessment

In collaboration with volcanologists, disaster-preparedness officials should develop a range of scenarios involving the smallest to the largest possible eruptions, together with the most foreseeable likely event. This latter scenario should be used as the basis for emergency planning. This tactic is preferable to the usual advice to produce a "hazard map" that may become falsely regarded either as the most accurate or as the only version of a future eruption. In reality, of course, the extent of an eruption can never be exactly foretold, and volcanologists may disagree over interpretations of the findings of field surveys. The scenarios should be used by disaster planners in making risk assessments of the impact the eruption will have on the community and its economy. In particular, the vulnerability of structures (e.g., homes, hospitals, and buildings used as shelters) and infrastructure (e.g., communications, power lines) should be assessed. Community vulnerability (i.e., social and economic factors that can lead to increased risk) also needs to be included in future assessments. Using geographical information systems to develop scenarios and map risks is only now beginning.

Emergency Planning

Using the different scenarios, all the usual disaster planning measures, including evacuation plans and search-and-rescue planning, need to be established with civil protection authorities and emergency services personnel. Warning systems and evacuation criteria are the most important and difficult measures to establish for use during a volcanic crisis.

Community Preparedness

Risk perception of communities is almost always at variance with that of volcanologists. Communities should be instructed on how to respond to warnings of an impending eruption and what to do if an eruption occurs before an evacuation has been completed. Search-and-rescue skills and first-aid training on the special types of injuries that may be incurred need to be included in the training, at least for those special groups capable of mobilizing themselves to deal with casualties in an emergency.

Specific Pre-eruption Measures

The renewal of activity in an explosive volcano is a public health emergency, and the most appropriate initial response is to consider the worst type of event that could happen and plan accordingly (34, 35). A disaster planning committee that includes health care professionals should be established. The committee should undertake the following steps when planning to assist those living in the vicinity of the volcano:

- Designate areas for evacuation and identify at-risk areas. These key preventive measures are essentially decisions made by government officials after consultation with volcanologists. Information from health officials (e.g., on the feasibility of evacuating the sick, the aged, and the very young on short notice) also needs to be considered. The health and welfare of people evacuated either temporarily or for long periods is also a public health matter. The safety of specific groups of workers who may be permitted into dangerous areas needs careful, unbiased assessment, and information on the risks and benefits associated with working in these areas should be disseminated to all workers.
- Develop search-and-rescue plans for locating and retrieving the dead and any marooned survivors after the eruption. These plans should also include designating the sites for emergency field casualty stations and morgues and determining which personnel will staff these sites.
- Stage mock disaster drills to test the efficacy of local hospital emergency plans, especially for a sudden influx of victims with (1) body surface burns and lung damage from inhalation of hot ash in pyroclastic flows or surges and (2) various kinds of trauma from lahars, building collapses in earthquakes, ashfalls, and pyroclastic surges.
- Provide emergency air-monitoring equipment for detecting toxic gases inside houses (from soil gas) and in the ambient air.
- Establish an epidemiologic surveillance system.

In addition, planning for heavy ashfalls over a wide area, if applicable, should include these arrangements:

- Provide laboratory facilities for collecting and analyzing ash for leachable toxic elements and for monitoring drinking water quality. Special laboratories should be made available for measuring the particle size and crystalline silica content of the ash.

- Provide equipment for monitoring exposures to airborne ash in the community and among people who work outdoors.
- Stockpile lightweight, disposable, high-efficiency masks, if indicated, for distribution to the public after an ashfall. Eye shields and more robust respiratory protection may be needed for emergency workers and other outdoor workers.
- Prepare for possible temporary breakdowns of water supplies and sewage-treatment plants. Such preparation should ensure that adequate chlorination of water occurs or that advisories recommending that residents boil their water are issued.
- Maintain emergency health services and hospitals.
- Provide emergency shelter and food relief.
- Advise residents of affected communities about protective measures to combat overloading and collapse of roofs in heavy ashfalls.

Post-eruption Measures

A small eruption of an explosive volcano may be the prelude to a much larger eruption in the ensuing days, weeks, or months. Conversely, large eruptions may be followed by a succession of small eruptions over the following days or weeks, during which time the volcano may remain extremely dangerous. Indeed, the hazardous behavior of the volcano may recur in the following months or years during dome formation, a process in which liquid magma is extruded at the top of the volcano as it rebuilds itself. Domes can collapse and produce pyroclastic flows. These uncertainties require that the volcano be monitored intensively by a team of volcanologists, although they may not always be able to predict its behavior.

During a volcanic crisis, the following requirements should be considered:

- Establish a national-level disaster committee whose members report to the head of state. A senior member of the Ministry of Health or a person with cabinet-level status is usually a member of the committee. Although the most prominent health issues discussed by the committee may revolve around concerns for evacuees and their health, and around ways to provide adequate relief supplies to affected areas, and although attention will also focus on the importance of predicting any future volcanic activity, the concerns of the population may go unheeded unless health professionals are involved in emergency relief efforts. For example, the most frequently asked questions in ashfall areas are whether it is safe for humans or animals to breathe the air, to ingest crops or grass on which ash has fallen, or to drink water from surface or deep sources around the volcano, and these concerns must be addressed by disaster-relief authorities.
- Authorities should establish an emergency health team with medical, epidemiologic, and community health skills before the eruption and should deploy the team

immediately afterward. Its function is to collaborate with other agencies and to give advice and information relating to all health concerns arising from the disaster. This team needs to establish epidemiologic surveillance through a network incorporating hospitals and emergency departments in affected areas. Rapid field surveys may be necessary to assess the nature of health problems in areas of heavy ashfall as soon as travel conditions permit. In particular, it is critical that ash be collected and tested for toxicity by performing leachate studies in water and by testing water samples from ground and surface sources for the presence of a wide range of cations and anions, particularly for fluoride and heavy metals.

- The emergency health team should communicate with volcanologists to determine whether the volcanic plume of a low-lying degassing volcano is likely to cause air pollution in populated areas downwind of the volcano. Normally, an assessment can be made by directly observing the crater from a helicopter or airplane or from a safe distance on the ground. Volcanologists also measure SO_2 flux from craters using the correlation spectrometer (COSPEC) technique.

- The public may need to be informed about the effects of ash on the eyes and respiratory system. Epidemiologic monitoring of visits to medical centers and hospitals will provide important information on outbreaks of asthma, for example, as well as on the occurrence of other health problems and injuries. People living in makeshift evacuation camps can be at high risk for infectious diseases such as measles, and special immunization programs also may be needed. (Such a situation occurred in 1991 after the eruption of Mount Pinatubo.)

- Veterinarians, preferably those with disaster experience, have an important role in the response phase. The health of outdoor grazing animals should be monitored and a reporting system of animal deaths established in order to exclude any toxic cause. Animals may suffer badly after eruptions as a result of burns and other injuries and may roam until they die from exhaustion. In addition, people may be unable to farm their land for prolonged periods if the depth of ashfall is in excess of 30 cm; long-term disruption can also be caused by the risk for lahars if large amounts of volcanic debris have built up on the volcanos flanks and are capable of being mobilized by heavy rains.

- Close communication between volcanologists and health care workers is necessary for advising the population about future volcanic activity and its impact. Regular dissemination of information is an essential part of posteruption activities, and health professionals need to be closely involved in the process. Radio and television will be essential for transmitting warnings and providing pre- and posteruption advice. Advice and equipment, including emergency warning systems, should be provided for people permitted to live or work in restricted or high-risk areas near a volcano. Examples of brochures sent to households and workers at the time of the Mount St. Helens eruptions in 1980 are given elsewhere (*35*).

Critical Knowledge Gaps and Research Recommendations

Our limited knowledge of the acute and long-term impact of eruptions on human health needs urgent augmentation, particularly because such a wide range of eruptive phenomena and adverse consequences to health and safety can occur. The lack of well-conceived epidemiologic studies to examine both the acute- and long-term impact of volcanic eruptions on populations limits our understanding of the various natural phenomena at work and hampers our ability to provide appropriate and timely emergency assistance to affected areas. More epidemiologic studies are needed immediately after eruptions, particularly those involving pyroclastic flows, lahars, and ashfalls, to record injuries and health problems and to relate them to actual injury agents.

Health professionals need to collaborate with volcanologists, engineers, and emergency planners in developing disaster preparedness in at-risk areas. Whenever possible, opportunities should be taken to study volcanoes during their dormancy periods in order to obtain information that would be immediately useful should volcanic activity recommence. This type of research is still embryonic and to be successful requires a multidisciplinary approach.

Hazard assessment of the worlds most dangerous volcanoes is proceeding at a disappointingly slow pace, for despite the stimulus given by the IDNDR, few volcanoes have been adequately studied. Hazard mapping is an academic task that requires adequate funding, but the research bodies of developed countries are reluctant to fund work that they regard as applied and less worthy than studies on mechanisms. The methodologies used in hazard mapping need to be standardized. For volcanologists, there are few more depressing experiences than being proudly shown a crude map of an at-risk area and being told that hazard planning has been completed. Generally, the map displays a few curved lines at various distances from a volcano, each marking the predicted limit of an erupted product. Unfortunately, these predictions have usually been based on little, if any, fieldwork. Thus far, taking scientifically based and realistically constructed hazard maps and turning them into useful risk assessments (analyzing what lies inside those deceptively curved lines) is not being done routinely anywhere in the world. Undoubtedly, important advances will be made when numerical simulation modeling of pyroclastic flows, lahars, and ashfalls becomes more available and capable of being applied routinely to vulnerability assessments. Geographical information systems will need to be developed to simplify the handling of the large and disparate data sets required for mapping and scenario development purposes around an active volcano.

Public health and primary health care workers in volcanic areas need to be educated about the risks of explosive volcanism so that they can understand the importance of disaster preparedness and act as communicators to local populations. Not only is research needed on devising methods for improving communication of disaster risks, including the study of risk perceptions in at-risk communities, but traditional medical models need to be expanded to include social and behavioral causes of vulnerability.

Burgeoning populations and economic forces appear to result in the exploitation of all available land capable of sustaining agricultural and industrial development, including tourism. The economies of volcanic islands are especially vulnerable. Unfortunately, long-term land-use planning to minimize risk in volcanic areas is still in its infancy. Today, the emphasis is on adaptive living, or coexistence, with volcanic threats and on an ideal of sustainable development, which, for most parts of the world, will remain remote until the risk profiles of many more volcanoes are completed and the lessons learned are accepted by governments and citizens alike.

Summary

By the year 2000, more than 500 million people will be living in active volcanic areas around the world, and an urgent need exists to incorporate volcanic disaster planning into sustainable development policies in those countries at risk. A wide range of devastating and lethal-injury phenomena occur in volcanic eruptions, and their impact is poorly understood. The most hazardous phenomena are pyroclastic flows and surges and lahars. Heavy ashfalls may have a wide impact, including deaths from collapsing buildings, respiratory effects in humans, and fluoride intoxication in grazing animals, across large areas hundreds of kilometers from a volcano. Carbon dioxide and hydrogen sulfide can cause asphyxia near vents on a volcano, whereas irritant gases, in particular sulfur dioxide and acid aerosols, and other constituents of volcanic plumes from degassing volcanoes may cause air pollution in communities downwind of the volcano. Other hazardous or environmentally damaging eruptive phenomena include earthquakes, lava flows, tsunamis, and avalanches from slope collapses.

Preventing the worst consequences of explosive eruptions requires the active collaboration of health workers in disaster planning. Volcano hazard maps need to be applied to risk assessment and scenario development for different eruption types. In the post-eruption phase, public health workers may need to undertake rapid public health surveillance and must provide advice on a wide range of health issues, and their role should be integral to the disaster planning process.

References

1. Tilling RI, Lipman PW. Lessons in reducing volcanic risk. *Nature* 1993;364:277–280.
2. Simkin T, Siebert L. *Volcanoes of the world*, 2nd edition. Washington, D.C.: Smithsonian Institution, 1994.
3. Francis P. *Volcanoes. A planetary perspective*. Oxford: Oxford University Press, 1993.
4. McCormick MP, Thomason LW, Trepte CR. Atmospheric effects of the Mt. Pinatubo eruption. *Nature* 1995;373:399–404.

5. Tilling RI, editor. *Volcanic hazards: short course in geology.* Washington, D.C.: American Geophysical Union, 1989.

6. Blong RJ. *Volcanic hazards: a source book on the effects of eruptions.* Sydney: Academic Press, 1984.

7. Eisele JW, O'Halloran RL, Reay DT, *et al.* Deaths during the May 19, 1980, eruption of Mount St. Helens. *N Engl J Med* 1981;305:931–936.

8. Parshley PF, Kiessling PJ, Antonius JA, et al. Pyroclastic flow injury, Mount St. Helens, May 18, 1980. *Am J Surg* 1982;143:565–568.

9. Bernstein RS, Baxter PJ, Falk H, *et al.* Immediate public health concerns and actions in volcanic eruptions: lessons from the eruptions of Mount St. Helens, May 18–Oct. 18, 1980. *Am J Public Health* 1986;76(Suppl.):25–38.

10. Baxter PJ. Medical effects of volcanic eruptions. 1. Main causes of death and injury. *Bulletin of Volcanology* 1990;52:532–544.

11. Lipman PW, Mullineaux DR, editors. *The 1980 eruptions of Mount St. Helens, Washington.* U.S. Geological Survey Professional Paper 1250. Washington, D.C.: U.S. Geological Survey, 1981.

12. Voight B. The 1985 Nevado del Ruiz volcano catastrophe: anatomy and retrospection. *Journal of Volcanological and Geothermal Research* 1990;44:349–386.

13. Saarinen TF, Sell JL. *Warning and response to the Mount St. Helens eruption.* Albany: State University of New York Press, 1985.

14. Spence RJS, Pomonis A, Baxter PJ. Building damage in the Mount Pinatubo eruption. In: Newhall C, editor. *The 1991 eruption of Mount Pinatubo, Philippines.* Reston, VA: U.S. Geological Survey, 1995.

15. Rubin CH, Noji EK, Seligman PJ, *et al.* Evaluating a fluorosis hazard after a volcanic eruption. *Arch Environ Health* 1994;49:395–401.

16. Baxter PJ, Ing R, Falk H, *et al.* Mount St. Helens eruptions, May 18–June 12, 1980: an overview of the acute health impact. *JAMA* 1981;246:2585–2589.

17. Baxter PJ, Ing R, Falk H, *et al.* Mount St. Helens eruptions: the acute respiratory effects of volcanic ash in a North American community. *Arch Environ Health* 1983;38:138–143.

18. Dollberg DD, Bolyard ML, Smith DL. Crystalline silica in Mount St. Helens volcanic ash. *Am J Public Health* 1986;76(Suppl.):53–58.

19. Shore JH, Tatum EL, Vollmer WM. Evaluation of mental health effects of disaster. *Am J Public Health* 1986;76(Suppl.):76–83.

20. Baxter PJ, Tedesco D, Miele G, *et al.* Health hazards of volcanic gases. *Lancet* 1990;336:176.

21. Olsen KB, Fruchter JS. Identification of hazards associated with volcanic emissions. *Am J Public Health* 1986;76(Suppl.):45–52.

22. Baxter PJ, Stoiber RE, Williams SN. Volcanic gases and health: Masaya Volcano, Nicaragua. *Lancet* 1982;2:150–151.

23. Bernstein RS, Falk H, Greenspan J, *et al.* Assessment of respiratory hazards associated with air pollutants from volcanic eruptions, Kilauea Volcano, Hawaii. Internal report (EPI-83-23-2). Atlanta, GA: Centers for Disease Control 1984.

24. Advisory Group on the Medical Aspects of Air Pollution Episodes. *Sulphur dioxide, acid aerosols and particulates*, 2nd report. London: HMSO Department of Health, 1992.

25. World Health Organization. *Air quality guidelines for Europe.* Copenhagen: World Health Organization, 1987.

26. Le Guern F, Tazieff H, Faiure PR. An example of health hazard: people killed by gas during a phreatic eruption: Dieng Plateau (Java, Indonesia), February 20, 1979. *Bulletin of Volcanology* 1982;45:153–156.

27. Williams SN, Moore JG. *Man against volcano: the eruption on Heimaey, Vestmannaeyjar, Iceland.* Washington, D.C.: U.S. Geological Survey, 1983.

28. Baxter PJ, Kapila M, Mfonfu D. Lake Nyos disaster, Cameroon, 1986: the medical effects of large scale emission of carbon dioxide? *Br Med J* 1989;298:1437–1441.

29. Tazieff H. An exceptional eruption: Mount Nyiragongo, January 10, 1977. *Bulletin of Volcanology* 1976–77;40(3):188–200.

30. Barberi F, Villari L. Volcano monitoring and civil protection problems during the 1991–1993 Etna eruption. *Acta Vulcanologica* 1994;4:1–16.

31. Siebert L. Threats from debris avalanches. *Nature* 1992;356:658–659.

32. Crandell DR, Booth B, Kazumadinata K, *et al. Source book for volcanic hazards zonation.* Paris: UN Educational, Scientific and Cultural Organization, 1984.

33. Office of the United Nations Disaster Relief Coordinator (UNDRO). *Volcanic emergency management.* New York: United Nations, 1985.

34. Baxter PJ, Bernstein RS, Falk H, *et al.* Medical aspects of volcanic disasters: an outline of the hazards and emergency response measures. *Disasters* 1982;6:268–276.

35. Baxter PJ, Bernstein RS, Buist AS. Preventive health measures in volcanic eruptions. *Am J Public Health* 1986;76(Suppl.):84–90.

III

···

WEATHER-RELATED
PROBLEMS

10

Tropical Cyclones

JOSEPHINE MALILAY

Background and Nature of Tropical Cyclones

Tropical cyclones are among the most destructive weather systems *(1–3)*. The impact from cyclones generally extends over a wide area, with mortality, injury, and property loss that result from strong winds and heavy rains. Often secondary events such as storm surges, flooding, landslides, and tornadoes exacerbate effects of these systems *(4)*. Although improved warning systems in most cyclone-prone areas of the world today prevent or reduce deaths, meteorological elements, increased population growth, and the development of human settlements along coastal areas continue to present risks associated with cyclone-related mortality and morbidity.

Tropical cyclones are meteorological depressions, or low pressure systems, that develop over open water in the tropics, usually between the latitudes of 30° N and 30° S *(5)*. They originate at locations where an unstable atmosphere causes differences in the amount of energy received by the earth's poles. A rotating disturbance forms around a center of calm atmosphere, or *eye*, usually 30–50 kilometers in diameter, with air circulating counterclockwise in the Northern Hemisphere and clockwise in the Southern Hemisphere. From energy obtained through oceanic evaporation, cyclones may move at speeds of 10 to 50 kilometers per hour within the zone of trade winds *(1)*. Each year about 80 tropical cyclones with an average duration of 9 days develop, travel a distance of over 10, 000 kilometers, and then lose force overland *(1, 5)*. Known as *hurricanes* in the North Atlantic, Caribbean Gulf, eastern north Pacific, and western coast of Mexico, they are called *typhoons* in the western Pacific and *cyclones* in the Indian Ocean and Australasia *(5)*.

The life cycle of tropical cyclones consists of development, intensification, maturity, decay, or modification *(6)*. In this cycle, tropical cyclones may originate from *subtropical cyclones*, defined as low-pressure systems over tropical waters. As they develop, other tropical cyclones may lose their tropical characteristics altogether and become *extratropical cyclones*, or *"nor'easters"* *(6)*.

By definition, a tropical cyclone is a term assigned to cyclonic circulations that originate over tropical waters *(7)*. A circulation is further classified by the following levels and may be upgraded or downgraded at any time, depending on form and intensity: (1) tropical wave; (2) tropical disturbance; (3) tropical depression; (4) tropical storm; and (5) hurricane, typhoon, or cyclone *(8)*. Table 10-1 lists the definitions of each of these terms. In the United States, hurricanes are ranked on the Saffir/Simpson Hurricane Scale, which relates hurricane intensity to damage potential. The scale accounts for size, coastal configuration, astronomical tides, terrain features, urbanization, and industrialization *(6)*. The conditions for wind speeds and storm surges that describe each storm category are shown in Table 10-2.

Scope and Relative Importance of Tropical Cyclones

Worldwide, 150 million people were affected by cyclones from 1967 to 1991. Of these tropical cyclones an estimated 900 killed approximately 900, 000 people and injured more than 240, 000 *(2)*. In the United States during this century, hurricanes have resulted in more than 14, 600 deaths and have caused property damage of more than $94 billion, when adjusted to 1990 dollars *(9)*. In the continental United States, an annual average of two hurricanes develops sufficiently to make landfall on the coastline of the Atlantic and the Gulf of Mexico *(8)*, although many more develop in the course of a year, as shown in Table 10-3 *(6)*. The National Weather Service estimates that of approximately 70 million people at risk from hurricanes, 50 to 100 people on average are killed per

Table 10-1 Definitions of Tropical Cyclonic Circulations

Tropical wave	A trough of low pressure in the trade-wind easterlies.
Tropical disturbance	A moving area of thunderstorms in the tropics that maintains its identity for 24 hours or more.
Tropical depression	A tropical cyclone in which the maximum sustained surface wind is 38 miles per hour (33 knots*) or less.
Tropical storm	A tropical cyclone in which the maximum sustained surface wind ranges from 39 to 73 miles per hour (34–63 knots).
Hurricane	A tropical cyclone in which maximum sustained surface wind is 74 mph (64 knots) or greater.

*A knot is one nautical mile per hour; a nautical mile is approximately 1.15 statute miles.

Source: U.S. Department of Commerce, National Oceanic and Atmospheric Administration, National Weather Service (8).

Table 10-2 The Saffir/Simpson Hurricane Scale*

Category	Description
1	Winds 74–95 miles per hour Damage primarily to shrubbery, trees, foliage, and unanchored mobile homes. No damage to other structures. Some damage to poorly constructed signs. Storm surge 4–5 feet above normal Low-lying coastal roads inundated, minor pier damage, some small craft in exposed anchorage torn from moorings.
2	Winds 96–110 miles per hour Considerable damage to shrubbery and tree foliage; some trees blown down. Major damage to exposed mobile homes. Extensive damage to poorly constructed signs. Some damage to roofing materials of buildings; some window and door damage. Storm surge 6–8 feet above normal Coastal roads and low-lying escape routes inland cut by rising water 2 to 4 hours before arrival of hurricane center. Considerable damage to piers. Marinas flooded. Small craft in unprotected anchorages torn from moorings. Evacuation of some shoreline residences and low-lying island areas required.
3	Winds 111–130 miles per hour Foliage torn from trees; large trees blown down. Practically all poorly constructed signs blown down. Some damage to roofing materials of buildings; some window and door damage. Some structural damage to small buildings. Mobile homes destroyed. Storm surge 9–12 feet above normal Serious flooding at coast and many smaller structures near coast destroyed; larger structures near coast damaged by battering waves and floating debris. Low-lying escape routes inland cut by rising water 3 to 5 hours before hurricane center arrives. Flat terrain 5 feet or less above sea level flooded inland 8 miles or more. Evacuation of low-lying residences within several blocks of shoreline possibly required.
4	Winds 131–155 miles per hour Shrubs and trees blown down; all signs down. Extensive damage to roofing materials, windows, and doors. Complete failure of roofs on many small residences. Complete destruction of mobile homes. Storm surge 13–18 feet above normal Flat terrain 10 feet or less above sea level flooded inland as far as 6 miles. Major damage to lower floors of structures near shore due to flooding and battering by waves and floating debris. Low-lying escape routes inland cut by rising water 3 to 5 hours before hurricane center arrives. Major erosion of beaches. Massive evacuation of all residences within 500 yards of shore and of single-story residences on low ground within 2 miles of shore possibly required.
5	Winds greater than 155 miles per hour Shrubs and trees blown down; considerable damage to roofs of buildings; all signs down. Very severe and extensive damage to windows and doors. Complete failure of roofs on many residences and industrial buildings. Extensive shattering of glass in windows and doors. Some complete building failures. Small buildings overturned or blown away. Complete destruction of mobile homes. Storm surge greater than 18 feet above normal Major damage to lower floors of all structures less than 15 feet above sea level within 500 yards of shore. Low-lying escape routes inland cut by rising water 3 to 5 hours before hurricane center arrives. Massive evacuation of residential areas on low ground within 5 to 10 miles of shore possibly required.

*Conditions for wind speeds and/or storm surge determine the category of a hurricane.

Source: U.S. Department of Commerce, National Oceanic and Atmospheric Administration, National Weather Service, National Environmental Satellite Data, and Information Service. *(6)*

Table 10-3 Frequency of Hurricanes Making Landfall in the United States by Saffir-Simpson Category, 1982—1992

Area	Category 1	2	3	4	5	All	Major Hurricanes ≥ 3
United States (Texas to Maine)	11	7	9	2	0	29	11
Texas							
North	3	0	1	0	0	4	1
Central							
South							
Louisiana	3	0	1	0	0	4	1
Mississippi	0	0	1	0	0	1	1
Alabama	0	0	1	0	0	1	1
Florida							
Northwest	0	1	1	0	0	2	1
Northeast							
Southwest	1	0	1	0	0	2	1
Southeast	0	0	0	1	0	1	1
Georgia							
South Carolina	1	0	0	1	0	2	1
North Carolina	1	0	2	0	0	3	2
Virginia	1	0	0	0	0	1	1
New York	0	1	1	0	0	2	1
Connecticut	0	2	0	0	0	2	0
Rhode Island	0	1	0	0	0	1	0
Massachusetts	0	1	0	0	0	1	0
New Hampshire	0	1	0	0	0	1	0
Maine	1	0	0	0	0	1	0

Source: U.S. Department of Commerce, National Oceanic and Atmospheric Administration, National Weather Service, National Environmental Satellite Data, and Information Service. *(6)*

event, with property losses in the billions of dollars during a worse-than-average hurricane season *(9)*. The impact of Hurricane Andrew in Florida alone amounted to $25 billion in 1992 *(10)*.

Factors that Contribute to Tropical Cyclone Problem

Despite massive mortality and morbidity worldwide, early detection and warning systems leading to evacuation and sheltering have helped to reduce or prevent deaths in many areas, notably in the United States, the Caribbean countries, and the coastlines of Central and South America. In other countries, such as Bangladesh and the Philippines, technology to forecast storms is relatively modern and accurate; however, timely evacuation and safe sheltering have yet to improve for vast numbers of inhabitants in vulnerable areas *(11, 12)*.

In the United States, mortality peaked at 6,000 in the hurricane of 1900 in Galveston, Texas, and declined over the decades to 256 when Hurricane Camille struck the Gulf Coast and the Virginias in 1969 (see Table 10-4). In most instances, drowning from storm surges accounted for the majority of these deaths. Thereafter, the National Weather Service developed a forecasting model called the "Sea, Lake, and Overland Surges from Hurricanes," or SLOSH model, to compute storm surge from hurricanes *(13, 14)*. Because the models determine patterns of flooding and thus predict the most vulnerable areas to a hurricane's forces, occupants can be evacuated safely before a hurricane's landfall in areas subject to hazardous inundation *(14)*. For instance, advanced preparation, including the evacuation of more than 350, 000 people, in Alabama before Hurricane Frederic in 1979 resulted in a low death toll of 5 people for this event *(15)*. After Hurricane Andrew struck southeastern Florida in 1992, however, several deaths occurred outside inundation and evacuation zones and were attributed to winds that may have been unique to this disaster *(10)*. Wind-related issues are presently being incorporated into a comprehensive national hurricane program *(10)*.

Like most natural disasters, the nature of cyclones requires continued observation of their effects on public health and safety well into the response and recovery phases. Latent effects are often typified by deaths and injuries, such as electrocutions from loose or wet wiring, cleanup injuries, and burns from unattended flames *(16–18)*. Furthermore, surveillance of endemic illnesses and infectious diseases heralds the occurrence of epidemics that may arise, particularly after hydrometeorological disasters. Knowledge of these effects and others have yet to be reinforced and investigated, and appropriate public health strategies have yet to be devised.

Factors Affecting Tropical Cyclone Occurrence and Severity

Although property damage has increased considerably, deaths and injuries associated with tropical cyclones have been prevented or reduced in recent decades, largely because of improved forecasting, warning, evacuation, and sheltering of communities at risk. However, the hazards associated with tropical cyclones continue to present problems for public health, emergency management, and meteorological forecasting.

Meteorological events elsewhere in the world can precede the occurrence of tropical cyclones in a given region. The *frequency* of major hurricanes off the coast of the southeastern United States has been found to correlate with the wet and dry phases of rainfall in West Africa *(19)*. Of more than 100 tropical disturbances that develop in the Atlantic, the Caribbean, and the Gulf of Mexico in any given year, an estimated 10 become tropical storms, of which 6 mature into hurricanes. On the average, 2 of these hurricanes directly hit the United States annually *(8)*.

Table 10-4 Hurricane Events with Mortality ≥25 Deaths in the United States, by Saffir-Simpson Category, 1900–1992

Hurricane	Year	Category	No. of Deaths
1. Texas (Galveston)	1900	4	6,000
2. Florida (Lake Okeechobee)	1928	4	1,836
3. Florida (Keys)/South Texas	1919	4	600*
4. New England	1938	3[†]	600
5. Florida (Keys)	1935	5	408
6. Audrey (Southwest Louisiana/North Texas)	1957	4	390
7. Northeast United States	1944	3[†]	390[‡]
8. Louisiana (Grand Isle)	1909	4	350
9. Louisiana (New Orleans)	1915	4	275
10. Texas (Galveston)	1915	4	275
11. Camille (Mississippi and Louisiana)	1969	5	256
12. Florida (Miami)	1926	4	243
13. Diane (Northeast US)	1955	1	184
14. Southeast Florida	1906	2	164
15. Mississippi/Alabama/Florida (Pensacola)	1906	3	134
16. Agnes (Northeast US)	1972	1	122
17. Hazel (South Carolina/North Carolina)	1954	4[†]	95
18. Betsy (Southeast Florida/Southeast Louisiana)	1965	3	75
19. Carol (Northeast US)	1954	3[†]	60
20. Southeast Florida/Louisiana/Mississippi	1947	4	51
21. Donna (Florida/Eastern US)	1960	4	50
22. Georgia/South Carolina/North Carolina	1940	2	50
23. Carla (Texas)	1961	4	46
24. Texas (Velasco)	1909	3	41
25. Texas (Freeport)	1932	4	40
26. South Texas	1933	3	40
27. Hilda (Louisiana)	1964	3	38
28. Southwest Louisiana	1918	3	34
29. Southwest Florida	1910	3	30
30. Connie (North Carolina)	1955	3	25
31. Louisiana	1926	3	25

*Of 600–900 deaths, over 500 occurred among persons who were thought to be lost on ships at sea.

[†]Moving more than 30 miles an hour.

[‡]An estimated 344 were lost on ships at sea.

Source: U.S. Department of Commerce, National Oceanic and Atmospheric Administration, National Weather Service. *(8)*

Tropical cyclones have seasonal patterns in many regions of the world. In the Caribbean and the Pacific, hurricanes occur between June and November when atmospheric conditions are conducive to their development *(8)*. However, severe storms have been known to take place outside this period. In the Indian Ocean, cyclones normally occur during early summer (April–May) or late rainy season (October–November) when low atmospheric pressures favor their birth *(20)*. However, they have been known to strike the southern coast at any time between April and December *(21)*.

Elements that constitute tropical cyclones can lead to direct or indirect injuries or damages to humans and dwellings. Winds with velocities of as much as 210 miles per hour (336 kilometers per hour) cause structural collapse and force debris to be hurled through the air as high-velocity projectiles *(9)*. Accompanying torrential rains, as much as 30 inches in several days, can generate flash flooding and mudflows *(5, 9)*. Storm surges, the abnormal rising of water generated by a storm over and above the predicted astronomical tide, have been observed up to 25 feet in height; they typically last for several hours and generally affect an estimated 100 miles of coastline *(9, 15)*. Flooding occurs as strong winds or tides push sea waves created by a cyclone up the coastlines with destructive force. These storm surges are differentiated from *tsunamis*, which are seismic sea waves produced by movement of the earth's crust on the ocean's floor. Inland, cyclones can also prompt backwater surging in estuaries of water streams *(5)*.

Tropical cyclones may also be accompanied by secondary disasters that can create or exacerbate new or existing hazards. Under appropriate meteorological conditions, tornadoes can be created by hurricanes. The violent winds and erratic paths of hurricane-spawned tornadoes may require extraordinary responses on the part of the disaster-affected community *(10)*. Other secondary disasters, such as landslides or mudslides, also have the potential to develop. In October 1985, tropical storm Isabel caused widespread flooding and landslides in Puerto Rico; 127 deaths, 78 percent of all storm-related deaths, occurred in one landslide *(22)*.

Public Health Impact: Historical Perspective

The public health impact of cyclones has been examined in the context of the development of warning and forecasting systems. Before the introduction of warning systems that can result in timely evacuation and sheltering, drowning from storm surge accounted for an estimated 90 percent of all cyclone-related deaths *(5, 23)*. This percentage remains much the same today in areas where cyclone forecasting and warning, although improved, have yet to be disseminated to all public sectors. This pattern of death continues, for example, in Bangladesh and the Philippines, where other factors, such as inadequate housing and population density, exacerbate risks for drowning from storm surge *(24, 25)*.

Cyclone-related morbidity generally includes trauma, gastrointestinal illnesses, and dermal conditions *(17, 18, 22, 26–29)*. Structural collapse and wind-strewn debris account for many of the injuries observed during a tropical cyclone. In particular, blunt trauma due to structural collapse may cause mortality during the impact phase; occupancy of mobile homes was implicated in the deaths of several people after Hurricane Andrew in Florida *(30)*.

In areas where warning systems effectively interface with scientific forecasting and emergency management, such as in developed countries, community activities undertaken during the preparedness, response, and recovery phases are frequently associated with actions undertaken during the preparedness, response, and recovery phases. Data from hospital-based surveillance of people with cyclone-related conditions treated in emergency departments indicate that circumstances for mortality and morbidity differ for pre- and postimpact phases. For example, injuries and deaths related to attempts to secure potential projectile objects have been observed before a hurricane's landfall; deaths from falling trees, trauma related to use of chain saws, and burns from unattended flames and generators are commonly reported in the aftermath of a cyclone. Heart attacks, attributed to stress, are also observed during this time *(27)*.

Infectious Diseases

Concern about potential epidemics from infectious diseases generally arises after a disaster. Usually, the risk for increased communicable disease is affected by six conditions: (1) changes in preexisting levels of disease, (2) ecological changes as a result of the disaster, (3) population displacement, (4) changes in population density, (5) disruption of public utilities, and (6) interruption of basic public health services (31). However, with the exception of a malaria outbreak after Hurricane Flora in Haiti in 1963, few serious epidemics of infectious diseases have been documented after tropical cyclones *(32, 33)*. Despite the lack of disease outbreaks to date, the potential for communicable disease exists in situations where sanitation and hygiene are compromised by changes in the environment incurred during the disaster.

In past hurricanes surveillance systems have been implemented to monitor communicable diseases, injuries, and other hurricane-related conditions. According to information from hospital emergency departments and care sites in both active and passive surveillance systems, serious disease outbreaks have yet to be documented during surveillance periods lasting as much as 1 month after a hurricane's impact *(17, 18, 22, 26, 34)*.

One study, however, showed a delayed increase in the incidence of typhoid and paratyphoid fever, infectious hepatitis, gastroenteritis, and measles after Hurricanes David and Frederick in the Dominican Republic on August 31 and September 3, 1979, respectively *(35)*. In another study, diarrheal morbidity rose by 17-fold during the 6 weeks after the cyclone in Bangladesh in 1991. The latter increase, however, was attributed to changes in reporting methods by the Bangladesh National Diarrhea Surveillance System *(36)*. Nevertheless, enteric and respiratory agents may contribute to the overall morbidity observed after cyclones. And because index conditions including gastrointestinal illnesses, respiratory illnesses, and dermal conditions make up the majority of postcyclone morbidity, they continue to be monitored after such events *(17, 22, 26)*.

Finally, the potential for vector-transmitted diseases may be exacerbated by a cyclone *(37)*. Human exposure to disease vectors may increase due to a damaged physical environment and due to migration to vector-borne-disease endemic areas (e.g., malaria and dengue). In addition, rains related to a cyclone may provide a breeding ground for nuisance mosquito populations. After Hurricane Andrew in Florida, emergency surveillance for mosquito-borne diseases such as St. Louis encephalitis, dengue, and malaria showed no marked increase, but in Louisiana, mosquito control was implemented for large nuisance populations that hampered disaster-recovery efforts after Hurricane Andrew *(37)*.

Animal Bites and Stings

Ecological disruptions after a cyclone may lead to changes in the natural habitat of wild animals. After Hurricane Hugo struck South Carolina in 1989, insect stings accounted for 21% of all hurricane-related cases that were treated inland; of these cases, 26% of people experienced generalized reactions *(38)*. Insect stings as a major source of morbidity were thought to result from destroyed insect nests caused by downed trees, the time of year in which the hurricane occurred (i.e., coincidental with the maturity phase of many species of biting or stinging insects), and the proximity of insects to people during cleanup activities. In areas where mosquito populations may increase as a result of storm-associated rains, secondary bacterial infections from mosquito bites may also occur, although no problem has been observed to date *(37)*.

Nutrition and Birth Defects

Long-term health outcomes due to a compromised nutritional status in the aftermath of hurricanes have been reported in the literature. The incidence of neural-tube defects (i.e., spina bifida cystica and encephalocele) among live-born infants increased in Jamaica 11 to 18 months after Hurricane Hugo occurred in 1988 *(39)*. The rise coincided with megaloblastic changes in sickle-cell patients at the time of conception and suggested a deficient intake of dietary folate.

Mental Health

As in most natural disasters, short- and long-term mental health effects are observed as long as 5 years after a hurricane's impact. Outcomes such as emotional and physical distress, nonpsychotic psychological disturbances, and post-traumatic stress disorders have been found in different subgroups of the population *(40)*. In one case study, psychological disturbances were documented in cyclone evacuees after Cyclone Tracy swept through Darwin, Australia, in 1974 *(41, 42)*. Post-traumatic stress disorder was observed among adolescents 1 year after Hurricane Hugo struck South Carolina *(43)*. A population-based study among these adolescents indicated the following risk factors for post-traumatic stress disorder: (1) exposure to the hurricane, (2) prior experience with violent trauma, (3) ethnicity (i.e., being white), and (4) gender (i.e., being female) *(43)*. Finally, increased mental problems were described during a 5-year period after Hurricane Agnes brought widespread flooding to Pennsylvania in 1972 *(44)*. (Psychosocial factors are further discussed in Chapter 6, ''Mental Health Consequences of Disasters''.)

Factors Influencing Mortality and Morbidity

Early epidemiologic studies focused primarily on descriptive accounts of deaths and injuries after cyclones, particularly as they related to accompanying storm surges, heavy rains, and violent winds. With advances in forecasting and warning technology, timely evacuation, and accessible and adequate shelters, more recent research has focused on behavioral factors such as adequate receipt of warning messages, appropriate safety responses by citizens, and the appropriate use of shelters during the impact phase. The few impact deaths from hurricanes in the United States are largely attributed to roof collapse.

Postimpact investigations have addressed deaths and injuries that may occur during specific activities, including cleanup and the use of alternate sources to generate electricity. Risk factors for psychosocial conditions are also observed during the postimpact phase, as long as 5 years after the disaster has occurred.

Finally, displaced populations, often temporarily sequestered in designated sites, may live under conditions where sanitation and hygiene may be compromised owing to the large numbers of people living in an evacuation site. Maintaining safe and adequate supplies of food and water and monitoring communicable diseases are priorities for health management during this period.

Natural Factors

The hazards associated with cyclones center primarily on the effects of storm surge, violent winds, and rains. Almost 90 percent of all cyclone-related deaths are attributed to drowning from accompanying storm surge, which results from the motion of high winds on water. The rise in sea levels due to the storm surge may also result in the flooding of areas far inland *(5)*. Violent winds result in flying debris and structural collapse. Of 14 deaths directly attributed to Hurricane Andrew in Florida in 1992, preliminary reports indicated that 11, or 79%, occurred when structures collapsed on occupants *(45)*. Heavy, torrential rains may lead to flooding of inland estuaries and streams and may precipitate riverine floods and flash flooding.

Cyclonic events can also weaken structures and vegetation, such as trees, in the surrounding environs. Injuries may then be caused when such objects fall on people. Of 38 fatalities associated with Hurricane Hugo in Puerto Rico and South Carolina in 1989, 3 deaths were associated with falling trees that either directly hit a victim or struck a structure or vehicle, killing the occupant *(46)*.

In some cases, hazards associated with a secondary natural disaster, such as a tornado, may accompany the main event, or the cyclone. Of 17 hurricane-related fatalities in Louisiana after Hurricane Andrew, 1 was caused by violent winds during a tornado that was spawned from the hurricane before landfall *(18)*.

Human-Generated Factors

Human-generated risk factors for morbidity and mortality from tropical cyclones in both developed and developing countries include poor building design or construction, insufficient lead times for warning and evacuation, noncompliance with timely evacuation, and the use of inadequate shelter.

In developed countries such as the United States, building codes for hurricane-resistant construction have yet to improve in hurricane-prone communities. An estimated 126, 000 single-family dwellings and 9,000 mobile homes were destroyed or damaged after Hurricane Andrew struck South Dade County in Florida in 1992. Of the 15 deaths directly caused by the hurricane, 12 were wind-related *(10)*. Although a building code had been implemented since 1957, damages from this hurricane underscored the need for developing better designs for wind safety *(47)*. Mobile homes continue to be popular, particularly along coastal areas of the warm sunbelt region. Although residents of mobile homes were warned to evacuate, several deaths directly attributed to the forces of the hurricane occurred in mobile homes within the evacuation zone *(30)*.

Land-use patterns also affect the severity of impact of tropical cyclones. Although much is known about the hazards of cyclones along vulnerable coasts, the settlement of barrier islands and other vulnerable locations has grown tremendously in recent years and has placed additional people at risk, many of whom have had little or no experience with hurricane preparedness *(8)*. The problem is further exacerbated during weekends, holidays, and peak vacation seasons when populations in coastal communities can increase by 10- to 100-fold or more *(8)*. For example, according to the 1990 U.S. Census, the permanent population of Worchester County, Maryland, is 35, 000. Ocean City, a major regional tourist hub located in the county, attracted an estimated 350, 000 visitors during the Memorial Day weekend in 1991 and approximately 3.8 million visitors during the Labor Day weekend *(45)*.

Among residents of nursing homes and hospitals, evacuation is a major problem because of the lack of mobility and special requirements for adequate care among such patients. Evacuation of nursing home patients during Hurricane Elena in Pinellas County, Florida, in 1985 raised issues related to timely patient transport, inappropriate medical care and facilities in shelters, and equipment and supply needs of caregivers during the impact and postimpact phases *(48)*. The risks for injury and illness during evacuation have yet to be fully determined among people with special needs.

Deaths related to preparedness measures undertaken by the population have been observed before a cyclone's landfall. Many deaths have been associated with electrocution or drowning while securing property such as television antennas or boats *(16, 27)*. One death resulted from an impact injury in a motor vehicle crash during evacuation from areas under hurricane watch or warning *(18)*.

The building of enough transportation routes to evacuate residents and visitors in the event of a hurricane has not kept pace with increases in the permanent population of hurricane-prone areas and increases in the number of visitors to such areas (8). For example, only one highway exists to provide for the safe evacuation of the population of the lower Keys in Florida.

In Bangladesh, non-use of shelters contributed to the overwhelming mortality observed after the cyclone in 1991. From a sample of 1,123 people, an estimated 22% of those who did not reach a block or concrete structure perished in the cyclone. Deaths were highest among women older than 40 years of age (31%) and among children younger than 10 years of age (26%) *(49)*.

Fatalities during posthurricane cleanup activities are largely attributed to electrocution from improper use of generators, trauma from weakened structures or trees, and asphyxiation while entrapped under uprooted trees.

Lacerations and punctures, mainly from operating chain saws while clearing debris, are often observed in the postimpact phase. Results from a study of morbidity related to Hurricane Andrew using data collected at a pediatric emergency department suggested the potential for increased hydrocarbon or bleach poisoning among children in households involved in cleanup activities *(34)*. Public health recommendations point to the importance of observing adequate injury prevention and control measures in the aftermath of a hurricane, such as exercising caution during any cleanup operation where heavy equipment is in use.

The lack of electricity, a common phenomenon after a hurricane, may result in increased injuries related to the use of candles and generators. Burns and smoke inhalation from fires due to unattended open flames were observed after Hurricane Hugo in 1989 *(27)*.

Prevention and Control Measures

Although prevention and control strategies for cyclones are similar to those used for most hydrometeorological disasters, preventive measures feature a "window of opportunity'' before a cyclone makes landfall. During this time, occupants of areas under watch or warning may evacuate in a timely manner to seek safe shelter. Coupled with advances in forecasting and warning technology in recent years, adequate warning times for evacuation have allowed for the clearance of areas that would otherwise be subjected to the forces of a hurricane, thus decreasing mortality and morbidity. To date, prevention focuses on disseminating information, making appropriate decisions, coordinating warnings, and crafting more understandable warning messages *(9)*.

Appropriate Building Design and Construction Materials

In countries that are frequently affected by cyclones, such as Bangladesh and the Philippines, local and international authorities currently are investigating the use of appropriate building design and construction materials that are culturally appropriate to the region and that can withstand gale forces of hurricanes *(50)*.

Appropriate Land-Use Planning

Effective land-use planning can mitigate the adverse public health effects of cyclones. For example, structures with occupants who have special needs, such as the hospitalized, the institutionalized, and elderly people, should be located away from low-lying coastal areas in hurricane-prone areas.

Preparedness

Hurricane preparedness continues to play a major role in offsetting mortality or morbidity associated with the hazards of hurricanes. In some cyclone-prone areas of the world, notably the Western Pacific, the seasonal occurrence of typhoons creates a ''disaster culture'' for which preparation is almost habitual. As a result, typhoon-related mortality and morbidity are generally low. In contrast, adequate preparedness may be difficult to achieve in some areas of the United States, where 80%–90% of people living in hurricane-prone areas have never experienced a major hurricane *(45)*.

Warning

The meteorologic properties of cyclones, such as well-defined paths, allow for more effective watch and warning systems, particularly in the southeastern United States. In 70% of hurricanes, paths can be forecasted 24 hours in advance on the basis of speed and direction during the previous 24 to 36 hours *(5)*.

Because predictions lead to expensive preparations and disruptive evacuations, however, the error factor becomes a dilemma for forecasters *(5)* and, ultimately, for public health officials. Those issuing warnings must balance safe and timely clearance of an area with the potential that such predictions have for causing economic losses incurred by the disruption of commercial and other business activities. However, a degree of "overwarning" (defined as the tendency to add more time to the regular "warning time") may be necessary due to (1) increased population densities, especially in high-risk coastal areas; (2) the limitations of forecasters to know the exact timing, strength, and location of impact of a storm; (3) public reluctance to evacuate (due in part to the costs mentioned above); and (4) the potential for loss of lives during a hasty evacuation due to heavily congested traffic. An estimated minimum of 30 hours is now needed to evacuate people from Galveston Island, Texas; the Florida Keys; New Orleans, Louisiana; and Ocean City, Maryland (9). Unfortunately, "overwarning" (i.e., long and frequent population clearance times) presents a dilemma because overwarning too often could eventually detract from the credibility of hurricane forecasters and result in delayed public evacuation.

Adequate forecasting is also based on the width of an area under hurricane watch or warning and changes in storm category (e.g., from Category 3 to 4). For example, expanding the width of the area under warning for Hurricane Elena in the Florida Panhandle in 1985 led to considerable loss of income—an estimated $10 million for every increase of 20% in the size of the area under warning. Raising the storm category from 3 to 4 in the Galveston-Houston, Texas, area would necessitate the evacuation of an additional 200, 000 people (8). It follows that overwarning by wide margins could reduce public credibility for evacuation warnings (8). Any changes in warning zones or storm categories that result in evacuation could result in substantial public health problems as a direct result of large-scale population movements. Likewise, decisions to remain in place rather than to evacuate potentially increase risks for injury, illness, or death in a hurricane.

Evacuation

Adequate emergency planning should allow for the safe evacuation of coastal and low-lying areas and adequate in-place sheltering for temporary increases in population. Using conventional horizonal evacuation to safer inland areas rather than vertical evacuation (e.g., in-place sheltering on higher floors of multistory buildings) is a possible mitigative strategy for ensuring the safety of people living in coastal communities (51).

Behavior

Given an impending cyclone, appropriate behavior invariably leads to greater safety. Compliance with evacuation orders from public officials obviously results in a greater chance for survival. Results of a study of 1,123 people after the cyclone of 1991 in Bangladesh showed that all people who sought refuge in brick or concrete shelters survived, whereas nearly 22% of those who did not seek refuge died (49).

Adequate Shelter

Shelters that are appropriately constructed and accessible to the public, particularly in developing countries, may enhance survival. The use of shelters in coastal villages in Bangladesh during the 1991 cyclone was a major determinant of survival. To prevent deaths and injuries in future cyclones, additional shelters have been planned for construction in coastal communities in Bangladesh *(49, 52)*.

Continuing Public Education

Perhaps the single most important prevention measure for cyclones is public compliance with evacuation orders. The public should also be informed of the margins of error in forecasting a cyclone's intensity and area of impact. Moreover, the public should be aware of the variability of a cyclone's intensity, which is subject to changing meteorological conditions.

In the aftermath of a hurricane, guidelines for preventing or reducing health effects are issued by local health departments, cooperative extension units, or emergency management agencies. Prevention guidelines for individuals and households in the aftermath of a hurricane are found in the CDC pamphlet *Hurricane: a Prevention guide for maintaining your personal health and safety (53)*.

Needs Assessment

Because a cyclone's strong forces can affect a large geographical area, the impact in the disaster zone tends to be widespread. Rapid needs assessments of areas affected by a hurricane should be conducted in order to determine appropriate health and medical requirements in the affected community. Results of these assessments would assist in directing appropriate resources and services to an area. A typical needs assessment would be repeated over time, since needs are likely to change when people relocate or move back and when services are restored in the areas of impact. Also, needs assessments may be performed to determine the adverse affects cyclones have on the public health infrastructure. Such assessments may also be modified as appropriate to the situation; in one postcyclone investigation epidemiologists assessed community nutritional status and agricultural and fishing potential in a developing country *(54)*.

Surveillance

Cyclone-related deaths, illnesses, and injuries and their circumstances should be monitored so that appropriate prevention or citizen-safety guidelines can be issued to the public. Active and passive surveillance systems should be based on a variety of reporting sources, including hospital emergency departments, shelters where medical care is provided, free-care sites, private health care providers, and medical examiners' and coroners' offices. Further, special surveys may be undertaken to identify any increases in postcyclone vector populations, particularly in areas where arboviral diseases may be endemic.

Response and Recovery

Appropriate response in the aftermath of cyclones is similar to that used in postflood situations and other hydrometeorological disasters *(55)*. Major issues involve the following: (1) water quality; (2) food safety; (3) sanitation and hygiene; (4) precautions during cleanup activities that may lead to injuries; (5) potential immunizations—for example, maintaining current tetanus immunization as determined by local officials; (6) protective measures against vectors, such as mosquitoes, rodents, and other wild animals; (7) chemical hazards; and (8) mental well-being, such as stress reduction and counseling, for both victims and responders. Issues such as water quality, food safety, sanitation, and hygiene are especially germane among displaced people who are temporarily housed in densely populated quarters where the potential for transmission of disease may be exacerbated *(56, 57)*.

Critical Knowledge Gaps

Although the cyclone literature describes postimpact mortality and morbidity and outlines risk factors, several important gaps in the epidemiologic knowledge base need to be addressed. Still needed are:

- description of needs in the aftermath of cyclones in inland and coastal communities
- identification of determinants of shelter use, particularly in cyclone-prone cultures
- identification of risk factors for mortality or injury among shelter-seekers
- identification of risk factors for death, illness, or injury among groups with special needs, such as hospitalized or elderly people
- association between mortality or injury and the major meteorological elements that typify a particular cyclone, such as degree of storm surge and wind strength
- association between mortality or injury and the structural integrity and relative wind resistance of buildings
- description of the long-term health effects of cyclones, such as nutritional deficiency and birth defects
- evaluation of the effectiveness of prevention and mitigation measures (e.g., coastal afforestation, the planting of trees on previously unforested land) on public health outcomes

Methodologic Problems of Epidemiologic Studies

The following methodologic problems have been identified in past cyclone-related studies:

- Case ascertainment for cyclone-related conditions. Defining a cyclone-related death, injury, illness, or condition has yet to be uniform and consistently applied to cyclone-related studies.
- Misclassification of cyclone-related health and medical conditions. Often, local officials such as medical examiners, coroners, and personnel in hospital emergency departments decide whether or not an event is ''hurricane-related.''
- Selection bias can be introduced when investigators monitor cyclone-related health effects. Results are often generalized from data sources that include several of the following: (1) hospital emergency departments, (2) temporary shelters that provide health and medical care, and (3) free-care sites operated by the American Red Cross and other private voluntary organizations. It is important to know what roles, if any, private health care providers and other parties such as the military are contributing to overall health effects when attending to cyclone-related illnesses and injuries, even if only for a limited time. Moreover, many external aid groups commonly enter affected areas to provide medical care and leave without reporting or even documenting the types of injuries and illnesses they treated.
- The time period for monitoring cyclone-related deaths, illnesses, or injuries must be standardized in order to ensure consistency when comparing health outcomes for different disaster events. Because most illnesses or injuries tend to be acute, local officials normally use a period of 1 month after a cyclone's impact in which to monitor medical conditions *(26, 35)*. In one extreme case, 1 death due to direct impact occurred approximately 6 months after Hurricane Andrew passed through South Dade County, Florida, in August 1992 *(58)*.

Research Recommendations

- Surveillance of cyclone-related deaths, diseases, and injuries should continue through the response and recovery periods. Gastrointestinal morbidity, respiratory illnesses, and injuries related to cleanup activities are among the common conditions that should be monitored, particularly after a hydrological disaster. Should any changes from precyclone conditions be detected, then investigations of risk factors related to the condition should be initiated.
- In areas where mortality occurs during the impact phase, systematic studies should be undertaken to determine the effectiveness of warning systems.
- Systematic studies should be undertaken to estimate the association between deaths

and injuries and the structural integrity and relative wind resistance of buildings. Because high winds are instrumental in causing morbidity and mortality in some hurricanes and because evacuation zones are primarily determined by the damage potential of storm surges, studies should address the association of structural collapse with deaths and injuries.

- Systematic studies should be conducted to determine risks for illness or injury during evacuation at different points in time during the population-clearance process.
- Among populations with special requirements, such as the institutionalized, systematic studies should be conducted to determine any adverse health outcomes during horizontal or vertical evacuation.
- Systematic studies should be undertaken to determine any differences between risks for injury or illness in coastal communities and inland communities (e.g., during both the impact and postimpact phases) *(38)*.
- Systematic studies should be conducted to assess the short- and long-term effects of cyclones on the mental health status of the affected community.

Summary

Tropical cyclones are among the most destructive of natural disasters. Because cyclonic storms tend to be wide, their effects after landfall may encompass a large area. Hazardous affects of cyclones arise from violent winds, torrential rains, and storm surges. Other hazards usually present themselves during the preimpact preparedness phase (e.g., securing potential high-velocity projectile objects) and after the passage of a tropical storm during cleanup activities (e.g., operating chain saws and electric generators).

Developments in forecasting and warning technology have contributed much to ameliorating the adverse health effects of tropical cyclones. Better and more understandable communication of information from meteorologists to the community may result both in more timely evacuations of inhabitants in areas under hurricane watch or warning and in subsequent more appropriate relocation to safe shelter.

To strengthen community hurricane preparedness, appropriate evacuation behaviors, given certain clearance times and storm categories, must be determined more fully. Safe shelters should also be identified both in areas for evacuees and in areas under hurricane watch or warning. Warning information must also be communicated clearly to the public.

After impact, the health effects of tropical cyclones, like those of floods, are dependent on water quality, food safety, sanitation and hygiene, precautions during cleanup activities, potential immunizations as determined locally, protective measures against vectors, potential release of toxic substances, and mental health sequelae.

Assessing health needs and services in affected communities; maintaining surveillance of deaths, illnesses, injuries, and, if necessary, vectors; and monitoring the quality of water and wastewater systems should continue in the aftermath of a cyclone until predisaster conditions are restored in the affected area.

References

1. Office of the United Nations Disaster Relief Coordinator. *Mitigating natural disasters; phenomena, effects and options*. Geneva: Office of the United Nations Disaster Relief Coordinator, 1991.
2. International Federation of Red Cross and Red Crescent Societies. *World Disasters Report 1993*. Norwell, MA: Kluwer Academic Publishers, 1993.
3. World Meteorological Organization. *The role of the World Meteorological Organization in the International Decade for Natural Disaster Reduction*, report no. WMO-745. Geneva: World Meteorological Organization, 1990.
4. Robinson A. *Earthshock: Hurricanes, volcanoes, earthquakes, tornadoes and other forces of nature*. London: Thames and Hudson Ltd., 1993.
5. Alexander D. *Natural disasters*. New York: Chapman & Hall, Inc., 1993.
6. National Environmental Satellite, Data, and Information Service. *Tropical cyclones of the North Atlantic Ocean, 1871–1992. Historical Climatology Series 6-2*. Silver Spring, MD: U.S. Department of Commerce, National Oceanographic and Atmospheric Administration, National Weather Service, 1993.
7. Gunn SWA. *Multilingual dictionary of disaster medicine and international relief*. Dordrecht, the Netherlands: Kluwer Academic Publishers, 1990.
8. National Weather Service. *Hurricane: a familiarization booklet*. NOAA PA 91001. Silver Springs, MD: U.S. Department of Commerce, National Oceanographic and Atmospheric Administration, National Weather Service, 1993.
9. National Research Council. *Facing the challenge. The US national report*. Washington, D.C.: National Academy Press, 1994.
10. National Weather Service. *Hurricane Andrew: South Florida and Louisiana, August 23–26, 1992. Natural Disaster Survey Report*. Silver Springs, MD: U.S. Department of Commerce. National Oceanic and Atmospheric Administration, National Weather Service, 1993.
11. Chowdhury AMR, Bhuyia AU, Choudhury AY, Sen R. The Bangladesh cyclone of 1991: why so many people died. *Disasters* 1993;17:291–303.
12. Delica ZG. Citizenry-based disaster preparedness in the Philippines. *Disasters* 1993;17:239–247.
13. Shaffer WA, Jelesnianski CP, and Chen J. Hurricane storm surge forecasting. *Preprints Oceans 86* 1986:September 23–26:1379–1385.
14. Jelesnianski CP, Chen J, Shaffer WA. *SLOSH: sea, lake, and overland surges from hurricanes*. NOAA Technical Report NWS 48. Silver Spring, MD: U.S. Department of Commerce, National Oceanic and Atmospheric Administration, National Weather Service, 1992.
15. National Hurricane Center. *Memorable Gulf Coast hurricanes of the 20th century*. Miami: U.S. Department of Commerce, National Oceanic and Atmospheric Administration, National Weather Service, National Hurricane Center, 1993.
16. Centers for Disease Control and Prevention. Update: work-related electrocutions associated with Hurricane Hugo—Puerto Rico. *MMWR* 1989;38:718–720,725.
17. Centers for Disease Control and Prevention. Hurricanes and hospital emergency room vis-

its—Mississippi, Rhode Island, Connecticut (Hurricanes Alicia and Gloria). *MMWR* 1986;34:765–770.

18. Centers for Disease Control and Prevention. Injuries and illnesses related to Hurricane Andrew—Louisiana, 1992. *MMWR* 1993;42:242–243,249–251.

19. Gray WM. Strong association between West African rainfall and U.S. landfall of intense hurricanes. *Science* 1990;249:1251–1256.

20. Khalil G. Cyclones and storm surges in Bangladesh: some mitigative measures. *Natural Hazards* 1992;6:11–24.

21. Hossain M, Aminul Islam ATM, Kumar Saha S. *Floods in Bangladesh: recurrent disaster and people's survival.* Dhaka, Bangladesh: Universities Research Centre, 1987.

22. Dietz VJ, Rigau-Perez JG, Sanderson L, Diaz L, Gunn RA. Health assessment of the 1985 flood disaster in Puerto Rico. *Disasters* 1990;14:164–170.

23. Organization of American States (OAS). *Disasters, planning, and development: managing natural hazards to reduce loss.* Washington, D.C.: Organization of American States (OAS), Department of Regional Development and Environment, Executive Secretariat for Economic and Social Affairs, 1990.

24. Chowdhury M, Choudhury Y, Bhuiya A, *et al.* Cyclone aftermath: research and directions for the future. In: Hossain H, Dodge CP, Abed FH, editors. *From crisis to development: coping with disasters in Bangladesh.* Dhaka, Bangladesh: The University Press Limited, 1992:101–133.

25. Diacon D. Typhoon resistant housing the Philippines: the core shelter project. *Disasters* 1992;16:266–271.

26. Lee LE, Fonseca V, Brett KM, Sanchez J, Mullen RC, Quenemoen LE, *et al.* Active morbidity surveillance after Hurricane Andrew—Florida, 1992. *JAMA* 1993;270:591–594.

27. Philen RM, Combs DL, Miller L, *et al.* Hurricane Hugo, 1989. *Disasters* 1992;15:177–179.

28. Alson R, Alexander A, Leonard RB, Stringer LW. Analysis of medical treatment at a field hospital following Hurricane Andrew, 1992. *Ann Emerg Med* 1993;22:1721–1728.

29. Longmire AW, Ten Eyck RP. Morbidity of Hurricane Frederic. *Ann Emerg Med* 1984; 13:334–338.

30. Centers for Disease Control and Prevention. Preliminary report: medical examiner reports of deaths associated with Hurricane Andrew—Florida, August 1992. *MMWR* 1992; 41:641–644.

31. Western K. *Epidemiologic surveillance after natural disaster.* Scientific Publication No. 420. Washington, D.C.: Pan American Health Organization, 1982.

32. Mason J, Cavalie P. Malaria epidemic in Haiti following a hurricane. *Am J Trop Med Hyg* 1965;14:533–539.

33. Pan American Health Organization. *Emergency health management after natural disaster.* Scientific Publication No. 407. Washington, D.C.: Pan American Health Organization, 1981.

34. Quinn B, Baker R, Pratt J. Hurricane Andrew and a pediatric emergency department. *Ann Emerg Med* 1994;23:737–741.

35. Bissell RA. Delayed-impact infectious disease after a natural disaster. *J Emerg Med* 1983; 1:59–66.

36. UNICEF Cyclone Evaluation Team. Health effects of the 1991 Bangladesh cyclone: report of a UNICEF evaluation team. *Disasters* 1993;17:153–165.

37. Centers for Disease Control and Prevention. Emergency mosquito control associated with Hurricane Andrew. *MMWR* 1993;42:240–242.

38. Brewer RD, Morris PD, Cole TB. Hurricane-related emergency department visits in an inland area: an analysis of the public health impact of Hurricane Hugo in North Carolina. *Ann Emerg Med* 1994;23:731–736.

39. Duff EMW, Cooper ES. Neural tube defects in Jamaica following Hurricane Gilbert. *Am J Public Health* 1991;84:473–475.
40. World Health Organization Division of Mental Health. *Psychosocial consequences of disasters: prevention and management.* Report No. WHO/MNH/PSF/91.3. Geneva: World Health Organization, 1992.
41. Grant WB, McNamara L, Bailey K. Psychiatric disturbance with acute onset and offset in a Darwin evacuee. *Med J Aust* 1975;1:652–654.
42. Parker G. Psychological disturbance in Darwin evacuees following Cyclone Tracy. *Med J Aust* 1975;1:650–652.
43. Garrison CZ, Weinrich MW, Hardin SB, Weinrich S, Wang L. Post-traumatic stress disorder in adolescents after a hurricane. *Am J Epidemiol* 1993;138:522–530.
44. Logue JN, Hansen H, Struening E. Emotional and physical distress following Hurricane Agnes in Wyoming Valley of Pennsylvania. *Public Health Rep* 1979;94:495–502.
45. Sheets RC. *The United States hurricane problem: an assessment for the 1990's.* Miami: National Hurricane Center, 1994.
46. Danis DM. Disaster-related deaths from Hurricane Hugo and the Northern California earthquake. *J Emerg Nursing* 1990;16:295–257.
47. Federal Emergency Management Agency, Federal Insurance Administration. *Building performance: Hurricane Andrew in Florida.* Report No. FIA-22 (2/93). Washington, D.C.: Federal Emergency Management Agency, 1993.
48. Mangum WP, Kosberg JI, McDonald P. Hurricane Elena and Pinellas County, Florida: some lessons learned from the largest evacuation of nursing home patients in history. *Gerontologist* 1989;29:388–392.
49. Bern C, Sniezek J, Mathbor GM, *et al.* Risk factors for mortality in the Bangladesh cyclone of 1991. *Bull World Health Organ* 1993;71:73–78.
50. Gupta SP. Core shelter assistance project in the Philippines for typhoon victims. *Disaster Management* 1990;3(1):14–20.
51. Salmon JD. Vertical evacuation in hurricanes: an urgent policy problem for coastal managers. *Coastal Zone Management Journal* 1984;12:287–300.
52. Siddique AK and Eusof A. Cyclone deaths in Bangladesh, May 1985: who was at risk. *Trop Geogr Med* 1987;39:3–8.
53. Centers for Disease Control and Prevention. *Hurricane: a prevention guide to promote your personal health and safety.* Atlanta: Centers for Disease Control and Prevention, 1994.
54. Sommer A, Mosley WH. East Bengal cyclone of November, 1970: epidemiological approach to disaster assessment. *Lancet* 1972;May 13:1029–1036.
55. French JG. Floods. In: Gregg MB, editor. *The public health consequences of disasters.* Atlanta: Centers for Disease Control, 1989:39–49.
56. Blake PA. Communicable disease control. In: Gregg MB, editor. *The public health consequences of disasters.* Atlanta: Centers for Disease Control, 1989:7–12.
57. Pan American Health Organization. *Assessing needs in the health sector after floods and hurricanes.* Technical Paper No. 11. Washington, D.C.: Pan American Health Organization, 1987.
58. Combs D, Parrish RG, McNabb SJN, Davis JH. Deaths related to Hurricane Andrew in Florida and Louisiana, 1992. *Int J Epidemiol.* In press.

11

Tornadoes

SCOTT R. LILLIBRIDGE

Background and Nature of the Problem

Tornadoes are funnel-shaped windstorms that occur when masses of air with differing physical qualities (e.g., density, temperature, humidity and velocity) collide *(1)*. These violent rotating winds converge to form a vortex, which is usually narrow at the base and which gives a tornado its typical funnel-shaped appearance. Air and debris are actively drawn into the base of the vortex as the tornado moves across the ground, resulting in a path of destruction. Tornadoes in the Northern Hemisphere rotate counterclockwise, while those in the Southern Hemisphere rotate clockwise *(2)*. Winds associated with tornadoes can reach speeds in excess of 250 miles per hour (mph) *(1, 3)*. Because weather conditions that create tornadoes may be present over a large geographic region, tornado outbreaks, defined as six or more tornadoes, may occur within a relatively short period of time *(2)*. For example, in 1974, an outbreak of 148 tornadoes throughout the eastern United States affected 13 states and resulted in approximately 300 deaths and 6,000 injuries *(4)*. The cost of property damage caused by a single outbreak can be in excess of $200 million *(5)*.

As shown in Table 11-1, tornadoes are rated by the Fujita-Pearson Tornado Scale (F0 through F5) on the basis of the estimated wind speed of their vortices and the width and length of their paths *(3, 6)*. Most tornadoes (60%) are considered weak (F0,F1), with wind speeds less than 113 mph; these have limited potential to cause injury or destroy property. However, 1%–2% of all tornadoes are considered violent (F4–F5), with wind speeds greater than 206 mph; these tornadoes are highly destructive and account for more than 50% of all tornado-related deaths in the United States (Table 11-

Table 11-1 Fujita-Pearson Tornado Scale

Tornado Class	Wind Speed (miles per hour)	Path Length (in miles)	Path Width	Severity of Destruction
Class 0	<73	<1.0	< or = 17 yards	—
Class 1	73–112	1.0–3.1	18–55 yards	Minimal
Class 2	113–157	3.2–9.9	56–175 yards	Mild
Class 3	158–206	10.0–31.9	0.34–0.9 miles	Moderate
Class 4	207–260	32.0–99.0	1.0–3.1 miles	Severe
Class 5	>260	100.0–999.0	3.2–9.9 miles	Total

Source: National Climatic Data Center.

2). Because the force of a tornado is strongly associated with its potential to cause injury and death, the number of violent tornadoes (F4,F5) per area of landmass may provide a more accurate representation of a state's public health risk from tornadoes. States with high concentrations of F4 and F5 tornadoes include Oklahoma, Indiana, Iowa, and Kansas *(2)*. Among all states, Florida has the highest concentration of tornadoes (tornadoes per 100,000 sq km) (Table 11-3), although tornadoes in Florida tend to be weak (F0,F1) and thus to have limited public health impact. When the size of a state is not controlled for (number of tornadoes divided by 100, 000 sq km), however, Texas is consistently the most tornado-prone state in terms of the total number of all classes of tornadoes (Table 11–3) and the number of tornado-related deaths per geographical area.

Table 11-2 Frequency of Tornadoes and Tornado-Related Deaths by Fujita Class in the United States from 1985 through 1993

Tornado Strength by Fujita Class	Total Number (%) of Tornadoes by Fujita Class	Total Number (%) of Deaths by Fujita Class
Weak		
F0	4,305 (51.3%)	3 (0.7%)
F1	2,860 (34.1%)	31 (7.5%)
Strong		
F2	907 (10.8%)	76 (18.4%)
F3	250 (3.0%)	85 (20.5%)
Violent		
F4	64 (0.8%)	152 (36.7%)
F5	6 (0.1%)	67 (16.2%)
Total number of tornadoes	8,392 (100.0%)	414 (100%)

Source: National Severe Storms Forecast Center.

Table 11-3 Tornado Frequency by State from 1953 through 1991

Absolute Number of Tornadoes by State (all classes of tornadoes)*		States with Most Frequent Number of Tornadoes Adjusted for Area (tornadoes per 100,000 sq km)
State	Number of Tornadoes	
1. Texas	(4,949)	1. Florida
2. Oklahoma	(2,042)	2. Oklahoma
3. Florida	(1,762)	3. Indiana
4. Kansas	(1,735)	4. Iowa
5. Nebraska	(1,449)	5. Kansas
6. Iowa	(1,229)	6. Delaware
7. Missouri	(1,044)	7. Louisiana
8. Illinois	(1,042)	8. Mississippi
9. South Dakota	(970)	9. Nebraska
10. Louisiana	(949)	10. Texas

*Total number of tornadoes in U.S. from 1953 to 1991 was 29,993.

Source: National Climatic Data Center.

In the United States, most tornadoes (59%) travel toward the Northeast at an average ground speed of 40 mph *(2)*. However, tornadoes have been noted to move along the ground at velocities up to 75 mph, remain stationary, or even reverse course. The average length of a tornado is 4.4 miles and the average width of a tornado is 128 yards. Most tornadoes last for only a few short minutes; however, maximum-strength

Table 11-4 Tornadoes with Longest Path Lengths

States	Dates	Path Length (Miles)
Missouri-Illinois-Indiana	March 18, 1925	219
Texas-Oklahoma-Kansas	April 9, 1947	170
Missouri	February 21, 1971	160
Louisiana-Mississippi	April 24, 1908	155
Illinois	May 26, 1917	155
Alabama	May 27, 1973	135
Mississippi-Alabama	April 20, 1920	130
Mississippi-Tennessee	April 29, 1909	125
Indiana	April 3, 1974	121
Illinois	March 30, 1938	115

Source: Grazulis TP. *Significant tornadoes 1680–1991.* St. Johnsbury, VT: The Tornado Project of Environmental Films, 1993. *(2)*

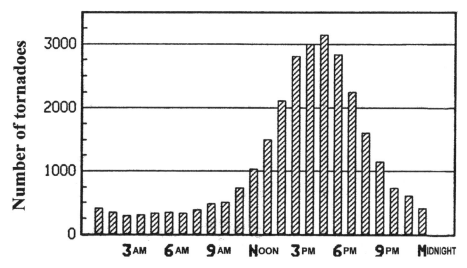

Figure 11-1. United States tornadoes by hour of day, 1950–1989. *Source*: Grazulis TP. *Significant tornadoes 1680–1991*. St. Johnsbury, VT: The Tornado Project of Environmental Films, 1993. (2)

tornadoes have been known to travel more than 200 miles (Table 11-4), persist for hours, and span 3 miles in width *(2, 3)*. In the United States, the peak time of day for the occurrence of tornadoes is between 5 and 6 P.M. (Fig. 11-1). The time of year is also an important factor related to the development of tornadoes (Fig. 11-2). April, May, and June are the peak months for the occurrence of tornadoes in the United States; however, the months of peak occurrence vary considerably from state to state. For example, the peak season for tornadoes in North Dakota is actually June, July, and August. Although tornadoes occur most frequently in certain geographical regions, at certain times of days, and during certain months, tornadoes have actually been recorded at all hours of the day and in all months of the year. Tornadoes have also been recorded in Alaska and Hawaii.

The property destruction that accompanies a tornado is directly related to the strength of its destructive winds. These forces can be sufficient to sweep houses off their foundations and carry debris hundreds of miles. Tornado outbreaks with multiple simultaneous tornadic storms may create substantial and wide-ranging demands on state and local emergency services and health departments *(5)*. The disruption of electrical power and telephone services and the financial losses due to tornadoes can be catastrophic to a community *(3)*. Because of the highly localized path of destruction that accompanies a tornado, the infrastructure of an affected community usually remains intact. However, these storms can result in mass-casualty situations for emergency responders and local medical facilities *(7–9)*.

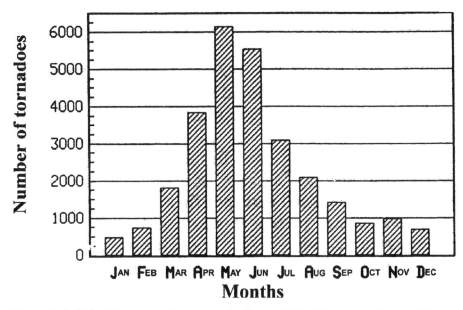

Figure 11-2. United States tornadoes by month of year, 1950–1989. *Source*: Grazulis TP. *Significant tornadoes 1680–1991*. St. Johnsbury, VT: The Tornado Project of Environmental Films, 1993. (2)

Scope and Relative Importance of Tornadoes

North America is the most tornado-active continent and is known for particularly forceful and destructive tornadoes *(2)*. In North America most of these destructive storms occur within the continental United States *(10)*. Among all natural hazards in the United States, only floods and lightning result in more weather-related deaths *(11)*. Other countries, such as Canada, Russia, Australia, China, India, and Bangladesh, are also tornado-prone and have recorded significant tornado-related disasters *(2)*. The worst European tornado occurred on August 19, 1845, when between 70 and 200 people were killed in Moneuil, France. The world's deadliest tornado occurred on April 26, 1989, in Bangladesh near Dhaka when approximately 1,300 people were killed and more than 12,000 were injured. Worldwide, tornadoes are probably underreported because many developing countries lack adverse weather reporting systems. Consequently, the global impact of tornadoes on public health is not known.

Factors that Contribute to Tornado Disasters

Tornadoes pose their greatest danger to public health as they move through heavily populated areas *(5, 8)*. Unlike other disasters, such as hurricanes, which are preceded by a lengthy warning period that allows response officials to evacuate the vulnerable population, tornadoes occur suddenly. Therefore, unless disaster-mitigation steps are undertaken prior to the tornado, preventing death and injury from these storms may be impossible. Inadequate warning and a lack of suitable sheltering for the population at risk are the main contributing factors to the adverse public health effects of tornadoes. Multiple and even redundant sources of warning dissemination are needed to ensure that everyone in the potential path of a tornado is informed of the danger *(12, 13)*. For example, during the Wichita-Andover tornado (1991) in Andover, Kansas, the town's only outdoor tornado siren failed to sound as the storm approached *(5)*. However, nearly 81% of the population whose homes were destroyed were able to receive at least 5 minutes of warning through other sources, such as the media or telephone, thus significantly limiting loss of life.

Unfortunately, many community residents do not have access to appropriate storm shelters *(5)*. A suitable storm shelter for people threatened by tornadoes is usually defined as a subgrade (underground) structure such as a basement or a structure specifically designed to provide temporary protection from adverse weather conditions. People in multiple-family dwellings and other tornado-vulnerable communities such as mobile home parks pose a special storm sheltering challenge for disaster-management officials, particularly when no community storm shelters are located nearby. In addition, the lack of tornado-shelter drills for tornado-vulnerable communities may significantly contribute to residents' risk from tornadoes.

Factors Affecting Problem Occurrence and Severity

Because of recurrent weather patterns favorable to the formation of tornadoes, certain geographic regions are at higher risk for the development of tornadoes than other areas. For example, from 1953 through 1991, five states (Texas, Oklahoma, Florida, Kansas, and Nebraska) accounted for 11, 935 (40%) of the 29, 953 tornadoes that occurred in the United States *(2)* (Fig. 11-3). Throughout the world, agricultural areas (e.g., the midwestern United States and farming regions within other countries like Brazil and Argentina) tend to be at higher risk for the development of tornadoes because certain weather patterns that promote good crop yields may also contribute to the development of tornadoes *(10)*. In addition to geographic factors, the time of day and the time of year also affect a population's risk from tornadoes. For example, late afternoon is the time of day when tornadoes are most likely to occur. Seasonal variation associated with the development of tornadoes means that the risk from tornadoes to the population at any given location is not constant throughout the year. In the United States, January is the month when the fewest tornadoes occur, and May is the month when the most tornadoes occur *(10)*. Other natural factors that promote the development of tornadoes include weather phenomena such as hurricanes. Hurricane Beulah, for example, which

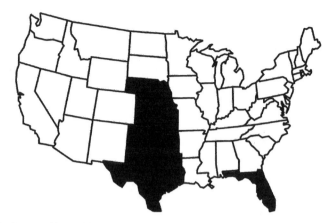

Figure 11-3. States with the highest number of tornadoes from 1953 to 1991. *Source*: Grazulis TP. *Significant tornadoes 1680–1991*. St. Johnsbury, VT: The Tornado Project of Environmental Films, 1993. (2)

struck in 1967, is credited with spawning 115 tornadoes in the coastal region of Texas *(2)*.

Public Health Impacts: Historical Perspective

From 1953 through 1991, the United States averaged 768 tornadoes per year *(14)*. During that period, an average of 93 people were killed each year by tornadoes in the United States. In 1882, in one of the earliest and most comprehensive accounts of U.S. tornadoes, U.S. Army Sergeant J. P. Finley reported on 600 tornadoes that occurred from 1860 through 1880 *(15)*. While stationed in the midwestern region of the United States, he investigated many reports of tornadoes. He traced their paths and recorded their patterns of damage. Sergeant Finley also established in the midwestern United States a tornado surveillance network composed of more than 1,000 people who routinely collected and reported details concerning the occurrence and effects of local tornadoes. The program was the first comprehensive and systematic weather reporting system, and it set the stage for the development of a modern national meteorological observational system. Many of Sergeant Finley's original observations and safety recommendations have stood the test of time. For example, he recommended that "persons residing in tornado-prone regions should build underground shelters" to provide protection from these storms *(15)*. However, other observations, such as the recommendation that "tornadoes can be safely observed from a distance of 300 yards," were not as prudent. (Current recommendations are that anyone threatened by a tornado should take shelter immediately.)

Interestingly, although the annual number of tornadoes reported in the United States generally increased from 1921 through 1990, the annual number of tornado-related deaths actually decreased (Fig. 11-4) *(2, 14)*. One reason for the decrease in mortality associated with tornadoes is the increasing effectiveness of the National Weather Service's (NWS's) severe storm warning systems. Since 1952, when the NWS first began broadcasting tornado warnings, the number of tornado-related deaths has been declining steadily *(2)*. Increased reporting of tornadoes is also thought to have been facilitated by the combination of improvements in NWS storm-detection technology (e.g., Next Generation Weather Radar or NEXRAD) and the development of a national system of NWS volunteer weather spotters.

People are injured or killed by tornadoes when they are struck by energized debris or when their bodies are thrown into stationary objects. Head injuries have been observed to be the most likely cause of death among tornado victims *(16, 17)*. For every person who dies as a result of a tornado, an estimated 20 people are injured *(8)*. Immediate public health relief needs of survivors include medical care, shelter, and assistance in collecting dispersed property and disposing of debris.

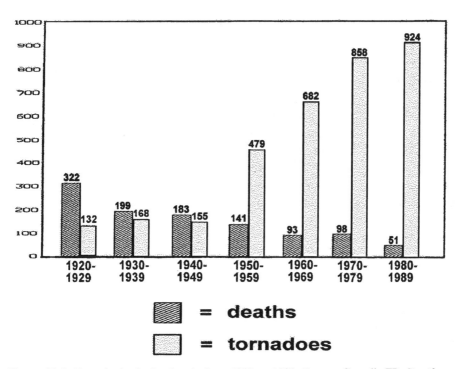

Figure 11-4. Tornado deaths by decade from 1920 to 1989. *Source*: Grazulis TP. *Significant tornadoes 1680–1991*. St. Johnsbury, VT: The Tornado Project of Environmental Films, 1993. (2)

Factors Influencing Morbidity and Mortality Associated with Tornadoes

Natural Factors

As shown in Table 11-2, a population's risk for injury and death from a tornado increases with the tornado's strength. Fortunately, violent (F4 and F5) tornadoes are rare *(2)*. Another factor related to the risk from a particular tornado is the length of its path. However, the association between the length of a tornado's path and its destructive power is somewhat confounded by the fact that tornadoes with long paths also tend to be the most powerful and destructive *(10)*. Another factor that influences morbidity and mortality from a tornado is the time of day that it occurs. For example, in 1947, in Compton, Kansas, 78 people were killed by a tornado that struck at night without warning *(2)*. Tornadoes that occur at night, when people are sleeping, are more dangerous because people are less likely to hear any warnings. Another factor that can contribute to morbidity and mortality are adverse weather conditions, such as hail or rain, that obscure the presence of tornadoes, making their detection by weather spotters more difficult.

Human Factors

Human factors also contribute to the severity of the adverse public health consequences associated with tornadoes. Epidemiologic studies have identified several risk factors for injury and death during tornado disasters, including the following: (1) residing in mobile homes; (2) being more than 60 years old; (3) remaining in a vehicle; (4) failing to seek shelter during a tornado warning; and (5) being unfamiliar with tornado-warning terminology *(2, 5, 8, 9, 16, 18, 19)*. Although the number of tornado-related deaths in the United States is decreasing, the number of tornado-related deaths among people residing in "mobile homes" may be growing at an alarming rate *(5)*. In addition, people with disabilities such as decreased vision or hearing may not be aware of tornado warnings. Elderly people are also at risk from tornadoes for reasons that may relate to both sensory and physical disabilities *(5, 8, 18)*.

Several myths concerning proper actions to take following a tornado warning may increase people's risk for injury or death. The belief that one can outrun a tornado or accurately judge its direction while driving in an automobile is extremely hazardous. For example, during the 1979 Wichita Falls tornado, 40% of people who died were attempting to flee in automobiles *(8)*. Ironically, many of these vehicular occupants had left areas of relative safety and moved directly into the path of the storm. Another belief that has no scientific basis is that tornadoes will not repeatedly strike the same geographical location. This belief is belied by the experience of Codell, Kansas, which was struck by a tornado for 3 straight years—1916, 1917, and 1918 *(2)*. Although such repeat strikes are rare, they serve to remind us that the direction and path of any given tornado is purely a matter of chance. Yet another dangerous myth is that opening or closing windows may mitigate tornado damage; in fact, such actions only serve to delay a person's seeking safe shelter.

As consistently demonstrated in several studies, tornado-related morbidity and mortality rates are higher when no effective storm warnings are issued and when no suitable storm shelters are available. Furthermore, the effectiveness of official warning-dissemination systems is limited if populations are unable to understand the warnings because they are delivered in a culturally inappropriate manner *(20)*. For example, during a tornado disaster in 1987, the unincorporated rural community of Saragosa, Texas (population 200–415, largely Hispanic), was struck by a single, violent, maximum-strength tornado (F5) that killed 30 people and injured 131 more *(20)*. Results of a postdisaster investigation suggested that, in addition to an inadequate number of storm shelters for the town's population, the adverse public health impact of the disaster was exacerbated by the warnings not being disseminated in Spanish as well as in English *(21)*.

Prevention and Control Measures

Warning

One of the most important prevention tools that NWS warning meteorologists use to reduce a population's risk from tornadoes is the NEXRAD (Next Generation Weather Radar) Doppler radar weather system *(22)*. This new technology provides tornado detection that is from 30% to 60% more sensitive than conventional radar at distances of more than 200 miles *(23)*. Doppler weather radars are able to detect the movement of tornadoes an average of 20 minutes before touchdown. Unfortunately, in 1990, Doppler radar coverage had not yet extended to include the region of Plainfield, Illinois. The Plainfield tornado (F5) resulted in 28 fatalities and 274 injured people *(22)*. The extremely short time period between the tornado warning and the tornado's arrival in Plainfield and the odd shape of this particular tornado's funnel cloud made it difficult for observers to recognize the approaching storm as a tornado. The resulting tragedy illustrates the importance of expanding the availability of new technology, such as Doppler radar, to all tornado prone regions. In addition to improvements related to tornado detection, the NWS is undergoing a major nationwide modernization program to improve the dissemination of weather hazard information through radio, television, and telephone. Storm warnings are increasingly being incorporated into the commercial news media (e.g., television's 24-hour ''Weather Channel'') *(24)*. Continued improvements in tornado detection and warning dissemination are credited with the decrease in the annual number of observed tornado-related deaths in the United States *(2)*.

Epidemiology: Assessment and Surveillance

Epidemiologists may be required to provide technical assistance in the conduct of emergency health assessments of populations affected by tornado disasters *(25, 26)*. Such assessments following tornado disasters are usually conducted by following the path of the storm in a simple door-to-door fashion or by assessing the needs of people who have been displaced from their homes into temporary shelters. Because tornadoes have their greatest adverse effect on public health when they move into populated areas, assessment teams should initially focus on highly urbanized residential areas when resources are limited. Two important logistical requirements influence the success of a disaster assessment conducted in the wake of a tornado:

- Highly detailed maps. Such maps are extremely important tools for those organizing geography-based field surveys in highly urbanized areas. These are best obtained from state and local authorities.
- Aerial reconnaissance. The earliest and most reliable information concerning the path of the tornado storm is usually obtained from aerial reconnaissance. If the ground-based assessment is not guided by such aerial visual surveys, it will be delayed and its effectiveness reduced.

Postdisaster public health surveillance of a population affected by a tornado may be an important component of the emergency public health response *(27)*. Information obtained from such surveillance can be used to detect epidemics of infectious disease, injuries, and environmentally related illness that occur within a population as a result of a tornado disaster *(28, 29)*. To be effective, postdisaster surveillance activities for health and medical conditions should be based at clinical sites and at both official and unofficial shelters where displaced persons have collected. In addition, using a standard shelter surveillance form,

relief agencies such as the American Red Cross collect data on the status of victims living in shelters *(30)*. Therefore, epidemiologists conducting postdisaster surveillance should coordinate surveillance and other data-collection activities with all relief agencies and with state and local public health authorities.

Engineering and Legal Controls

Residents of ''mobile homes'' have been identified as being at especially high risk for death and injury from tornadoes *(8, 18)*. The most graphic example occurred in Andover, Kansas, in 1991, when an F5 tornado struck a mobile-home community and destroyed 205 residential units. Of the 38 unsheltered residents who remained within the mobile-home community, 11 (29%) were killed, 17 (45%) were hospitalized, and 9 (24%) sustained injuries that were treated on an outpatient basis. Incredibly, only one unsheltered person escaped injury. In contrast, none of the approximately 150 residents of the mobile-home community who were able to obtain shelter in the community's single underground storm shelter were killed or injured. Unfortunately, at the time of this disaster, 40% of all mobile-home parks surveyed in the affected county did not have a community storm shelter.

Although tornado-related mortality in the United States has been steadily decreasing from 1985 through 1993, 151 (36.5%) of the 414 tornado deaths that occurred in the United States during that period were among mobile-home residents, even though only 7% of the U.S. population lives in mobile homes *(31)*. This population is thus an important one to target for tornado disaster mitigation *(32)*. Apart from enhancements in warning, the most effective prevention and control measure for reducing tornado-related injuries and deaths is to provide adequate sheltering options for this population *(23)*.

Medical Treatment and Rehabilitation

Because tornadoes create destruction along paths that may span many miles, quickly determining where the majority of casualties occurred can be difficult. Following a major tornado, communication systems are frequently disrupted and highways are often blocked with debris. Many patients with minor injuries may suddenly converge on local hospital emergency departments and overwhelm available staff and material resources. This may hinder efforts by the hospital staff to prepare for more severely injured patients who may arrive later because of their need for extrication, field stabilization, and ambulance transport. Effective hospital disaster planning should ensure that casualties are effectively triaged and distributed throughout the local medical system *(33)*.

Studies have shown that tornado-related injuries tend to be severe soft-tissue injuries in the form of contusions, complex lacerations, and multiple fractures, particularly of long bones *(7, 8, 34)*. Because people with these tornado-related soft-tissue injuries also tend to develop wound infections caused by gram-negative bacilli commonly found in soil *(7, 35)*, tornado-related wounds should be considered highly contaminated and handled appropriately. Wound management may include debridement, secondary closure, and appropriate tetanus prophylaxis (e.g., passive or active immunization, depending on a patient's immunization status). Antibiotic treatment for tornado-related wound infections should include coverage for gram-negative bacterial organisms *(36)*. In addition to infectious-disease problems associated with tornadoes, mental health problems among both responders and victims may be a significant public health issue and should be considered during disaster planning (see Chapter 6, ''Mental Health Consequences of Disasters'').

Public Awareness and Education

Tornado watches and warnings issued by the NWS to the media and to community organizations are the primary means of alerting the public about an approaching tornado *(4)*. An NWS Tornado Watch means that weather conditions are conducive to the development of tornadoes. An NWS Tornado Warning means that a tornado has been sighted by ground observers or has been detected by advanced technology. One limitation to this nomenclature is that the local population may not understand the difference in meaning between the two terms. For example, after the North/South Carolina tornado outbreak of 1986, a field survey of people in the path of the tornadoes revealed that only 40% of them understood the difference between a "watch" and "warning" *(9)*. Community programs such as maintaining a volunteer system of weather spotters may increase rates of local tornado detection and improve warning dissemination. Because of the strong association between the strength of tornadoes and their potential to cause death or serious injury, tornado-related disaster preparedness should concentrate on those parts of the country that have high numbers of violent tornadoes (Fujita classes F4 and F5). Another important component of disaster preparedness is to educate the public to seek appropriate shelter, particularly in public buildings such as schools. Improved hazardous weather awareness can also be promoted by encouraging households located in tornado-prone parts of the country to have National Oceanic and Atmospheric Administration (NOAA) "Weather Radios," which provide 24-hour information to the public concerning adverse weather conditions.

Critical Knowledge Gaps

Given the frequency of tornadoes within the United States, far too little investigation has been done to determine risk factors for injury and death in order to develop more effective strategies for protecting the public from the hazardous effects of tornadoes. Further epidemiologic studies are clearly needed. Numerator data describing the age, sex, and race of people injured or killed and denominator data describing the population at risk are necessary to develop rates of tornado-related morbidity and mortality *(37)*. Epidemiologists' attempts to locate victims (case finding) in the wake of a tornado can be greatly facilitated by their working with county health officials, local hospitals, law-enforcement agencies, the American Red Cross and disaster-management officials. Several sources of data on tornado-related injuries may be available. Local emergency medical service (EMS) officials may have information on ambulance transport and field medical activities. Patient records from physician offices, hospital emergency departments, and medical records departments may be an excellent source of injury data. County medical examiners, coroners, law-enforcement officials, and the media may also provide additional information on tornado-related deaths. Local census information can be extremely useful in developing an estimate of the size of the affected population

Current severe-weather morbidity and mortality surveillance systems (e.g., the National Climatic Data Center) collect only limited information on the circumstances associated with tornado-related injuries or deaths. Medical records and coroner reports are usually not examined by those collecting information on the effects of adverse weather events in order to obtain further data on the mechanism of injury or the cause of death. Little information is collected on the shelter-seeking behavior of victims at the time of injury or death or on whether victims had been adequately warned that a tornado was approaching. In part because of this lack of data, most epidemiologic studies have concentrated on tornado-related deaths, which are more easily measured and less numerous than tornado-related injuries. Morbidity studies following tornadoes have been limited because victims seek medical care in many diverse locations and because patient-care documentation during a disaster may not be a priority for emergency responders *(38)*. In addition, very little research has been done to relate the physical characteristics of a given tornado (e.g., wind speed, width, duration, etc.) with the tornado's public health effects. Studies to determine optimal tornado-warning dissemination strategies are lacking, and the potential for new media technologies such as satellite transmission and cable television to disseminate storm warnings effectively has not been thoroughly evaluated.

Methodologic Problems of Epidemiologic Studies

Like most natural disasters, tornadic storms create situations in which the size of the affected population is difficult to determine. Estimating the size of populations affected by tornadoes is especially difficult because tornadoes often take meandering paths of destruction across a community and, thus, the entire community may not be uniformly affected. Another key element of any epidemiologic investigation of a community affected by a tornado is determining the amount of warning time that population had prior to the tornado's impact. However, estimating precise times is difficult in retrospect (e.g., estimates may be based only on a person's recall), and estimates are therefore subject to considerable bias. In addition, it is impossible to establish the exact mechanism of death for many victims because autopsies are not performed on most people killed by tornadoes. Locating or following up on survivors is also difficult because many victims relocate to temporary shelters or the homes of relatives. Another difficult task in comparing injuries and deaths associated with any specific tornado is determining the extent to which various building types (e.g., wood frame, brick) tend to resist wind damage. Highly resistant structures would be expected to protect their occupants better. In addition, the wind speed gradient associated with a tornado may differ significantly at distances of only a few meters from the funnel cloud. Therefore, the extent to which a person's injuries reflect the full effect of the winds associated with a particular tornado is often unclear. As mentioned above, the NWS conducts nationwide surveillance for tornado-related injuries and deaths, but this system collects very little additional information on personal safety-seeking behavior, the degree of warning that occurred, or people's access to shelter. Although some case-control studies of risk factors associated with tornado-related death and injury have been done, most have lacked the type of multidisciplinary approach needed for good epidemiologic studies, with few incorporating contributions from epidemiology, wind engineering, and meteorology.

Research Recommendations

- Conduct research to define the optimum use of new warning technology. Although the NWS has developed improved tornado prediction and detection methods *(2, 22)*, the communication of this information to the public can still be improved. Automatic telephone warning systems and NWS storm warning radios show great promise. In addition, research to develop storm-warning technology that is specific for both indoor and outdoor populations is required if communities are to be fully protected.
- Develop methods to protect our increasingly aging population from tornadoes. Because of hearing or vision loss, elderly people may be unable to benefit from new technological developments in warning systems that depend on one's being able to see or hear well. Research is required to determine the best methods to warn and shelter this vulnerable segment of the population.
- Standardize the collection of data by medical examiners or coroners following natural disasters.
- Develop standard definitions for tornado-related injury and death.
- Ensure that teams investigating the effects of tornadoes contain multidisciplinary components. Because tornado disasters involve the correlation of physical and meteorological information with epidemiologic data, multidisciplinary research teams are necessary to optimally study the health effects of tornadoes.
- Conduct further research into the best use of the new technology and modern media resources for disseminating weather warnings. Concerns have arisen that frequent "false positive" tornado watches might make people less likely to seek shelter when warned in the future.

Summary

Tornadoes remain the most frequent adverse weather event likely to result in a disaster in the United States. Unfortunately, preventing tornadoes is currently beyond our technical capabilities. Research results have illustrated the lifesaving importance of providing adequate warning and shelter to populations at risk. These prevention measures are particularly important in states with large numbers of violent tornadoes (e.g., Kansas, Iowa, Illinois, Indiana, and Oklahoma) and in locations where many people live in mobile homes *(5, 39)*. The National Weather Service continues to modernize its nationwide adverse weather warning system. As a result, communities are relying less on warning systems that depend solely on outdoor warning sirens and more on a variety of technologically advanced warning systems, including weather scanners, cable television override, and automatic telephone alerting. Tornado-related morbidity and mortality should continue to decrease in the United States if efforts to warn and shelter vulnerable populations, such as the elderly and residents of mobile homes, become part of routine community emergency preparedness.

References

1. National Weather Service. *Tornadoes: nature's most violent storms. A preparedness guide* (NOAA/PA 92052). Washington, D.C.: Department of Commerce, National Oceanic and Atmospheric Administration, National Weather Service, 1992.
2. Grazulis TP. *Significant tornadoes 1680–1991*. St. Johnsbury, VT: The Tornado Project of Environmental Films, 1993.
3. Sanderson LM. Tornadoes. In: Gregg MB, editor. *The public health consequences of disasters*. Atlanta: Centers for Disease Control, 1989:39–49.
4. National Weather Service. *Tornado safety: surviving nature's most violent storms* (NOAA/PA 82001). Washington, D.C.: Department of Commerce, National Oceanic and Atmospheric Administration, National Weather Service, 1982.
5. Centers for Disease Control. Tornado disaster—Kansas, 1991. *MMWR* 1992;41:181–183.
6. National Climatic Data Center. *Storm data and unusual weather phenomena with late reports and corrections, 1993*. Asheville, NC: National Climatic Data Center, 1993;35:71.
7. Harris LF. Hospitalized tornado victims. *Ala Med* 1992;61:12–16.
8. Glass RI, Craven RB, Bregman DJ. Injuries from the Wichita Falls tornado: implications for prevention. *Science* 1980;207:734–738.
9. Centers for Disease Control. Tornado disaster—North Carolina, South Carolina, March 28, 1984. *MMWR* 1985;34:205–213.
10. Fujita TT. *U.S. tornadoes. Part I. 70-year statistics*. Chicago: University of Chicago, 1987.
11. Kremkau L. Severe weather fatalities. In: Kremkau L, editor. *Hazard Awareness Report*. Silver Spring, MD: Warning Coordination Branch, National Weather Service, 1993:25.
12. Mileti DS, Sorensen JH. Planning and implementing warning systems. In: Lystad M, editor. *Mental health response to mass emergencies*. New York: Brunner/Mazel, 1988.
13. Lindell MK. Warning mechanisms in emergency response systems. *Int J Mass Emergencies and Disasters* 1987;5:137–153.
14. National Climatic Data Center: *National summary of tornadoes, 1991. Storm data with annual summaries and unusual weather phenomena with late reports and corrections*. Asheville, NC: National Climatic Data Center, 1991;33:66–79.
15. Finley JP. *Character of six hundred tornadoes*. Professional papers of the Signal Service No.7. Washington (DC): U.S. War Department, 1882.
16. Carter AO, Millson ME, Allen DE. Epidemiologic study of deaths and injuries due to tornadoes. *Am J Epidemiol* 1989;130:1209–1218.
17. Brenner SA, Noji EK. Head and neck injuries from 1990 Illinois tornado [letter]. *Am J Public Health* 1992;82:1296.
18. Eidson M, Lybarger JA, Parsons JE, *et al*. Risk factors for tornado injuries. *Int J Epidemiol* 1990;19:1051–1056.

19. Duclos PJ, Ing RT. Injuries and risk factors for injuries from the 29 May 1982 tornado, Marion, Illinois. *Int J Epidemiol* 1989;18:213–219.
20. Centers for Disease Control: Tornado disaster—Texas. *MMWR* 1988;37:454–456,461.
21. Aguirre BE. Feedback from the field: the lack of warning before the Saragosa Tornado. *Int J Mass Emergencies and Disasters* 1988;6:65–74.
22. Centers for Disease Control: Tornado disaster—Illinois, 1990. *MMWR* 1991;40:33–36.
23. Eilts MD. Severe weather warning tools. *Storm, the World Weather Magazine* 1993; September:28–34.
24. Belville JD. The National Weather Service warning system. *Ann Emerg Med* 1987;16:1078–1080.
25. Lillibridge SR, Noji EK, Burkle FM. Emergency health assessment of a population affected by a disaster. *Ann Emerg Med* 1993;22:1715–1720.
26. Centers for Disease Control. Rapid health needs assessment following Hurricane Andrew—Florida and Louisiana, 1992. *MMWR* 1992;41:685–688.
27. Glass RI, Noji EK. Epidemiologic surveillance following disasters. In: Halperin WE, Baker E, editors. *Textbook of epidemiologic surveillance.* New York: Van Nostrand Reinhold, 1992:195–205.
28. Toole MJ. Communicable disease epidemiology following disasters. *Ann Emerg Med* 1992; 21:418–420.
29. Binder S, Sanderson LM. The role of the epidemiologist in natural disasters. *Ann Emerg Med* 1987;16:1081–104.
30. Patrick P, Brenner SA, Noji EK, Lee J. The American Red Cross-Centers for Disease Control Natural Disaster Morbidity and Mortality Surveillance System [letter]. *Am J Public Health* 1992;82:1690.
31. Brooks H, Purpura J. Mobile home tornado fatalities: some observations. In: Kremkau L, editor. *Hazard awareness report.* Silver Spring, MD: Warning Coordination Branch, National Weather Service, 1994:25.
32. Bureau of the Census. *1990 U.S. Census.* Washington, D.C.: Department of Commerce, Bureau of the Census, 1990.
33. Waeckerle JF. Disaster planning and response. *N Engl J Med* 1991;324:819.
34. Centers for Disease Control and Prevention. Tornado disaster—Alabama, March 27, 1994. *MMWR* 1994;43:356–359.
35. Gilbert DN, Sanford JP, Kutscher E, *et al.* Microbiologic study of wound infections in tornado casualties. *Arch Environ Health* 1973;26:125–130.
36. Brenner SA, Noji EK. Wound infections after tornadoes [letter]. *J Trauma* 1992;33:643.
37. French JG, Falk H, Caldwell GG. Examples of CDC's role in the health assessment of environmental disasters. *The Environmental Professional* 1982;4:11–14.
38. Lillibridge SA, Noji EK. The importance of medical records in disaster epidemiology research. *J Am Health Information Management Assoc* 1992;63:137–138.
39. National Weather Service. *Wichita/Andover, Kansas tornado, April 26, 1991. Natural disaster survey report.* Washington, D.C.: Department of Commerce, National Oceanic and Atmospheric Administration, National Weather Service, 1991.

12

Heat Waves and Hot Environments

EDWIN M. KILBOURNE

Hot weather is an important determinant of human mortality. In the United States, a major heat wave can cause literally thousands of excess deaths in a given summer. Yet, for purposes of public health, the term "heat wave" is not easily defined. "Hot" is a relative term, and periods of hot weather (heat waves) vary greatly in intensity and duration. Ambient temperatures may change rapidly, and they have marked diurnal fluctuations. Their effect on human beings is not the same in different geographic areas. Moreover, the microclimates, behaviors, and preexisting medical conditions of individual human beings dramatically affect the biological consequences of macroenvironmental heat. Thus, at the present time, a precise description of conditions constituting a heat wave of public health importance eludes description. Determining the precise hot weather conditions leading to an adverse impact on public health remains an important area for scientific investigation.

Physics and Physiology of Heat

Although there may be considerable fluctuation of the temperature of the extremities and outer body surfaces of human beings, thermal homeostatic mechanisms attempt to maintain a relatively constant inner body or "core" temperature. For practical purposes, there are four physical processes involved in thermal homeostasis: (1) heat gain from metabolism, (2) heat loss from evaporation, (3) heat gain or loss from conduction and convection, and (4) gain or loss of radiant heat energy. The body gains metabolic heat from the myriad biochemical reactions that are essential to life. The body loses heat, however, when perspiration evaporates from the skin or secretions evaporate from the respiratory epithelium. If the temperature of the body surface is different from that of substances with which it is in contact, then the body gains or loses heat by means by conduction. If the substance with which it is in contact is a fluid medium such as air or water, then conduction is hastened by the flow of fluid over body surfaces (convection). Finally, regardless of the ambient temperature, if a person is in the presence of objects or surfaces hotter or colder than the body, then body heat is gained from or lost to those objects by means of radiation *(1)*.

Four meteorological variables significantly impact the physical processes mediating thermal homeostasis. These are (1) air temperature (measured by shaded dry-bulb thermometer), (2) humidity (measured either as the dewpoint temperature or by comparison of dry-bulb and wet-bulb temperatures), (3) air motion (wind speed), and 4) solar radiant heat energy (measured in a variety of ways). When the dry-bulb air temperature is low, metabolically generated heat is more easily lost from the body to the air via conduction/convection. As air temperature increases, convective heat loss occurs less readily until, at temperatures above body temperature, convective heat loss is no longer possible and heat may be gained from the air. High humidity limits the cooling effect of the evaporation of perspiration and secretions, and, therefore, leads to increased heat stress. Increased air speed facilitates convective heat transfer and the evaporation of sweat. Radiant heat energy adds to heat stress, independent of other variables. For example, radiant heat causes one to feel hotter in direct sunlight than in the shade, even under identical air temperature, humidity, and air speed *(2–4)*.

Thus, the stress that hot weather places on thermal homeostasis is not a simple function of temperature alone. Other meteorological variables come into play. A number of indices have been developed for the purpose of yielding a single number expressing the combined effects of the environmental variables relevant to heat stress. One such index is the *Effective Temperature* (ET) *(4)*. An empirical index developed during the early part of the twentieth century, it was based on actual observations of human subjects under a variety of conditions, temperature, humidity, and air movement. The effective temperature of any given combination of temperature, humidity, and air movement is the temperature of still, saturated air that would yield the same subjective thermal sensation. Because of concern that the original scale was too sensitive to the effect of humidity at low temperatures and not sensitive enough to humidity at high temperatures, a reformulated version of ET has been published *(5, 6)*.

Another index, currently favored by U.S. meteorologists, is the *Apparent Temperature* scale of Professor R. G. Steadman. Apparent Temperature was derived mathematically and is based on physical and physiological principles *(7)*. The *Heat Index* currently reported by the U.S. National Weather Service is based on the Apparent Temperature index of Steadman.

The *Wet-Bulb Globe Temperature* (WBGT) is frequently used to assess heat exposure in occupational situations. This index is calculated as a weighted average of dry-bulb, wet-bulb, and globe thermometer temperatures. (The globe thermometer is a dry-bulb thermometer with the bulb located at the center of a 6-inch-diameter thin copper sphere painted matte black on the outside. Among the factors influencing the globe thermometer reading is radiant heat). The formula weighting was chosen so that WBGT values would approximate those of ET *(8)*.

Because WBGT requires the measurements of three separate instruments, its use in the field is problematic. The *Botsball* or wet globe thermometer (basically a thermal probe located within a wet, black sphere) is a single instrument designed to take into account the combined effects of dry-bulb temperature, humidity, air movement, and radiant heat energy. The Botsball temperature reading can be related to that of the WBGT by means of a simple linear function *(9)*.

Heat stress indices have significant limitations. Most indices involve implicit assumptions about metabolic heat production, clothing, and body habitus. Since these parameters vary among people, the predicted value of heat stress for any single person is, at best, an approximation. Certain heat indices are difficult to use because the raw data required for their calculation (e.g., globe temperatures) are not easily available. Finally, it should be recognized that the value of an index calculated from the results of meteorologic observations at a weather station may differ greatly from the values obtained if one could measure the microclimates to which individuals are exposed.

Health Effects of the Heat

Spectrum of Illness Recognized as Heat-Related

Illnesses recognizable as the direct result of exposure to prolonged periods of high environmental temperature are heatstroke, heat exhaustion, heat syncope, and heat cramps. Heat waves may also increase morbidity and mortality due to other illnesses that occur even in the absence of heat stress (e.g., myocardial infarction; see below). Burns, which result from the local application of intense heat, are not considered here.

Heatstroke occurs when perspiration and the vasomotor, hemodynamic, and adaptive behavioral responses to a heat stress are insufficient to prevent a substantial rise in core body temperature. Some authors distinguish between ''classical'' and ''exertional'' heatstroke. Classical heatstroke is said to occur largely in sedentary elderly people who are exposed to a prolonged (days to weeks) period of heat stress. Exertional heatstroke affects younger, relatively fit persons who exert themselves in a hot environment (as in a summer road race) beyond their capacity to maintain thermal equilibrium. Anhidrosis (absent or greatly diminished perspiration) is reportedly more common in the presentation of classical heatstroke *(10)*.

Classical and exertional heatstroke are not distinct clinical entities. Rather, they represent two ends of a spectrum of circumstances under which heatstroke occurs. Anyone, young or old, can develop heatstroke if subjected to a sufficiently prolonged and intense heat stress. Exercise increases the production of metabolic heat, predisposing persons of all ages to the development of heatstroke.

Although standardized diagnostic criteria do not exist, a patient's condition is usually designated as heatstroke when rectal temperature rises to ≥105°F (40.6°C) as a result of high environmental temperatures. Mental status is affected, and the patient may be delirious, stuporous, or comatose. Anhidrosis may or may not be present.

Heatstroke is a medical emergency. Rapid cooling—usually by means of ice massage, ice-water bath, or special facilities for evaporative cooling—is essential to prevent permanent neurological damage or death. Further treatment is supportive, and admission to an intensive-care unit is often required. The outcome is often fatal, even with expert care. The death-to-case ratio in reported case series generally varies from 0% to 40%, averaging about 15% *(11–19)*.

Heat exhaustion is a much less severe disease than heatstroke. Patients may complain of dizziness, weakness, or fatigue. Body temperature may be normal or slightly to moderately elevated. The cause of heat exhaustion seems to be fluid and electrolyte imbalance due to increased perspiration in response to intense heat. Therefore, treatment is directed toward the normalization of fluid and electrolyte status, and the prognosis is generally good *(10)*.

Heat syncope refers to the sudden loss of consciousness by persons who are not acclimatized to hot weather. Consciousness returns promptly with assumption of a recumbent posture. The cause is thought to be circulatory instability due to superficial vasodilation in response to the heat, and the disorder is benign *(20)*.

Heat cramps occur as the result of fluid and electrolyte imbalances following strenuous exercise done in the heat. Cramps tend to occur in the muscles that have been exercised most. They are common in athletes who must perform in the heat or in workers in "hot" industries. Such persons may be highly acclimatized to hot weather and therefore able to lose great quantities of fluid and electrolytes in their perspiration. Disproportionate repletion of fluid and salt leads to the imbalances *(10)*.

Public Health Impacts: Historical Perspective

Heat-Wave Associated Mortality

Currently in the United States, in years during which no major heat wave occurs, approximately 270 deaths are recorded on death certificates as having been caused by the heat *(21)*. A few such deaths occur during winter and the cooler months of the year, indicating that not all of them are caused directly by meteorologic conditions. However, the great majority occur during summer. In years in which prolonged periods of abnormally high temperatures (heat waves) affect large areas of the country, the number of deaths attributed to heat may rise greatly. In 1980, when summer temperatures reached all-time high levels in much of the central and southern United States, some 1,700 deaths were diagnosed as heat-related, over six times the number expected if there had been no heat wave *(21)*.

Such figures, however, do not reflect the full extent of the problem. In July 1980, some 5,000 deaths over the number expected occurred in the United States, far more than the 1,700 documented as having been caused by the heat *(21)*. This finding is consistent with those of many other studies that show that only a portion of the increase in mortality during heat waves is documented on death certificates as having been caused by the heat *(22)*. Totals of diagnoses of heat-related death have regularly underestimated heat-wave-associated excess mortality by from 22% to 100% (Table 12-1) *(23, 29)*. (In this chapter, "excess mortality" and "excess deaths" during a heat wave refer to the difference between the number of deaths observed and the number expected based on the crude death rate in the same geographic area during some appropriate control period during which neither a heat wave nor any epidemic was present.) Mortality figures give no indication of the substantial number of nonfatal illnesses that occur as a result of the heat.

Causes of Death

Of the syndromes whose sole cause is environmental heat, heatstroke is the only one with a substantial death-to-case ratio. Thus, one might suppose that the great majority of deaths diagnosed as caused by heat represent mortality due to heatstroke. Some studies support this supposition. Henschel and others reviewed the hospital charts of 120 persons whose deaths had been certified as heat-related during the 1966 heat wave in St. Louis. They found that virtually all had a temperature of $\geq 103°F(39.4°C)$ upon hospital admission, a fact that they interpreted as showing that most of these deaths were due to heatstroke *(29)*. However, in another series only 60% of 57 persons hospitalized for physician-diagnosed heat-related illness and who later died met the authors' strict definition of heatstroke *(26)*. During the heat waves in Detroit in May 1962 and June–July 1963, as well as during the June–July 1976 heat wave in Birmingham, England, no deaths were classified as having been caused by the heat, despite substantial "excess" mortality of from 17% to 32% (Table 12-1) *(23, 24)*.

Current death-certificate coding practices at the national level in the United States make it difficult to evaluate the precise clinical diagnoses leading to heat-related death. Deaths are coded by their external cause, environmental heat (*International Classification of Diseases*, 9th Revision, Code E900), rather than by the specific illness that the heat produces.

Mortality associated with a heat wave is often so great that it appears as a sudden and substantial increase in the total number of deaths occurring in a given area (Fig. 12-1). Increases of over 50% in the crude mortality rate are not uncommon. Moreover,

Table 12-1 Numbers of Total Deaths Observed, Total Deaths Expected, Excess Deaths, and Deaths Attributed to the Heat in Specific Locations During Selected Heat Waves, 1872–1980

Location/Period	Reference	Observed Deaths	"Expected" Deaths	Excess Deaths	Excess deaths (as a percentage of expected)	Deaths Classified as Related to Heat	Deaths Related to Heat (as a percentage of excess deaths)
Birmingham, England							
June 24–July 8,1976	24	491	384*	107	27.9	0	0.0
Detroit, Michigan							
May 12–May 18, 1962	25	429	325†	104	32.0	0	0.0
June 23–July 6, 1963	25	783	669‡	114	17.0	0	0.0
Illinois, State of							
July 1–July 31, 1966	26	9,617	8,469‡	1,148	13.6	80	7.0
July 1–July 31, 1936	26	9,423	6,727‡	2,696	40.1	1,193	44.3
Kansas City, Missouri							
July 1–July 31, 1980	27	598	362‡	236	65.2	157	66.5
Memphis, Tennessee							
July 1–July 31, 1980	28	817	711‡	106	14.9	83	78.3
New York, New York							
July 22–July 28, 1972	29	2,319	1,592‡	727	45.7	10	1.4
August 31–Sept 7, 1973	29	2,242	1,808§	434	24.0	22	5.1
June 30–July 6, 1892	29	1,569	769‖	800	104.0	212	26.5
July 24–July 30, 1892	29	1,434	1,081‖	353	32.7	231	65.4
Aug 9–Aug 15, 1986	29	1,810	809‖	1,001	123.7	671	67.01
St. Louis, Missouri							
July 1–July 31, 1980	27	850	542‡	308	56.8	122	39.6
July 9—July 14, 1966	30	543	240#	303	126.2	182	60.1

*Deaths during previous 2 weeks.
†Deaths during same period the following year.
‡Deaths during same period the previous year.
§Eight times the daily average of September 1973 deaths.
‖Deaths during previous week.
#Based on deaths during previous 8 days.

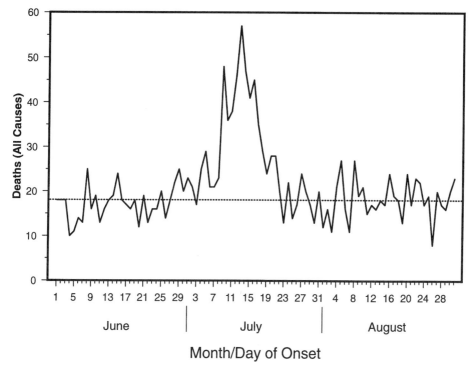

Figure 12-1. Trends in daily deaths showing the increase in numbers of deaths associated with the July 1980 heat wave, St. Louis, June 1–August 31, 1980.

despite the increased use of air-conditioning, there has been no clear and substantial decrease in the death toll taken by heat waves in recent years (Table 12-1).

Schuman and others found stroke (brain infarction or hemorrhage) to be an important cause of heat-wave-associated death; they found that deaths due to "cerebrovascular accident" rose 82% and accounted for 52% of the excess mortality caused by a heat wave in Detroit, Michigan, in 1963. During another Detroit heat wave in May of the previous year, they observed a 104% rise in deaths from stroke (26% of all heat-wave-associated deaths) (24). When Schuman studied the July 1966 heat wave in New York City, he found a far less dramatic increase of 27%, accounting for a little over 6% of an estimated 1,181 excess deaths caused by the heat. He felt, however, that the coding of stroke deaths in New York was different from that of other cities and tended to underestimate the problem (30).

Other investigators have observed that certified stroke deaths increase during severe heat (Table 12-2). However, the magnitude of the increase has been less than that noted in the Detroit studies. Increases have ranged from 25% to 55%, accounting for about 5% to 20% of heat-wave-associated mortality (25, 31). An increase in hospital admissions for persons with nonfatal strokes has also been reported (32).

Table 12-2 Percentage Increase in Selected Causes of Death and Percentage of Excess Deaths Attributable to these Causes During Heat Waves, Selected Heat Waves, United States, 1934–1983

Heat Wave Location & Period	Reference	Condition (Author's words)	Percentage Increase over Control Period	Percentage of Heat Wave Deaths Attributable to This Cause
Cerebrovascular				
Kansas State, July 1–31, 1934	32	Cerebral hemorrhage and softening	54.2	11.1
Illinois State, July 1–31, 1936	32	Cerebral hemorrhage and softening	39.2	6.0
Detroit, Michigan, May 12–18,1962	25	Cerebrovascular accident	103.8	26.0
Detroit, Michigan, June 23–July 6, 1963	25	Cerebrovascular accident	81.9	51.8
Illinois State, July 1–31, 1966	26	Vascular lesions of central nervous system	26.3	20.1
New York, New York, July 2–15, 1966	31	Cerebrovascular accident	27.2	6.4
St. Louis, Missouri, July 9–14, 1966	30	Cerebral accident	53.3	7.0
Cardiac				
Kansas State, July 1–31, 1934	32	Diseases of the heart	22.5	12.5
Illinois State, July 1–31, 1936	32	Diseases of the heart	40.8	25.2
Detroit, Michigan, May 12–18, 1962	25	Heart disease	14.0	18.3
Detroit, Michigan, June 23–July 6, 1963	25	Heart disease	6.9	15.8
Illinois State, July 1–31, 1966	26	Arteriosclerotic heart disease	13.3	36.1
New York, New York, July 2–15, 1966	31	Arteriosclerotic heart disease	40.8	41.5
St. Louis, Missouri, July 9–14, 1966	30	Cardiovascular disease	55.4	20.0
Memphis, Tennessee, July 1–31, 1980	28	Cardiovascular*	40.0	84.9
Latium, Italy, July 1–31, 1983	41	Cardiovascular disease[†]	58.7	90.4
Respiratory				
Kansas State, July 1–31, 1934	32	Pneumonia, all forms	74.6	2.5
Illinois State, July 1–31, 1936	32	Pneumonia, all forms	21.9	2.0
Detroit, Michigan, May 12–18, 1962	25	Respiratory	0.0	0.0
Detroit, Michigan, June 23–July 6, 1963	25	Respiratory	42.9	5.3

Table 12-2 (Continued)

Heat Wave Location & Period	Reference	Condition (Author's words)	Percentage Increase over Control Period	Percentage of Heat Wave Deaths Attributable to This Cause
New York, New York, July 2–15, 1966	31	Respiratory	84.2	13.5
St. Louis, Missouri, July 9–14, 1966	30	Pulmonary disorders	27.8	3.3

*May include cerebrovascular deaths.

†Includes cerebrovascular deaths.

The variability in the magnitude of heat-wave-related increases in stroke mortality relative to other causes suggests that some deaths attributed to stroke are misclassified. However, there is evidence for increased coagulability of blood in heat-stressed persons, and such increased coagulability may be the biological basis for an increase in thrombotic and embolic stroke in hot weather (33, 34). Moreover, the relative consistency of the finding of excess stroke mortality during heat waves in different years and in different locations argues that the association is a real one.

The frequency of deaths attributed to heart disease also increases during heat waves (Table 12-2), mainly due to an increase in deaths attributed to ischemic heart disease. The cause-specific death rate has increased in different heat waves by amounts ranging from about 7% to 55%, accounting for approximately 10%–40% of heat-wave-associated deaths (24, 25, 27, 29–31).

A recent investigation of heat-wave-associated mortality during the July 1993 heat wave in Philadelphia showed that cardiovascular deaths increased more than 100% over baseline. Excess cardiovascular deaths outnumbered hyperthermia (heatstroke) deaths by about 5 to 1. Interestingly, the investigators found no increase in cerebrovascular (stroke) deaths. This investigation underlines the importance of heat as an exacerbating factor for persons with preexisting heart disease and reinforces the point that heatstroke is not always the principal cause of excess death during a heat wave (Centers for Disease Control & Prevention, unpublished data).

The evidence mentioned above regarding increased coagulability of blood in heat-stressed persons lends plausibility to the idea that hot weather causes an increase in deaths from ischemic heart disease, since thrombosis or embolism may exacerbate cardiac ischemia (33, 34). Moreover, the increase in cardiac deaths occurs consistently during heat waves. Thus, the link between heat and death from ischemic heart disease is strong.

It is nevertheless possible that some of the heat-wave-associated deaths attributed to stroke or ischemic heart disease are actually misclassified heatstroke deaths. This situation could arise because of problems in postmortem diagnosis. The recognition of heatstroke in a living patient who has characteristic neurologic findings and a very high body temperature presents few difficulties for the average clinician, especially if anhidrosis (greatly diminished sweating) is present. However, heatstroke can progress rapidly to death, often within few hours of the onset of symptoms. In one study of 90 fatal heatstrokes, duration of illness was less than 24 hours for 70% of patients (35). Thus, many persons who develop heatstroke die before they can be found and brought to medical attention. In the United States such relatively sudden out-of-hospital deaths are usually referred to the local coroner or medical examiner for a determination of cause of death. Frequently, however, no detailed postmortem examination of the body is done, and the determination of the cause of death is based principally on a description of the circumstances under which the body was found. Thus, the possibility exists that some heatstroke victims examined because of relatively sudden, unattended death are diagnosed as having died from other, more common causes (e.g., stroke, myocardial infarction) that can appear to be similar (36).

Postmortem temperature measurement can be useful in the diagnosis of heatstroke. During hot weather in some jurisdictions, the temperature of each body referred to the medical examiner is routinely measured, either by an investigator in the field or by the morgue attendant. A postmortem temperature of $\geq 106°F$ measured soon after death is a useful indicator of heatstroke, because core temperature changes relatively little during the first 1 to 3 hours after death, especially if the ambient temperature is not particularly low. The possibility of false-positive and false-negative results must be considered, however, since the core temperature of a cadaver eventually approaches that of its surroundings. In time, the body of a person who died of heatstroke will cool if the ambient temperature is lower than that of the body core and can rise if ambient temperature exceeds core temperature (37–39).

Stroke and other types of cardiovascular disease taken together may account for as much as 90% of the excess mortality noted during heat waves (27, 40). Nevertheless, numbers of deaths from other causes have also been reported to rise. A clearly defined period of excess death due to respiratory causes corresponding to the July 1966 heat wave in the United States is apparent from national mortality statistics (41). In New York City, respiratory deaths rose 84% and accounted for 14% of the excess mortality attributed to the heat wave (30). However, in other heat waves respiratory deaths have not contributed substantially to excess mortality, generally accounting for 5% or less of such deaths (24, 31). Currently, there is no clear pathophysiologic explanation for how an increase in respiratory deaths could occur from a heat wave.

During a 2-week period of hot weather in New York City in 1966, there was a striking increase of 139% in the number of homicides committed. However, increases of similar magnitude have not been demonstrated subsequently, and, in any case, increased numbers of homicides accounted for less than 2% of the mortality excess during the 1966 heat wave *(30)*.

Many heat-wave-associated deaths are not a clear and direct result of an overwhelming heat stress (heatstroke), nor do they fall into any of the other categories of disease mentioned above. They are seen in the form of apparently excess deaths from a broad variety of underlying causes (e.g., nephritis, diabetes) that do not have any obvious relationship to the heat. Mortality excesses in each of these categories do not occur consistently during heat waves. Moreover, each specific diagnosis tends to account for a relatively small proportion of the excess death *(24, 30, 31)*. It has been suggested that heat-wave-related mortality in this broad group of categories may reflect an ability of heat stress to precipitate death for debilitated persons who are ill from a wide variety of chronic diseases and would die in the near future anyway.

As evidence of this assumption, Lyster presented weekly totals of deaths occurring in Greater London and the rest of England's southeast region before, during, and after the summer heat waves in 1975 and 1976. Mortality increased during both periods of severe heat in both geographic areas, but the increases were followed by several weeks of seemingly lower-than-normal mortality *(42)*. In heat waves before and since, however, such a phenomenon has been sought but not observed. Henschel presented data showing that the average daily death rate in St. Louis was about the same before and after the 1966 heat wave, and Ellis *et al.* reported the absence of a deficit of deaths following a heat wave in New York in 1972 *(28, 29)*. Similarly, there was no substantial fall in mortality following the excess deaths resulting from the 1980 heat wave in St. Louis and Kansas City, Missouri *(26)*. Thus, a depression in the crude mortality rate following a heat-wave-induced elevation is not always found.

Heat-Wave-Associated Morbidity

Nonfatal illness resulting from heat waves has been less well quantified than has heat-wave-related mortality. During the July 1980 heat wave, hospitals in St. Louis and Kansas City, Missouri, admitted 229 and 276 patients, respectively, with nonfatal illnesses thought by the attending physicians to be related to the heat *(26)*. In Memphis during the same period, there were 483 visits to emergency rooms for heat-related illness. Loss of consciousness was a frequent complaint, affecting almost half of the patients seen at City Hospital in Memphis. Dizziness, nausea, and cramps were other common symptoms. The proportions of the illnesses diagnosed for the 471 patients for whom diagnosis was known were as follows: heatstroke, 17%; heat exhaustion, 58%; heat syncope, 4%; heat cramps, 6%; and other heat-related illness, 15% *(27)*.

Indirect measures of morbidity also arise with the heat. In July 1980 in St. Louis and Kansas City, Missouri, emergency room visits rose 14% and 8%, respectively. The respective increases in overall hospital admissions were 5% and 2% *(26)*.

Factors Influencing Morbidity and Mortality: Determinants of Risk

Variation in Heat-Related Health Effects over Time

The public health impact of heat at any given time depends not only on the weather conditions at that time but also on previously existing conditions. That this is true can be seen in the fact that there is a delay between the onset of the heat wave and the appearance of substantial adverse effects on public health. Unusually high temperatures on several days in succession are required to produce a noticeable increase in mortality, and heat waves lasting less than 1 week result in relatively few deaths. The importance of sustained hot conditions is also illustrated by the observation that heat waves in which relatively little nighttime cooling occurs (i.e., those in which daily minimum temperatures are especially elevated) are particularly lethal *(28, 42, 43)*.

Over greater periods of time, however, hot weather seems to lose some of its virulence. Acclimatization of individuals to heat stress is a phenomenon that has been well documented by means of physiologic experimentation *(44, 45)*. Populations, too, seem to acclimatize to the heat over the course of a summer *(46)*. Thus, heat waves in the Northern Hemisphere occurring in August and September seem to be less lethal than those occurring in June and July *(47)*. During a sustained heat wave, after an initial dramatic increase, the number of deaths tends to return toward baseline, even though the temperature may remain elevated *(46)*. This fall in crude mortality may result not only from acclimatization, but also from earlier deaths of susceptible persons, decreasing their number in the population at risk *(24)*.

Urbanization and Risk

Heat waves cause a disproportionately severe health impact in cities, to a large extent sparing more rural and suburban areas. In July 1980, deaths in St. Louis and Kansas City, Missouri, were 57% and 65% higher, respectively, than in July 1979. In contrast, there was an excess mortality of only 10% in the remainder of Missouri, which is largely suburban and rural *(26)*. This trend is not a recent development. In a review of deaths caused by heat and registered in the United States from 1900 to 1928, Shattuck and Hilferty found that the rate of heat-related deaths was substantially higher in urban than in rural areas *(48)*. In a later work, the same investigators found that the effect of heat on death rates increased markedly with increase in the size of a city, suggesting a sort of "dose-response" effect of urbanization *(49)*.

One reason health effects of hot weather may be more extensive in cities is that temperatures there may actually be somewhat higher than in surrounding rural and suburban areas. During the 1980 heat wave, the daily maximum temperature averaged 2.5°C higher and the daily minimum temperature averaged 4.1°C higher at the Kansas City downtown airport than at the suburban Kansas City International Airport *(26)*.

The concept of the urban "heat island" has also been invoked to explain the disproportionate severity of the health impact of heat in cities. The masses of stone, brick, concrete, asphalt, and cement that are typical of urban architecture absorb radiant heat energy from the sun during the day and radiate that heat during nights that would otherwise be cooler. In many cities there are relatively few trees to provide shade. Tall city buildings may effectively decrease wind velocity, thereby decreasing the contribution of moving air to evaporative and convective cooling *(3, 50, 51)*.

The relative poverty of some urban areas is another factor that may contribute to the severity of urban heat-related health effects *(26)*. Poor people are less able to afford cooling devices and the energy needed to run them.

One report from Italy suggests that an urban predominance of heat-related health effects may not be universal. During a heat wave in July 1983 in the Latium region, one of 20 regions into which Italy is divided, mortality recorded at various inpatient facilities (hospitals and clinics) increased 49% over the previous year in the area outside of Rome, but only 25% in Rome itself *(40)*. The reasons for this anomalous finding are unclear.

There is considerable variation among different cities with regard to susceptibility to hot-weather-related health effects. For example, summer temperatures that would not be considered unseasonably high in Phoenix, Arizona, have occurred in St. Louis, Missouri, and caused a severe, adverse impact on public health. In July 1980 in St. Louis, 122 deaths, 229 hospitalizations, and an increase in total mortality of 57% over the previous year were attributed to the heat *(26)*. During that period, however, the average daily maximum temperature in St. Louis was 95.4°F—12.2°F lower than the normal July daily maximum temperature in Phoenix—and the average daily minimum temperature in St. Louis was 74.5°F—3°F lower than Phoenix's normal daily minimum temperature. The highest temperature recorded in St. Louis during the heat wave was 107°F, only 2.2°F higher than the expected (normal) maximum temperature of 104.8°F on any given July day in Phoenix *(52)*. Even after taking the higher humidity of St. Louis into account, its July 1980 temperatures were approximately those of an average July in Phoenix *(7)*.

The reasons for the differences in heat sensitivity of various cities have not been studied extensively. Possible explanations include differences in age structure and acclimatization of the population, architectural style, building materials, and use of air-conditioning.

High-Risk Groups

The overall mortality increases observed during heat waves disproportionately affect the elderly. During a heat wave in July 1983, deaths in Rome, Italy, increased 23% overall, but increased 35% among persons more than 64 years of age *(40)*. The increase in mortality in Greater London resulting from a heat wave in 1975 occurred almost exclusively among persons 65 years of age or older *(53)*. In New York City in the summer of 1966, deaths among persons age 45–64 increased substantially, but the increase in deaths of persons more than 80 years of age was far greater. Investigators also judged that excess deaths among persons 80 years of age or older began earlier in the heat wave than those among persons ages 45–64 years, possibly indicating greater heat sensitivity of the older group *(30)*.

Deaths specifically designated by physicians as having been caused by the heat also occur with a disproportionately high frequency among the elderly. This trend is easily seen in Figure 12-2, a graph of age-specific rates for heat-related mortality in the United States in the period 1979–91. Infancy and early childhood are periods of relative sensitivity to the heat. The rate of heat-related mortality is lowest in late childhood. It then increases monotonically throughout the teenage and adult years, with the slope of the curve increasing rapidly as old age is approached. This pattern is not a new finding; Shattuck and Hilferty observed essentially identical trends associated with heat-related deaths in Massachusetts in 1900–1930, in New York in 1900–1928, and in Pennsylvania in 1906–1928 *(49)*.

The elderly are also at increased risk of acquiring nonfatal heatstroke. A 1980 study of heatstroke survivors in St. Louis and Kansas City revealed that 71% were more than 65 years of age, although this group made up only about 15% of the population at risk *(26)*. Other studies have consistently confirmed the susceptibility of the elderly *(27, 29, 47)*.

The predisposition of the elderly to health effects of the heat may partially reflect impaired physiologic responses to heat stress. Vasodilation in response to the heat requires increased cardiac output, but persons more than 65 years of age are less likely to have the capacity to increase cardiac output and decrease systemic vascular resistance during hot weather *(54)*. Moreover, the body temperature at which sweating begins increases with increasing age *(55)*. The elderly are more likely than younger persons to have chronic diseases or to be taking medications (e.g., major tranquilizers and anticholinergics) that can increase the risk of heatstroke *(56, 57)*.

Finally, old people perceive differences in temperature less well than do younger persons *(58)*. They may, therefore, less effectively regulate their thermal environments.

At the other extreme of age, the rate of physician-diagnosed heat-related death is higher for babies and young children, as shown in Figure 12-2. However, the magnitude of this increased risk is nowhere near as great as it is for elderly persons. There was no detectable increase in mortality for the age group 0–4 years in Greater London during the June–July 1975 heat wave *(53)*. Only one of the 83 persons who died of heat-related causes in Memphis, Tennessee, in July 1980 was less than 20 years of age (a baby in the first year of life) *(27)*. No cases of fatal or nonfatal heatstroke were found to have occurred among persons aged 0–18 years in St. Louis or Kansas City during the July 1980 heat wave, despite careful case-finding efforts in pediatric hospitals and medical examiners' offices *(26)*. Nevertheless, Henschel and others found that four of 182 persons who died of heat-related illness during the July 1966 heat wave in St. Louis were babies less than 1 year of age *(29)*. The small but definitely increased risk of death from heat for babies and young children is most clearly seen in summaries of state and national data compiled over a number of years (as in Fig. 12-2) than in studies of specific heat waves in individual cities.

Other observations document the sensitivity to heat of the very young. Healthy babies kept in hot areas have been found to run temperatures as high as 103°F, and mild fever-causing illnesses of babies may be tipped over into frank heatstroke by heat stress. Children with congenital abnormalities of the central nervous system and with diarrheal illness appear to be particularly vulnerable *(59, 60)*. Parents may contribute to risk by failing to give enough hypotonic fluid during the heatwave and by dressing the child too warmly *(60, 61)*.

U.S. national figures show that in the teenage years and during early and middle adult life, males have an increased risk of heat-related death compared with females (Table 12-3). This difference may reflect a tendency toward greater heat exposure and exertional heat stress among males from occupational and leisure activities, but definitive epidemiologic data on this point are lacking. At the extremes of age, there is less difference between the sexes in rates of heat-related deaths.

Interestingly, many studies of heat waves have demonstrated greater numbers of heat casualties among women than among men. During the 1966 heat wave in New York City, deaths among women were 50% greater than expected, but deaths of men in-

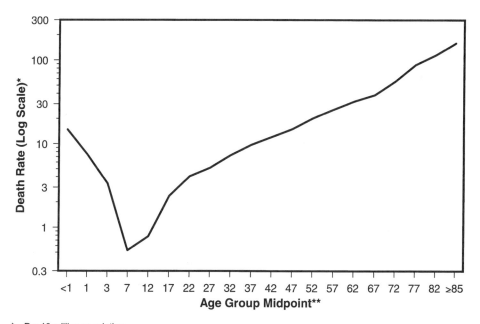

* Per 10 million population.

** 5 year age groups except for first three groups; which are <1, 1, and 2-4 years old.

Figure 12-2. Rates of death attributed to heat (ICD E900), by age, United States, 1979–1991.

Table 12-3 Rates* of Death Attributed to the Heat (Underlying Cause Coded as E900, ICD-9) by Age Group and Sex with Age-Specific Male/Female Rate Ratios, United States, 1979–1991

Age Group	Male	Female	Rate Ratio
1	15.60	13.99	1.12
1	9.16	5.68	1.61
2–4	3.34	3.34	1.00
5–9	0.60	0.45	1.33
10–14	1.11	0.45	2.47
15–19	3.95	0.73	5.41
20–24	6.88	1.23	5.59
25–29	8.60	1.73	4.97
30–34	12.59	2.09	6.02
35–39	16.43	3.23	5.09
40–44	19.98	4.44	4.50
45–49	22.70	7.71	2.94
50–54	30.12	10.97	2.75
55–59	37.16	15.34	2.42
60–64	43.83	22.20	1.97
65–69	49.43	29.71	1.66
70–74	68.29	47.43	1.44
75–79	99.25	81.22	1.22
80–84	130.28	107.40	1.21
85+	202.90	142.01	1.43

*Per 10 million population/year.

creased by only 25% *(30)*. In July of the same year in St. Louis, 59% of heat-related deaths occurred among women *(29)*. In July 1980 in Memphis, 61% of 83 persons who were diagnosed by a physician as having died from the heat were women *(28)*. In Latium Region, Italy, women accounted for 65% of fatal cases meeting specific diagnostic criteria for heatstroke *(40)*.

The probable reason for an apparent excess of women among heat fatalities despite the generally higher age-specific rates of heat-related mortality among men is that age confounds the association of female sex with death due to heat. Elderly populations are the ones at greatest risk, and there are substantially more women than men among the elderly *(62)*. The existence of such confounding was demonstrated in a heat-wave study in which age-adjusted rates of heatstroke were virtually identical for the two sexes despite a predominance of female study subjects *(26)*.

Heat-related health effects are disproportionately severe in areas of low socioeconomic status. In 1966 in St. Louis, the death rate rose most dramatically in areas of low median family income in which there was substantial crowding (high numbers of persons/room) *(30)*. In 1980 in St. Louis and Kansas City, Missouri, the heatstroke rate in census tracts in the highest socioeconomic quartile was about one-sixth that in tracts in the lowest quartile. The rates were intermediate in the tracts of intermediate socioeconomic status *(26)*. Factors leading to the relatively low incidence of heat-related health effects in well-to-do areas may include availability of air-conditioning, abundance of trees and shrubs that provide shading, and access to health care.

In several studies, the rates of heat-related illness have been higher for blacks than for whites. In 1980 in Texas, the heat-related death rate was 21.1/million for blacks and 8.1/million for whites *(47)*. Age-adjusted heatstroke rates were three to six times higher for minority races (principally blacks) in St. Louis and Kansas City in July 1980 *(26)*. The association of black race and relatively low socioeconomic status may well account for the disproportionately high heatstroke rate for blacks in the United States. No biologically based vulnerability of any particular race has been shown.

Persons with a history of prior heatstroke have been shown to maintain thermal homeostasis in a hot environment less well than otherwise comparable volunteers *(63)*. Whether a heatstroke damages the brain's thermoregulatory apparatus or thermoregulatory abnormalities antedate the first heatstroke is not known. However, persons with a history of heatstroke should be considered at risk of a recurrence.

Obesity is an important factor affecting heat tolerance. Obese subjects exercising in a hot environment show a greater increase in rectal temperature and heart rate than do lean subjects *(64, 65)*. The insulating effect of subcutaneous fat impedes the transfer of metabolic heat from core to surface. Soldiers in the U.S. Army who died of heatstroke during basic training during World War II were much more obese than their peers *(66)*. However, obesity may not importantly influence the rate of heatstroke for the largely sedentary elderly population that is at greatest risk during a heat wave *(56)*.

Persons with other less common conditions may also tolerate the heat poorly. These conditions include congenital absence of sweat glands and scleroderma with diffuse cutaneous involvement. In both conditions, perspiration is markedly diminished, resulting in impaired thermoregulation in a hot environment *(67, 68)*.

Some drugs predispose to heatstroke. Neuroleptic drugs (e.g., phenothiazines, butyrophenones, and thioxanthenes) have been particularly strongly implicated. Phenothiazine-treated animals survive in a hot environment for shorter periods than controls, and heatstroke occurs with increased frequency among patients taking these drugs *(56, 69)*. Neuroleptics appear to sensitize both to cold and heat *(69)*.

In laboratory tests of human volunteers, anticholinergic drugs decrease heat tolerance. Persons treated with anticholinergics while exposed to heat have been reported to have a decrease or cessation of sweating and a rise in rectal temperature *(70)*. Many commonly used prescription drugs (e.g., tricyclic antidepressants, some antiparkinsonian agents) and nonprescription drugs (e.g., antihistamines, sleeping pills) have prominent anticholinergic effects, and in one study the use of such drugs was more common among cases than controls *(56)*. The likely mechanism of action appears to be inhibition of the ability to perspire.

Certain stimulant and antidepressant drugs taken in combination or in overdose situations may induce the syndrome of heatstroke. Severe hyperthermia has been reported to result from an amphetamine overdose, an amphetamine taken with a monoamine oxidase inhibitor, and a tricyclic taken in combination with a monoamine oxidase inhibitor *(71–73)*.

Methodologic Problems of Epidemiologic Studies

The literature on heat-wave-related morbidity and mortality has been complicated by the fact that different researchers have studied different health outcomes. In some heat waves that cause substantial excess mortality, relatively few or none of these deaths are certified as having been caused by heat. Since physician-designated heat-related deaths are often so few in comparison to the magnitude of the total increase in mortality, some investigators have chosen to study the total increase in mortality itself as the health outcome of importance. In such studies the number of deaths has been studied in relation to the results of meteorologic measurements made at a local weather station. Since the administrative mechanisms for recording the mere occurrence of a death on a given date are fairly dependable in developed countries, the measure of the health outcome being studied (death on a particular day) is almost exact. Nevertheless, the weather station from which the data are taken may be at a site, such as an airport, miles away from the area in which most deaths occur. Even if readings are taken within the area inhabited by the population at risk, they are outdoor measurements that do not necessarily reflect the variable conditions within dwellings and other buildings in which most of the deaths occur. Since such studies also fail to take into account other host and environmental risk factors, only very limited conclusions can be drawn from their findings.

A number of studies of heat-wave-associated mortality have used information provided on death certificates, comparing deaths occurring during a heat wave with those during a control period. Apparent excess death attributed to a variety of diagnostic entities (e.g., stroke, ischemic heart disease) has been studied, not just those deaths corresponding to clear-cut heat-related illness (e.g., heatstroke). These studies have yielded interesting findings, but the well-known imprecision in certain of the data listed on death certificates leads to corresponding imprecision in study results. In particular, physicians' criteria for diagnosing various causes of death vary over time and in different locations.

In an attempt to deal specifically with morbidity and mortality that are clearly due to the heat—excluding cases of illness and death that could have occurred even in the absence of heat—some investigators have limited their studies of disease to cases classified as "heat-related." This term generally refers to a physician's determination that an illness or death was in some way related to environmental heat (this is how the term is used in this chapter). But even defined in this way, the term is somewhat ambiguous. Heat can produce several distinct syndromes, all of which are "heat-related." Moreover, heat-related death in some studies refers only to deaths in which environmental heat is judged to be the underlying cause of death, but in other reports, deaths for which heat was only a contributing factor are also included. Moreover, the use of this categorization in diagnosis and coding of the cause of death may vary greatly from region to region. Writing about the 1966 heat wave, which caused severe health consequences in New York City and St. Louis, Schuman observed that 130 deaths in St. Louis were attributed to "excessive heat and insulation" but that in New York City "only a handful of deaths were coded, preference being assigned . . . to underlying circulatory and degenerative conditions" *(30)*. Variation among physicians regarding the determination of heat "relatedness" continues to complicate studies of heat-related health effects *(74)*.

In an effort to limit parts of their investigation to the study of a clear-cut illness caused by heat, researchers investigating the effects of the 1980 heat wave in St. Louis and Kansas City, Missouri, defined the following people as having heatstroke:

> Patients with a presenting temperature (measured anywhere on the body) greater than or equal to 41.1°C (106°F); patients with documented temperature greater than or equal to 40.6°C (105°F) if altered mental status or anhidrosis was also present; and those pronounced dead on arrival at the hospital or medical examiner's office if the body temperature . . . was greater than or equal to 41.1°C (106°F). *(56)*

Other studies undertaken since that time have defined heatstroke similarly *(14, 75)*. Strict definitions could also be developed for the study of other outcomes whose direct cause is the heat (i.e., heat exhaustion, heat syncope, heat cramps). Such definitions do not necessarily help the clinician attempting to diagnose the case of an individual patient. Their usefulness lies in their value as entry criteria for epidemiologic studies of groups of patients, enabling the investigator to explain precisely which clinical entities have been studied when "heat-related" illness is the subject of the study. In this manner, future investigators will be better able to clarify and quantify the health consequences of heat.

Prevention of Adverse Health Effects Caused by Heat

Timing of Preventive Measures

In most parts of the United States, heat waves severe enough to threaten health do not occur every year, and several relatively mild summers may intervene between major heat waves. The erratic occurrence of heat waves hinders effective planning of prevention efforts. It may be administratively difficult for health departments to plan for adequate resources that will be available if needed but that will not be wasted if no heat wave occurs.

Although long-term weather forecasts (i.e., those done some months in advance of the event) cannot reliably predict periods of severe heat, near-term forecasts of hot weather several days in advance are becoming increasingly accurate. Could one also forecast the extent of mortality and morbidity expected to result from anticipated hot weather? Even 1 or 2 days of advance warning regarding the probable extent of heat-related adverse health effects would be of use in planning for their prevention.

Apparent Temperature, also known as *heat index* (one of the indices of human heat stress discussed above), has been proposed as a guide to classifying how hazardous to health the anticipated weather may be. However, the index was not developed for this specific use. The hazard posed by heat stress depends not only on its magnitude at a given moment but also on how it has varied over time. Moreover, this index in no way takes into account the variation in heat sensitivity of different regions. Thus, Apparent Temperature by itself, independent of geographical location and antecedent weather conditions, will probably not be found to be a very useful predictor of the extent of heat-related health effects to be expected in a population at risk *(2, 3, 7)*.

Several authors have attempted to develop mathematical models to quantify the increase in numbers of deaths to be expected for a given degree of temperature increase. These formulae have taken into account such factors as the usual seasonal trends in mortality, acclimatization, and the age structure and previous hot weather exposure of the population at risk. Currently available mathematical models have been fitted retrospectively to past mortality and meteorologic data. They are reasonably in accord with the observations from which they were developed. However, none of these models has yet demonstrated its usefulness in the prospective prediction of heat-related adverse health effects *(43, 46, 51)*. This is an important area for further research.

In the absence of reliable prediction, early detection of important adverse health consequences of heat could provide public health professionals with useful information, allowing them to mobilize resources for prevention relatively early in an epidemic of heat-related illness. A large increase in the caseload of the local medical examiner that is unexplained by any other disaster has been proposed as an early indicator of severe heat-related health effects in a community. This proposal was based on 1980 data from two midwestern cities showing that the number of cases reported to medical examiners increased to a proportionately greater extent than did other indirect measures of the heat's impact on public health, including total mortality, emergency room visits, and hospital admissions. Moreover, the total number of medical examiner cases is much more easily and rapidly available than these other statistics. Even the time required for postmortem diagnosis does not delay data collection *(36)*. Although prospective evaluation has not yet established the degree of utility of this sort of surveillance, this fact should not discourage state and local health departments from further evaluation of the method within their jurisdictions. There are as yet no firm criteria regarding just how much of an increase in caseload should trigger implementation of prevention programs.

Content of Prevention Programs

Programs to prevent heat-related illness should concentrate on measures whose efficacy is supported by empirical data. Many heat-illness prevention efforts have centered around the distribution of electric fans to persons at risk. However, study of the 1980 heat wave in Missouri did not show a significant protective effect of fans (56). This finding is consistent with theoretical predictions and empirical data showing that as air temperature rises toward about 99°F—the exact value depends on the humidity and other factors—increased air movement ceases to lessen heat stress. At even higher temperatures, increased movement of air may actually exacerbate heat stress (2–4, 7). Although further epidemiologic studies are required to evaluate the preventive efficacy of fans, fans probably should not be used in situations in which established indices of heat stress suggest they might be harmful.

Air-conditioning effectively prevents heatstroke and may decrease the incidence of other adverse health effects of heat waves. In one study, the presence of 24-hour air-conditioning in the home reduced heatstroke risk by 98%. In addition, just spending more time in air-conditioned places (regardless of whether there was a home air conditioner) was associated with a 4-fold reduction in heatstroke (56). These findings suggest that air-conditioned shelters are an effective means of preventing heatstroke. Persons at high risk who do not have home air-conditioning may benefit from spending a few hours each day in an air-conditioned environment.

The maintenance of adequate hydration is important in preventing heat-related illness. Increases in body temperature of heat-stressed volunteers were lessened when fluid losses were frequently replaced (76). Moreover, taking extra liquids has been associated with decreased risk of heatstroke (56). More fluid than the amount dictated by thirst may be required to fully offset the increased fluid losses that occur during hot weather (76, 77). Thus, unless there is a medical contraindication, persons at risk from the heat should be advised to make a special effort to increase the amount of liquid they consume.

Adequate intake of salt with meals is important. Although salt supplementation with tablets may be important in preventing electrolyte imbalances for carefully selected individuals who must tolerate intense heat for prolonged periods (20), it is of doubtful benefit in preventing heat-related illness in the general population (56). Furthermore, such supplementation may be harmful for persons with certain chronic illnesses in which a high sodium intake is undesirable (e.g., persons with hypertension, congestive heart failure). Therefore, salt tablets should not be recommended for consumption by the general population during a heat wave.

Persons at high risk should be advised to reduce activity in the heat, since such behavior appears to have protected against heatstroke in one study *(56)*. Conversely, athletic exertion in the heat substantially increases risk, although risk does not increase as much for persons who have become acclimatized by training in a hot environment *(66)*.

Target Groups

To be maximally effective, programs for the prevention of heat-related illness should be directed toward groups known to be at particularly high risk. Cities—especially low socioeconomic-status, inner-city areas—are particularly appropriate targets for prevention efforts. The elderly should receive special attention, since old age is one of the factors most strongly associated with increased risk of heatstroke or death from other causes during a heatwave. As much as possible, special living facilities for the elderly and institutions such as nursing homes and hospitals in which many elderly persons are to be found should be air conditioned during severely hot weather. The elderly living at home should not be forgotten, however, since they may be at even greater risk than those in institutions *(78)*. Parents should be made aware of the increased heat sensitivity of babies and children less than 5 years of age. Patients taking neuroleptic or anticholinergic drugs should be counseled regarding their possible increased sensitivity to heat.

Acknowledgement
Portions of this chapter have been excerpted or adapted from: Kilbourne EM. Illness due to thermal extremes. In: Last JM, Wallace RB. *Maxcy-Rosenau-Last Public Health & Preventive Medicine.* 13th ed. Norwalk, Connecticut: Appleton & Lange, 1992;491–501. Used with permission.

References

1. Collins KJ. *Hypothermia: the facts.* New York: Oxford University Press, 1983.
2. Steadman RG. The assessment of sultriness. Part I: a temperature-humidity index based on human physiology and clothing science. *J Appl Meterology* 1979:18:861–873.
3. Steadman RG. The assessment of sultriness. Part II: effects of wind, extra radiation, and barometric pressure on apparent temperature. *J Appl Meterology* 1979:18:874–885.
4. Yaglou CP. Temperature, humidity, and air movement in industries: the effect temperature index. *Journal of Industrial Hygiene* 1927;9:297–309.
5. American Society of Heating, Refrigerating, and Air Conditioning Engineers (ASHRAE). *Handbook of Fundamentals.* Atlanta: ASHRAE, 1981.
6. American Society of Heating, Refrigerating, and Air Conditioning Engineers (ASHRAE). *1989 ASHRAE Handbook: Fundamentals* (I-P ed.). Atlanta: ASHRAE, 1989.
7. Steadman RG. A universal scale of apparent temperature. *J Climate and Appl Meteorology* 1984;23:1674–1687.
8. Lee DHK. Seventy-five years of searching for a heat index. *Environ Res* 1980;22:331–356.

9. Beshir MY, Ramsey JD, Burford CL. Threshold values for the Botsball: a field study of occupational heat. *Ergonomics* 1982;25:247–254.

10. Knochel JP. Heat stroke and related heat stress disorders. *Dis Mon* 1989;35:301–378.

11. Hart GR, Anderson RJ, Crumpler CP, Shulkin A, Reed G, Knochel JP. Epidemic classical heat stroke: clinical characteristics and course of 28 patients. *Medicine* 1982;61:189–197.

12. Gauss H, Meyer KA. Heat stroke: report of one hundred and fifty-eight cases from Cook County Hospital, Chicago. *Am J Med Sci* 1917;154:554–564.

13. Shibolet S, Coll R, Gilat T, Sohar E. Heatstroke: its clinical picture and mechanism in 36 cases. *Q J Med* 1967;36:525–548.

14. Steinzeig SM. Heat stroke: experience at the Windfield State Training School during a record heat wave. *J Kan Med Soc* 1955;56:426–429.

15. Graham BS, Lichtenstein MJ, Hinson JM, Theil GB. Nonexertional heatstroke: Physiologic management and cooling in 14 patients. *Arch Intern Med* 1986;146:87–90.

16. Al-Aska K, Abu-Aisha H, Yaqub B, Al-Harthi SS, Sallam A. Simplified cooling bed for heatstroke [letter]. *Lancet* 1987;1:381.

17. Vicario SJ, Okabajue R, Haltom T. Rapid cooling in classic heatstroke: effect on mortality rates. *Am J Emerg Med* 1986;4:394–398.

18. Katsouyanni K, Trichopoulos D, Zavitsanos X, Touloumi G. The 1987 Athens heatwave. *Lancet* 1988;2:573.

19. Costrini, A. Emergency treatment of exertional heatstroke and comparison of whole body cooling techniques. *Med Sci Sports Exerc* 1990;22:15–18.

20. National Institute for Occupational Safety and Health. *Criteria for a recommended standard . . . occupational exposure to hot environments*. Revised Criteria 1986. Washington, D.C.: U.S. Government Printing Office, 1986.

21. National Center for Health Statistics. *Mortality public use computer data tapes for the years 1979–1991*. Hyattsville, MD: National Center for Health Statistics, 1994.

22. Ellis FP. Mortality from heat illness and heat-aggravated illness in the United States. *Environ Res* 1972;5:1–58.

23. Ellis FP, Prince HP, Lovatt G, Whittington RM. Mortality and morbidity in Birmingham during the 1976 heat wave. *Q J Med* 1980;49:1–8.

24. Schuman SH, Anderson CP, Oliver JT. Epidemiology of successive heat waves in Michigan in 1962 and 1963. *JAMA* 1964;180:131–136.

25. Bridger CA, Helfand LA. Mortality from heat during July 1966 in Illinois. *Int J Biometeorol* 1968;12:51–70.

26. Jones TS, Liang AP, Kilbourne EM, *et al*. Morbidity and mortality associated with the July 1980 heat wave in St. Louis and Kansas City, Missouri. *JAMA* 1982;247:3327–3331.

27. Applegate WB, Runyan JW Jr, Brasfield L, Williams ML, Konigsberg C, Fouche C. Analysis of the 1980 heat wave in Memphis. *J Am Geriatr Soc* 1981;29:337–342.

28. Ellis FP, Nelson F, Pincus L. Mortality during heat waves in New York City July, 1972 and August and September, 1973. *Environ Res* 1975;10:1–13.

29. Henschel A, Burton LL, Margolies L, Smith JE. An analysis of the heat deaths in St. Louis during July 1966. *Am J Public Health* 1969;59:2232–2242.

30. Schuman SH. Patterns of urban heat-wave deaths and implications for prevention: data from New York and St. Louis during July, 1966. *Environ Res* 1972;5:59–75.

31. Gover M. Mortality during periods of excessive temperature. *Public Health Rep* 1938; 53:1122–1143.

32. Fish PD, Bennett GCJ, Millard PH. Heat wave morbidity and mortality in old age. *Age Ageing* 1985;14:243–245.

33. Keatinge WR, Coleshaw SRK, Easton JC, Cotter F, Mattock MB, Chelliah R. Increased

platelet and red cell counts, blood viscosity, and plasma cholesterol levels during heat stress, and mortality from coronary and cerebral thrombosis. *Am J Med* 1986;43:353–360.

34. Strother SV, Bull JMC, Branham SA. Activation of coagulation during therapeutic whole body hyperthermia. *Thromb Res* 1986;43:353–360.

35. Malamud N, Haymaker W, Custer RP. Heat stroke: a clinicopathologic study of 125 fatal cases. *Military Surgeon* 1946;99:397–449.

36. Centers for Disease Control. Medical examiner summer mortality surveillance—United States, 1979–1981. *MMWR* 1982;31:336–343.

37. Marshall TK, Hoare FE. Estimating the time of death: the rectal cooling after death and its mathematical expression. *J Forensic Sci* 1962;7:56–81.

38. Marshall TK. Estimating the time of death: the use of the cooling formula in the study of postmortem body cooling. *J Forensic Sci* 1962;7:189–210.

39. Marshall TK. Estimating the time of death: the use of body temperature in estimating the time of death. *J Forensic Sci* 1962;7:211–221.

40. Centers for Disease Control. Heat-related mortality—Latium Region, Italy, Summer 1983. *MMWR* 1984;33:518–521.

41. Housworth J, Langmuir AD. Excess mortality from epidemic influenza, 1957–1966. *Am J Epidemiol* 1974;100:40–48.

42. Lyster WR. Death in summer [letter]. *Lancet* 1976;2:469.

43. Oechsli FS, Buechley RW. Excess mortality associated with three Los Angeles September hot spells. *Environ Res* 1970;3:277–284.

44. Bonner RM, Harrison MH, Hall CJ, Edwards RJ. Effect of heat acclimatization in intravascular responses to acute heat stress in man. *J Appl Physiol* 1976;41:708–713.

45. Wyndham CH, Rogers GG, Senay LC, Mitchell D. Acclimatization in a hot humid environment: cardiovascular adjustments. *J Appl Physiol* 1976;40:779–785.

46. Marmor M. Heat wave mortality in New York City, 1949 to 1970. *Arch Environ Health* 1975;30:130–136.

47. Greenberg JH, Bromberg J, Reed CM, Gustafson TL, Beauchamp RA. The epidemiology of heat-related deaths Texas—1950, 1970–79 and 1980. *Am J Public Health* 1983;73:805–807.

48. Shattuck GC, Hilferty MM. Sunstroke and allied conditions in the United States. *Am J Trop Med Hyg* 1932;12:223–245.

49. Shattuck GC, Hilferty MM. Causes of death from heat in Massachusetts. *N Engl J Med* 1933;209:319.

50. Clarke JF. Some effects of the urban structure on heat mortality. *Environ Res* 1972;5:93–104.

51. Buechley RW, Van Bruggen J, Truppi LE. Heat island = death island? *Environ Res* 1972;5:85–92.

52. National Climatic Center. Local climatological data: annual summaries for 1980. Asheville, NC: National Climatic Center, 1981.

53. MacFarlane A, Waller RE. Short term increases in mortality during heat waves. *Nature* 1976;264:434–436.

54. Sprung CL. Hemodynamic alterations of heat stroke in the elderly. *Chest* 1979;75:362–366.

55. Crowe JP, Moore RE. Physiological and behavioral responses of aged men to passive heating. *J Physiol* 1973;236:43–45.

56. Kilbourne EM, Choi K, Jones TS, Thacker SB, and the Field Investigation Team. Risk factors for heatstroke: a case-control study. *JAMA* 1982;247:3332–3336.

57. Adams BE, Manoguerra AS, Lilja GP, Long RS, Ruiz E. Heatstroke associated with medications having anticholinergic effects. *Minn Med* 1977;60:103–106.

58. Collins KJ, Exton-Smith AN, Dore C. Urban hypothermia: preferred temperature and thermal perception in old age. *Br Med J* 1981;282:175–177.

59. Cardullo HM. Sustained summer heat and fever in infants. *J Pediatr* 1949;35:24–42.

60. Danks DM, Webb DW, Allen J. Heat illness in infants and young children: a study of 47 cases. *Br Med J* 1962;2:287–293.

61. Bacon C, Scott D, Jones P. Heatstroke in well-wrapped infants. *Lancet* 1979;1:913–916.

62. U.S. Bureau of the Census. *Computer tapes containing population data for the years 1970 and 1980*. Washington, D.C.: U.S. Bureau of the Census, 1980.

63. Shapiro Y, Magazanik A, Udassin R, Ben-Baruch GG, Shvartz E, Shoenfeld Y. Heat intolerance in former heatstroke patients. *Ann Intern Med* 1979;90:913–916.

64. Bar-Or O, Lundegren HM, Buskirk ER. Heat tolerance of exercising obese and lean women. *J Appl Physiol* 1969;26:403–409.

65. Haymes EM, McCormick RJ, Buskirk ER. Heat tolerance of exercising lean and obese prepubertal boys. *J Appl Physiol* 1975;39:457–461.

66. Schickele E. Environment and fatal heat stroke: an analysis of 157 cases occurring in the army in the U.S. during World War II. *Military Surgeon* 1947;98:235–256.

67. MacQuaide DHG. Congenital absence of sweat glands. *Lancet* 1944;2:531–532.

68. Buchwald I. Scleroderma with fatal heat stroke. *JAMA* 1967;201:270–271.

69. Kollias J, Ballard RW. The influence of chlorpromazine on physical and chemical mechanisms of temperature regulation in the rat. *J Pharmacol Exp Ther* 1964;145:373–381.

70. Littman RE. Heat sensitivity due to autonomic drugs. *JAMA* 1952;149:635–636.

71. Ginsberg MD, Hertzman M, Schmidt-Nowara WW. Amphetamine intoxication with coagulopathy, hyperthermia, and reversible renal failure. *Ann Intern Med* 1970;73:81–85.

72. Stanley B, Pal NR. Fatal hyperpyrexia with phenelzine and imipramine. *Br Med J* 1964; 2:1011.

73. Lewis E. Hyperpyrexia with antidepressant drugs. *Br Med J* 1965;1:1671–1672.

74. Centers for Disease Control and Prevention. Heat-related deaths—Philadelphia and United States 1993–1994. *MMWR* 1994;43:453–455.

75. Centers for Disease Control. Illness and death due to environmental heat—Georgia and St. Louis, Missouri, 1983. *MMWR* 1984;33:325–326.

76. Dill DB, Yousef MK, Nelson JD. Responses of men and women to two-hour walks in desert heat. *J Appl Physiol* 1973;35:231–235.

77. Pitts GC, Johnson RE, Consolazio FC. Work in the heat as affected by intake of water, salt and glucose. *Am J Physiol* 1944;142:253–259.

78. Centers for Disease Control. Heat-associated mortality—New York City. *MMWR* 1984; 33:430–432.

13

Cold Environments

EDWIN M. KILBOURNE

Background and Physical and Physiologic Aspects

Scope of the Problem

Unlike summer heat waves, sustained periods of unusually cold winter weather are not characteristically associated with a rise in numbers of deaths from all causes. Nevertheless, the cold causes mortality and severe morbidity of considerable public health importance. If one considers only U.S. deaths certified by physicians as being temperature-related, the average number of deaths attributed to the cold, approximately 770 yearly, is substantially higher than the average yearly number attributed to the heat, about 270 (1).

Air temperature, wind speed, humidity, and radiant heat energy are the four environmental measurements of greatest importance in assessing stress from heat and cold. Air movement facilitates convective heat loss from the body in cold conditions far more effectively than it does in warm ones. Changes in humidity do not affect cold stress as much as they do heat stress because perspiration is not an important physiologic mechanism for maintaining body temperature in the cold. Radiant heat emitted by indoor heating devices (e.g., stoves or radiators) may substantially ameliorate indoor cold stress; however, because the sun transmits radiant heat to the earth's surface less efficiently in winter than in summer, variations in outdoor radiant heat are not as important in the determination of cold stress. Thus, for most purposes, air temperature and wind speed are the two factors most important in determining thermal stress under cold conditions, particularly outdoors (2).

It is logical, then, that the widely used "windchill" index formulated by Siple and Passel in 1945 relies only on air temperature and wind speed to predict the cold stress resulting from specific meteorologic conditions (2). Although this index is widely applied and generally useful, it has inherent inaccuracies at the extremes of wind speeds, and alternative schemes have been proposed (3, 4). A relatively standard windchill equivalent temperature guide based on the Siple and Passel formula is shown as Table 13-1.

Adaptive Mechanisms

The principal immediate adaptive physiologic responses to cold are shivering and vasoconstriction. Muscular activity related to shivering causes increased metabolic heat production. Peripheral vasoconstriction causes a rerouting of some blood away from cutaneous and other superficial vascular beds toward deeper tissues, where the blood's heat can be more readily retained. In addition, blood returning from the limbs is rerouted from constricted superficial veins to the venae comitantes of the major arteries, thereby setting up a "countercurrent" mechanism for heat exchange. Arterial blood passing closely juxtaposed veins warms the venous blood returning to the core. Conversely, incoming venous blood cools outgoing arterial blood so that it gives up less heat when it reaches the periphery. The result is a fall in the temperature of superficial body parts in defense of core temperature. The difference between skin and core temperatures is thus an approximate measure of the efficacy of vasoconstriction (5, 6).

Cold Weather and Mortality

In the United States, mortality usually peaks in midwinter and reaches a low point in late summer (Fig. 13-1). Tens of thousands more deaths occur in January than in August, but the number of "excess" deaths in the winter substantially exceeds the number of deaths certified each year as having resulted from the cold (1). A similar seasonal rise and fall in death rate occurs in other countries in the temperate regions of both the Northern and Southern hemispheres. Of course, the seasonal patterns of these two hemispheres are 6 months out of phase, the death rate being maximal in winter in each hemisphere (5).

Nevertheless, for the most part, winter "cold snaps" (several days or more of unusually cold weather) generally do not seem to cause the sudden, striking increases in overall mortality that summer heat waves cause. An apparent exception was the doubling of the number of persons more than 65 years old dead on arrival (50 observed; approximately 25 expected) at Hope Hospital in Manchester, England, during the severe cold weather of January–February 1985 (7).

Nevertheless, investigators have had to rely on analyses of long series of daily temperature and mortality data to demonstrate both the existence and extent of day-to-day

Table 13-1 Windchill Equivalent Temperatures* for a Reference Wind Speed of 4 miles/hr (1.79 meters per second)

Temperature °F(°C)	Actual Wind Speeds in miles/hour (meters/sec)						
	4(1.79)	5(2.24)	10(4.47)	20(8.94)	30(13.41)	40(17.88)	50(22.35)
40(4.4)	40(4.4)	37(3.0)	28(−2.2)	18(−7.7)	13(−10.6)	10(−12.2)	9(−12.8)
35(1.7)	35(1.7)	32(0.1)	22(−5.6)	11(−11.7)	5(−14.9)	2(−16.6)	1(−17.3)
30(−1.1)	30(−1.1)	27(−2.9)	16(−9.0)	4(−15.6)	−2(−19.1)	−6(−21.0)	−7(−21.8)
25(−3.9)	25(−3.9)	22(−5.8)	10(−12.4)	−3(−19.6)	−10(−23.4)	−14(−25.4)	−15(−26.2)
20(−6.7)	20(−6.7)	16(−8.7)	4(−15.8)	−10(−23.5)	−18(−27.6)	−22(−29.7)	−23(−30.7)
15(−9.4)	15(−9.4)	11(−11.6)	−3(−19.2)	−18(−27.5)	−25(−31.8)	−29(−34.1)	−31(−35.1)
10(−12.2)	10(−12.2)	6(−14.5)	−9(−22.7)	−25(−31.5)	−33(−36.1)	−37(−38.5)	−39(−39.6)
5(−15.0)	5(−15.0)	1(−17.5)	−15(−26.1)	−32(−35.4)	−41(−40.3)	−45(−42.9)	−47(−44.1)
0(−17.8)	0(−17.8)	−5(−20.4)	−21(−29.5)	−39(−39.4)	−48(−44.6)	−53(−47.3)	−55(−48.5)
−5(−20.6)	−5(−20.6)	−10(−23.3)	−27(−32.9)	−46(−43.3)	−56(−48.8)	−61(−51.7)	−63(−53.0)
−10(−23.3)	−10(−23.3)	−15(−26.2)	−33(−36.3)	−53(−47.3)	−64(−53.1)	−69(−56.1)	−71(−57.4)
−15(−26.1)	−15(−26.1)	−20(−29.1)	−40(−39.8)	−60(−51.3)	−71(−57.3)	−77(−60.5)	−79(−61.9)
−20(−28.9)	−20(−28.9)	−26(−32.1)	−46(−43.2)	−67(−55.2)	−79(−61.5)	−85(−64.9)	−87(−66.4)

*Derived from the formula by Siple and Passel (2).

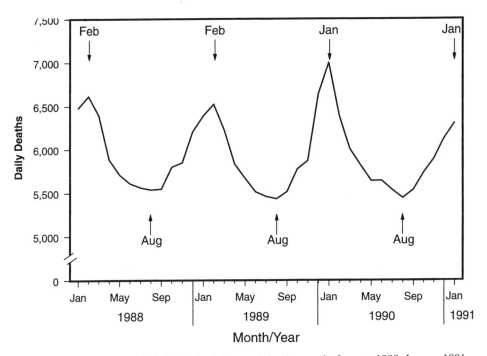

Figure 13-1. Average U.S. daily deaths (all causes) for the months January 1988–January 1991.

variation in numbers of deaths potentially explainable as having been caused by cold weather (8–12). These analyses are complicated greatly by the pattern of seasonal variation in mortality. Even differences in daily death totals for periods as short as 60–90 days may have a seasonal component that must be factored into an analysis for it to correctly assess how much of the day-to-day change in mortality is related to day-to-day changes in temperature.

The tendency for death to occur in the winter is most marked among the elderly and becomes more prominent with increasing age. However, for persons 44 years of age or younger, the trend is reversed. For this group, death is more likely to occur in summer than in winter. Many of the major causes of death are associated with increases in mortality in the winter, among them diseases of the heart, cerebrovascular disease, pneumonia, influenza, and chronic obstructive pulmonary disease. In contrast, deaths from malignant neoplasms remain virtually constant throughout the year (13).

Because of the seasonal fluctuation in mortality, regression analyses that are based on daily observations and that ignore seasonal effects show a significant inverse correlation between mortality and temperature—in other words, a direct association of high death rate with cold weather. The strength of this association reflects the seasonal pattern of mortality, but does not necessarily imply that cold weather is the direct cause of all of the wintertime death increase.

In fact, several observations tend to indicate that this seasonal increase is not completely attributable to temperature. One such observation is that the peaks and valleys in the U.S. mortality curve have not always appeared in January or February and September, respectively, as they do now. In the early part of this century, the peak was usually in February or March and the nadir in June (*14*). If seasonal mortality differences were completely temperature-dependent, one would not expect to see that pattern shift. Moreover, winter death increases occur even in states with relatively mild winters (e.g., Florida and Hawaii), and such increases are of approximately the same magnitude as those observed in states in which winter is characteristically harsh (e.g., Minnesota and Montana) (*11*).

One epidemiologic analysis sought to control for the confounding effect of seasonal fluctuations in mortality by limiting its observations to the months of November through February. The death rate for men less than 65 years of age increased modestly on days with mean temperatures below the monthly mean, but little change was observed in numbers of deaths among men and women 65 years of age or older, the group for which the seasonal mortality increase is most pronounced (*11, 15*).

Nevertheless, the ability of the cold to cause severe illness and death should not be underestimated. Deaths from stroke, ischemic heart disease, and pneumonia may all increase as a direct result of the cold (*9, 10*). Cold-related increases in blood pressure and coagulability may cause the reported increases in deaths from stroke and ischemic heart disease (*16, 17*). Low winter humidity (an indirect result of the cold) may augment the winter death excess, because it favors the transmission of certain infectious agents, most notably influenza (*18*).

Specific Clinical Syndromes

Hypothermia

The term *hypothermia* refers to either unintentional or purposeful lowering of core body temperature. For example, hypothermia has been purposefully induced to decrease oxygen consumption during certain surgical procedures (*5, 6*). Unintentional hypothermia (so-called ''accidental'' hypothermia) results from overexposure to ambient cold temperatures and is a problem of considerable public health importance. Unintentional hypothermia is the only type discussed further.

Hypothermia is the only known cold-related illness with a substantial death-to-case ratio. It is thus reasonable to suppose that cases of hypothermia account for the great majority of deaths for which exposure to cold is certified as the underlying cause (Code E901, *International Classification of Diseases*, 9th Revision). This supposition has not been verified, however.

Most authorities agree that hypothermia is clinically significant when core body temperature falls to 95°F (35°C) or lower. As body temperature drops, consciousness becomes clouded, and the patient appears confused or disoriented. Pallor results from intense vasoconstriction. Shivering occurs at first but decreases markedly in intensity as body temperature falls further and hypothermia itself impairs thermoregulation. With severe hypothermia (body temperature less than 86°F or 30°C), consciousness is lost, respiration may become imperceptibly shallow, and the pulse may not be palpable. At such low temperatures, the myocardium becomes irritable, and ventricular fibrillation is common. The patient may appear dead even though he or she may yet be revived with proper treatment (5).

Persons found apparently dead in circumstances suggesting hypothermia should be treated for hypothermia until death can be confirmed (19). The potential for hypothermia patients to recover after prolonged cardiopulmonary resuscitation should not be underestimated. One apparent victim of cold-water drowning recovered completely after being without an effective heartbeat for 2.5 hours (20). A 30-year-old man suffering from acute severe hypothermia (lowest body temperature 23°C (73.4°F) recovered without permanent sequelae after 4.5 hours of cardiopulmonary resuscitation (21).

Hypothermia can be a primary pathophysiologic event, or it can represent thermoregulatory failure secondary to other underlying illnesses, particularly sepsis, myocardial infarction, damage to the central nervous system, or metabolic derangements. Secondary hypothermia has a worse prognosis than does primary hypothermia, probably because of the severe nature of the associated concomitant illnesses (22).

There is controversy regarding the optimal method(s) for rewarming patients with hypothermia. Advocates of slow external rewarming contend that rapid rewarming causes an abrupt release of vasoconstriction in acral body parts, resulting in a sudden influx of cold, acidotic blood into the core, which exacerbates the metabolic derangements of hypothermia. Further, the release of vasoconstriction is said to result in a relative hypovolemia that may precipitate shock (6, 23). Advocates of rapid rewarming counter that volume deficits and acidosis can be corrected rapidly by infusion of fluids and sodium bicarbonate, and that the best way to treat any further deleterious effects of the cold is rewarming itself (24, 25).

There is less disagreement regarding treatment of hypothermia under extreme circumstances (e.g., when intractable ventricular fibrillation occurs). In such circumstances rapid, invasive "core" rewarming by such methods as peritoneal or open pleural or mediastinal lavage or cardiopulmonary bypass have been advocated (17, 26, 27). Norway has a system for the emergency management of hypothermia victims involving ambulance and rescue helicopters and a protocol for bypassing less advanced hospitals in order to fly patients directly to centers with facilities for extracorporeal circulation (28).

One recent review of hypothermia treatment offered a balanced view, arguing that the treatment of choice should depend on the clinical presentation of the patient.

Whether rewarming is active or passive and whether invasive and/or extracorporeal techniques are used should depend on such factors as the presence or absence of a perfusing heartbeat, the level of hypothermia, the success of initial treatment, and the availability of equipment required for specific types of extracorporeal rewarming (e.g., cardiopulmonary bypass).

No matter what method of rewarming is used, all but very mild hypothermia cases require intensive care, including respiratory support, electrolyte and acid-base disturbance correction, and intravascular volume optimization. The blood glucose level should be checked and hypoglycemia corrected, if present. In addition, the patient must be treated for any medical condition underlying the hypothermia.

Frostbite

Frostbite is local tissue damage caused by actual tissue freezing. At a cellular level, the precise determinants of tissue destruction from typical ''slow freezing'' frostbite have not been fully elucidated; however, formation of ice crystals (occurring first in the extracellular space) and consequent concentration of solutes in the remaining unfrozen fluid may play a role. Cellular damage may be caused by the resulting local hyperosmolar state (*29*). Subsequently, there is vasculopathy of the affected area, contributing to tissue damage. The vasoconstrictive and countercurrent heat-exchange mechanisms mentioned previously serve to lower the temperatures of acral body parts, particularly hands, feet, ears, and nose, making them particularly susceptible to frostbite. In mild cases, recovery is usually complete. In more severe cases, however, tissue viability is affected, gangrene develops, and amputation of affected tissues may be required (*30*).

Substantial clinical experience suggests that optimal treatment of frostbite includes rapid rewarming in a water bath with a temperature of from 37°C to 41°C and subsequent supportive care. Thawing with excessive heat and thawing followed by refreezing have been observed to have clear-cut deleterious effects, leading to the need for more extensive or unnecessary amputation (*31*).

Nonfreezing Local Tissue Injury

Prolonged exposure to cold conditions at above-freezing temperatures may also cause tissue injury. *Trench foot*, or *cold-water immersion foot*, results from prolonged (days to weeks) exposure to wet and cold conditions that are above freezing temperatures but below the usual temperature of the extremity. Damage to skin, muscle, nerve, and connective tissue can occur. Affected limbs are initially swollen and numb, but a painful hyperemic phase soon develops. Long-term (posthyperemic) effects may include persistent pain; hypesthesia; discomfort from the cold; and muscle weakness, atrophy, or fibrosis. In the early presentation of severe cases, there may be gangrene (*32–34*).

Prolonged exposure to warm-wet conditions produces a different and more benign syndrome which has been termed *warm-water immersion foot*. This syndrome also involves pain and swelling of the lower extremities. It responds to bed rest, elevation, and air drying of the feet and legs and typically resolves without lasting sequelae (*32*).

Pernio (*chilblains*) presents as pruritic or painful raised erythematous or violaceous plaques that tend to be distributed at acral body sites over the ears, nose, hands, and especially over the lower legs and feet. Severe lesions of pernio may blister or ulcerate. They are thought to result from a prolonged vasoconstrictive response to the cold and consequent circulatory inadequacy to affected body parts. The lesions improve or clear with vasodilator therapy (nifedipine or prazosin) and cause no long-lasting difficulty (*35–37*).

Determinants of Hypothermia Risk

Situational Factors

Unintentional hypothermia tends to arise in either of two sets of circumstances. One situation involves hypothermia affecting relatively young and generally healthy persons during outdoor sports or other activities typically done in cold weather (e.g., hiking, camping, or skiing). In this situation, an uncompromised host may be subjected to overwhelming cold stress. Hypothermia may develop rapidly, over a period of hours. Frostbite frequently accompanies hypothermia in this situation, because temperatures below freezing are generally involved. Factors that increase the likelihood of developing hypothermia include wearing insufficient clothing, getting clothing wet (which decreases its value as an insulator), and being immersed in cold water, in which case the relatively high heat-conducting capability of water results in rapid loss of heat from the body. Hypothermia may impair the judgment of recreationists, causing them to remain in situations of dangerous cold stress or not to protect themselves adequately (*5*).

The other situation in which hypothermia commonly occurs involves a particularly vulnerable person who is subjected to moderate, but prolonged, indoor cold stress. A common example is that of an elderly person living in an inadequately heated home. In such circumstances, hypothermia may not occur until days or weeks after the cold stress begins, and frostbite is not commonly involved (*5*). The risk factors in this situation are distinct from those involved in hypothermia among recreationists.

Hypothermia Involving the Elderly

The special vulnerability of elderly persons to hypothermia has been increasingly appreciated in recent years. After the first year of life, the rate of death due to effects of

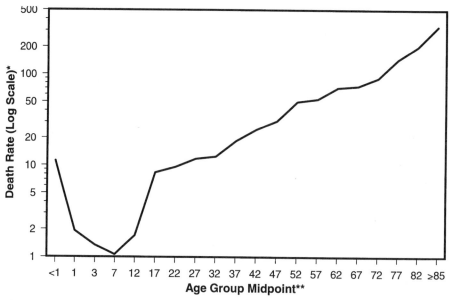

* Per 10 million population.

** 5 year age groups except for first three groups; which are <1, 1, and 2-4 years old.

Figure 13-2. Rates of death attributed to cold (ICD code: E901), by age, United States, 1979–1991.

the cold increases with advancing age (Fig. 13-2). In the United States, well over half of the (average) 770 persons who die each year because of cold exposure are 60 years of age or older, although persons in this age group represent only about 17% of the population (*1, 38*).

The extent of morbidity from hypothermia among the elderly is less easily measured. A national wintertime survey of 1,020 persons 65 years of age or older conducted in Great Britain found that few (0.58%) had hypothermic (35°C or less) morning deep-body temperatures. However, a substantial number (9%) had near-hypothermic temperatures (35.5°C or less but higher than 35°C) (*39*). In contrast, 3.6% of 467 patients more than 65 years of age admitted to London hospitals in late winter and early spring had hypothermia (*40*). The fact that hypothermia is relatively common among elderly persons admitted to hospitals—although virtually absent in the community— has been interpreted as showing that most elderly Britons with hypothermia are quickly hospitalized.

The apparent sensitivity to cold on the part of the elderly may be due to physiologic factors. Collins and others found that a high proportion of persons 65 years of age or older failed to experience physiologically significant vasoconstriction in response to a controlled cold environment and that the proportion of such persons increased with the age of the cohort examined. Elderly subjects with abnormal vasoconstriction tended to have relatively low core temperatures (41). Basal metabolic rate declines substantially with age, requiring elderly persons to battle cold stress from a relatively low level of basal thermogenesis (42), and the shivering mechanism of some older persons may be impaired (43). Voluntary muscular activity also releases heat, but the elderly are more prone than younger persons to debilitating chronic illnesses that limit mobility. Brown fat, a type of tissue whose principal purpose seems to be the generation of metabolic heat, is less abundant in elderly persons than in children and younger adults (44).

Elderly persons appear to perceive cold less well than younger persons and may voluntarily set thermostats to relatively low temperatures (45). In addition, the rising cost of energy in recent years, together with the relative poverty of some elderly people, may discourage their setting thermostats high enough to maintain adequate warmth.

Drugs Predisposing to Hypothermia

Ethanol ingestion is an important predisposing factor for hypothermia. The great majority of patients in many case series on hypothermia are middle-aged male alcoholics (46, 47). Ethanol produces vasodilatation, interfering with the peripheral vasoconstriction that is an important physiologic defense against the cold (6). Although ethanol-containing beverages are sometimes drunk in cold surroundings to obtain the subjective sense of warmth they produce, this practice is dangerous. Ethanol also predisposes persons to hypothermia indirectly by inhibiting hepatic gluconeogenesis, and it can cause healthy volunteers to develop hypoglycemia (48).

Ironically, ethanol treatment appears to improve survival from a hypothermic episode, a phenomenon that may account for the relatively low mortality observed among alcoholics with hypothermia (49). Ethanol appears to delay the harm produced by impaired circulation and respiration by decreasing cellular metabolism and, thus, the requirement for oxygen, especially in the central nervous system (50). In addition, ethanol may reduce the tendency to ventricular fibrillation associated with hypothermia (47).

Treatment with neuroleptics (e.g., phenothiazines, butyrophenones, and thioxanthenes) also predisposes to hypothermia. Chlorpromazine suppresses shivering, probably by a central mechanism, and causes vasodilatation (51, 52). The hypothermic action of drugs of this class becomes more pronounced with decreasing ambient temperature (53).

Other Risk Factors

Infants less than 1 year of age have a higher rate of death due to cold than do older children (Fig. 13-2). Neonates, especially premature or small-for-dates babies, are at particularly high risk. Although the mechanisms for maintaining thermal homeostasis (vasoconstriction and thermogenesis by shivering) are present at birth, they seem to function less effectively than in older children. Infants have a relatively large ratio of heat-losing surface to heat-generating volume, and the layer of insulating subcutaneous fat is relatively thin. Perhaps most important, babies lack the ability to control their own environment and are totally dependent on others to care for their thermal needs. If sufficient assistance is not forthcoming in a cold environment, hypothermia may result (5).

Hypothermia affecting infants can be a substantial public health problem in areas with severe winter weather. In December and January of the winters 1961–1962 and 1962–1963, 110 babies with severe hypothermia (temperature less than 90°F or 32.2°C) were admitted to hospitals in Glasgow, Scotland. Mortality in this group was 46% (54). Hypothermia affecting babies and young children can also be a winter problem in tropical climates, where it is associated with protein-calorie malnutrition (55).

Although not as high as the death rate for infants less than 1 year old, the death rate due to cold among 1-year-olds, and 2-, 3-, and 4-year-olds is still slightly elevated in comparison with children 5 to 9 years old, the age group with the lowest rate of cold-related mortality (Fig. 13-2).

After the age of 5 to 9 years, the rate of death due to cold begins a monotonic ascent with age. The rate is still relatively low in teenagers and young adults compared with the rates in middle-aged and elderly persons (Fig. 13-2). However, anyone in any age group is vulnerable to an overwhelming cold stress.

Deaths due to cold are more frequent among males than females in virtually all age groups (Table 13-2). The reasons for this difference between the sexes are not completely clear, but there are indications that differences in the occurrence of risk factors and in patterns of cold exposure play some role. A large, multicenter study of hypothermia showed that essentially equal numbers of male and female hypothermia victims were found indoors (86 and 83, respectively), but over four times as many men as women were found outdoors (208 and 47, respectively). The proportions of males and females developing hypothermia in association with illness or infection were 62% for each sex. However, some 22% of male but only 13% of female hypothermia cases involved injury (56).

Although adjustment for possible confounding factors is incomplete, these data suggest that premorbid behaviors of males (e.g., possibly spending more time outside or becoming involved in activities that lead to injury) may put them at greater risk of hypothermia. Behavioral differences seem less likely to play a role at the two extremes of the age spectrum, infancy and old age, where cases among males still predominate, although to a lesser degree (Table 13-2). The male predominance of hypothermia throughout life, even at ages where behavioral differences are probably few, suggests a biologically based vulnerability of males to the cold.

Hypothermia is common among persons with hypothyroidism. Persons with myxedema (severe hypothyroidism) may be hypothermic without having any unusual cold stress. Lack of thyroid hormone results in a low rate of metabolic heat production, leading to hypothermia (57).

Table 13-2 Rates* of Death Attributed to the Cold (underlying cause coded as E901, ICD-9) by Age Group and Sex with Age-Specific Male/Female Rate Ratios, United States, 1979–1991

Age Group	Male	Female	Rate Ratio
<1	12.93	9.32	1.39
1	2.50	1.31	1.91
2–4	1.60	1.06	1.51
5–9	1.47	0.63	2.33
10–14	2.89	0.45	6.42
15–19	14.33	2.10	6.82
20–24	16.19	2.85	5.68
25–29	18.55	4.97	3.73
30–34	21.09	3.95	5.34
35–39	31.66	5.65	5.60
40–44	41.35	8.58	4.82
45–49	51.46	10.85	4.74
50–54	85.24	17.29	4.93
55–59	94.07	16.80	5.60
60–64	123.82	25.67	4.82
65–69	126.57	31.92	3.97
70–74	147.39	49.06	3.00
75–79	237.97	86.53	2.75
80–84	306.36	146.18	2.10
85+	518.74	257.16	2.02

*Per 10 million population/year.

Risk Factors for Frostbite

Factors apparently associated with an increased risk for frostbite have been inferred from the apparently disproportionate occurrence of specific characteristics of patients in multiple case series. Frostbite cases occur predominantly among men. The proportion of males ranges from approximately 75% to 100% in several series (58–63).

Most frostbite cases are attributable to factors that diminish cerebral function, particularly alcohol ingestion and psychiatric disorders. The chief culprit is alcohol and alcoholism, accounting for 40%–80% of cases in some series (56, 57, 59–60). Alcohol may cause frank loss of consciousness in the cold, reduction in the physical capacity to seek shelter, or impaired judgment that adversely affects the decision to seek a warm environment. Psychiatric disorders are also frequent among frostbite victims with proportions of affected persons in case series ranging around 14%–22% (56, 57, 59, 60).

Persons having suffered trauma or vehicular failure under cold conditions made up 19% and 15%, respectively, of one case series (56).

None of these risk factors necessarily plays a role in the cases of workers whose jobs put them at increased risk of frostbite. Workers may be put at risk from indoor as well as outdoor cold. Indoor activities that may lead to frostbite include work in refrigerated rooms and the handling of cryogenic (cold-generating) substances, such as compressed gases.

The risk of frostbite to those working outdoors was shown to be substantial and to increase with both decreasing temperature and increasing wind speed, as would be expected from the observations on windchill by Siple and Passel (2, 58). In Ohio, a review of workers' compensation data found that 72 workers were injured during three 3-day cold snaps. Twenty-six of these workers injuries occurred during the coldest days, when the temperature fell to a record low of −27°F (−32.8°C). Most frostbite occurred outdoors when temperatures fell below 10°F (−12.2°C) and wind speeds exceeded 10 miles per hour (58).

Prevention of Illness Resulting from Cold

Because severe illness and death from hypothermia are not seen only in association with cold snaps, efforts to prevent hypothermia must be undertaken all winter long. Elderly persons are particularly vulnerable to hypothermia and form a prime target group toward which preventive efforts should be directed.

All dwellings, particularly those in which elderly persons reside, should be properly heated. Local governments can assist in this effort by adopting housing maintenance and occupancy ordinances that require each dwelling to have heating equipment that can safely maintain a reasonable room temperature under expected winter conditions (64). Maintenance of thermal standards is particularly important in nursing homes, hospitals, and other institutions that frequently house the elderly.

In the United Kingdom, there are health-based recommendations for minimum room temperatures in different rooms of the house (65). For protection of health, the World Health Organization recommends that indoor temperatures be at least 18°C (64.4°F) and that they be 2–3°C higher than the minimum (i.e., 20–21°C or 68–69.8°F) in rooms occupied by sedentary elderly persons, young children, and the handicapped (66).

Economically disadvantaged elderly persons may not make sufficient use of heating equipment because they are unable to pay the resulting fuel bills. In the United States in recent years, financial assistance has been made available by federal and certain state agencies to help needy elderly persons pay these bills. Publicity regarding the existence of such programs may enable these programs to better accomplish their purpose. Health education programs may be useful in informing elderly persons of their susceptibility to the cold.

Parents, pediatricians, and other health professionals involved in the care of babies in their first year of life should be aware that this age group is vulnerable to cold stress. Prevention of hypothermia among infants requires an adequate ambient air temperature and sufficient insulation by blankets or clothing.

Prevention of hypothermia, frostbite, and local nonfreezing cold injury among recreationists participating in winter sports also requires clothing with adequate insulating capacity. Teachers and trainers for cold-weather sports should inform their students and clients about the magnitude of the cold stress likely to be encountered and should teach them to dress accordingly. Care should be taken to keep clothing dry and to avoid immersion in cold water (67).

Workers exposed to conditions that put them at risk of hypothermia or frostbite should be educated about the type of hazard they face and told how to take steps to minimize the risk of cold-related injury. For example, the substantial proportion of frostbite cases related to vehicular failure suggests that truckers driving through cold country should be equipped with cold weather gear sufficient to maintain personal safety in the event of a mechanical breakdown.

Alcohol should not be used during periods of anticipated cold stress, and sedative drugs should be avoided to the extent possible. In particular, the time-honored practice of giving alcoholic beverages to persons suffering from cold exposure is dangerous and should be abandoned. Persons taking neuroleptic drugs (phenothiazines, butyrophenones, thioxanthenes, etc.) should be advised by their physicians of their increased susceptibility to the cold and taught to behave accordingly. The friends and family of alcoholics and persons with psychiatric disorders should check on these patients frequently during periods of particularly cold weather and attempt to discourage them from alcohol use and prolonged exposure to the cold.

Acknowledgement

Portions of this chapter have been excerpted or adapted from: Kilbourne EM. Illness due to thermal extremes. In: Last JM, Wallace RB. *Maxcy-Rosenau-Last Public Health & Preventive Medicine*, 13th ed. Norwalk, Connecticut: Appleton & Lange, 1992;491–501. Used with permission.

References

1. National Center for Health Statistics. *Mortality computer tapes for the years 1968–1985.* Hyattsville, MD: National Center for Health Statistics, 1985.
2. Siple PA, Passel CF. Measurement of dry atmospheric cooling in subfreezing temperatures. *Proc Am Philos Soc* 1945;89:177–199.
3. Steadman RG. Indices of windchill of clothed persons. *J Appl Meteorology* 1971;10:674–683.

4. Steadman RG. A universal scale of apparent temperature. *J Climate and Appl Meteorology* 1984;23:1674–1687.

5. Collins KJ. *Hypothermia: the facts*. New York: Oxford University Press, 1983.

6. MacLean D, Emslie-Smith D. *Accidental hypothermia*. Oxford: Blackwell Scientific Publications, 1977.

7. Randall PE, Heath DF, Little RA. How common is accidental hypothermia? [letter]. *Arch Emerg Med* 1985;2:174–175.

8. States SJ. Weather and death in Birmingham, Alabama. *Environ Res* 1976:12:340–354.

9. Anderson TW, Rochard C. Cold snaps, snowfall and sudden death from ischemic heart disease. *CMA Journal* 1979;121:1580–1583.

10. Rogot E. Associations between coronary mortality and the weather, Chicago, 1967. *Public Health Rep* 1974;89:330–338.

11. Bull GM, Morton J. Environment, temperature and death rates. *Age Ageing* 1978;7:210–224.

12. Kunst AE, Groenhof MA, Mackenbach JP. The association between two windchill indices and daily mortality variation in the Netherlands. *Am J Pub Health* 1994;84:1738–1742.

13. Feinlieb M. Statement of Manning Feinleib. In: *Deadly cold: health hazards due to cold weather*. Washington, DC: U.S. Government Printing Office, 1984.

14. Rosenwaike I. Seasonal variation of deaths in the United States, 1951–1960. *J Am Stat Assoc* 1966;61:706–1719.

15. Anderson TW, Rochard C. Cold snaps, snowfall, and sudden death from ischemic heart disease. *Can Med Assoc J* 1979;121:1580–1583.

16. Keatinge WR, Coleshaw SRK, Cotter F, Mattock M, Murphy M, Chelliah R. Increases in platelet and red cell counts, blood viscosity, and arterial pressure during mild surface cooling: factors in mortality from coronary and cerebral thrombosis in winter. *Br Med J* 1984;289:1405–1408.

17. Collins KJ, Easton JC, Belfield-Smith H, Exton-Smith AN, Pluck RA. Effects of age on body temperature and blood pressure in cold environments. *Clin Sci* 1985;69:465–470.

18. Schulman JL, Kilbourne ED. Experimental transmission of influenza virus in mice: II. Some factors affecting incidence of transmitted infection. *J Exp Med* 1963;118:267–275.

19. Althaus U, Aeberhard P, Schupbach P, Nachbur BH, Muhlemann W. Management of profound accidental hypothermia with cardiorespiratory arrest. *Ann Surg* 1982;195:492–495.

20. Young RSK, Zaineraitis EL, Dooling EC. Neurological outcome in cold water drowning. *JAMA* 1980;244:1233–1235.

21. Stoneham MD, Squires SJ. Prolonged resuscitation in acute deep hypothermia. *Anaesthesia* 1992;47:784–788.

22. Miller JW, Danzl DF, Thomas DM. Urban accidental hypothermia, 135 cases. *Ann Emerg Med* 1980;9:456–460.

23. Duguid H, Simpson RG, Stowers JM. Accidental hypothermia. *Lancet* 1961;2:1213–1219.

24. Ledingham IM, Mone JG. Treatment of accidental hypothermia: a prospective clinical study. *Br Med J* 1980;1:1102–1105.

25. Frank DH, Robson MC. Accidental hypothermia treated without mortality. *Surg Gynecol Obstet* 1980;151:379–381.

26. Maresca L, Vasko JS. Treatment of hypothermia by extracorporeal circulation and internal rewarming. *J Trauma* 1987;89–90.

27. Lonning PE, Skulberg A, Abyholm F. Accidental hypothermia; review of the literature. *Acta Anaesthesiol Scand* 1986;30:601–613.

28. Wisborg T, Husby P, Engedal H. Anesthesiologist-manned helicopters and regionalized extracorporeal circulation facilities: a unique chance in deep hypothermia. *Arctic Med Res* 1991;50(Suppl. 6):108–111.

29. Purdue GF, Hunt JL. Cold injury: a collective review. *J Burn Care Rehabil* 1986;7(4):331–342.

30. Mills WJ Jr. Frostbite. A discussion of the problem and a review of the Alaskan experience. 1973 [classical article]. *Alaska Med* 1993;35:29–40.

31. Mills WJ Jr. Comments on this issue of Alaska Medicine—from then (1960) until now (1993). *Alaska Med* 1993;35:70–87.

32. Mills WJ Jr, Mills WJ 3d. Peripheral non-freezing cold injury: immersion injury. *Alaska Med* 1993;35:117–128.

33. Parsons SL, Leach IH, Charnley RM. A case of bilateral trench foot. *Injury* 1993;24:680–681.

34. Wrenn K. Immersion foot. A problem of the homeless in the 1990s. *Arch Intern Med* 1991;151:785–788.

35. Goette DK. Chillblains (perniosis). *J Am Acad Dermatol* 1990;23:257–262.

36. Spittell JA Jr, Spittell PC. Chronic pernio: another cause of blue toes. *Int Angiol* 1992;11:46–50.

37. Rustin MHA, Newton JA, Smith NP, Dowd PM. The treatment of chilblains with nifedipine: the results of a pilot study, a double-blind placebo-controlled randomized study and a long-term open trial. *Br J Dermatol* 1989;120:267–275.

38. U.S. Bureau of the Census. *Computer files containing population data for years 1980 and 1990.* Washington, D.C.: U.S. Bureau of the Census, 1990.

39. Fox RH, Woodward PM, Exton-Smith AN, Green MF, Donnison DV, Wicks MH. Body temperatures in the elderly: a national study of physiological, social, and environmental conditions. *Br Med J* 1973;1:200–206.

40. Goldman A, Exton-Smith AN, Francis G, O'Brien A. A pilot study of low body temperatures in old people admitted to hospital. *J R Coll Physicians Lond* 1977;11:291–306.

41. Collins KJ, Dore C, Exton-Smith AN, Fox RH, MacDonald IC, Woodward PM. Accidental hypothermia and impaired temperature homeostasis in the elderly. *Br Med J* 1977;1:353–356.

42. Shock NW, Watkin DM, Yiengst MJ *et al.* Age differences in the water content of the body as related to basal oxygen consumption in males. *J Gerontol* 1963;18:1–8.

43. Collins KJ, Easton JC, Exton-Smith AN. Shivering thermogenesis and vasomotor responses with convective cooling in the elderly. *J Physiol* 1981;320:76.

44. Heat J. The distribution of brown adipose tissue in the human. *J Anat* 1972;112:35–39.

45. Collins KJ, Exton-Smith AN, Dore C. Urban hypothermia: preferred temperature and thermal perception in old age. *Br Med J* 1981;282:175–177.

46. Weyman AE, Greenbaum DM, Grace WJ. Accidental hypothermia in an alcoholic population. *Am J Med* 1974;56:13–21.

47. Centers for Disease Control. Exposure-related hypothermia deaths—District of Columbia, 1972–1982. *MMWR* 1982;31:669–671.

48. Haight JSJ, Keatinge WR. Failure of thermoregulation in the cold during hypoglycemia induced by exercise and ethanol. *J Physiol* 1973;229:87–97.

49. MacGregor DC, Armour JA, Goldman BS, Bigelow WG. The effects of ether, ethanol, propanol, and butanol on tolerance to deep hypothermia: experimental and clinical observations. *Dis Chest* 1966;50:523–529.

50. Miller DA, Miller J Jr. Interactions among ethanol, hypothermia, and asphyxia in guinea pigs. *Cryobiology* 1967;3:400–406.

51. Courvoisier S, Fournel J, Ducrot R, Kolsky M, Koetschet P. Proprietes pharmacodynamiques du chlorhydrate de cholor-3 (dimethylamino-3' propl)-10 phenothiazine (4.560 R.P.). *Arch Int Pharmacodyn* 1953;92:305–361.

52. Kollias J, Ballard RW. The influence of chlorpromazine on physical and chemical mechanisms of temperature regulation in the rat. *J Pharmacol Exp Ther* 1964;145:373–381.

53. Higgins EA, Iampietro PF, Adams T, Holmes DD. Effects of a tranquilizer on body temperature. *Proceedings of the Society for Experimental Biology and Medicine* 1964; 115:1017–1019.

54. Arneil GC, Kerr MM. Severe hypothermia in Glasgow infants in winter. *Lancet* 1963;2:756–759.

55. Cutting WAM, Samuel GA. Hypothermia in a tropical winter climate. *Indian J Pediatr* 1971; 8:752–757.

56. Danzl DF, Pozos RS, Auerbach PS, *et al*. Multicenter Hypothermia Survey. *Ann Emerg Med* 1987;16:1042–1055.

57. Forester CF. Coma in myxedema. *Arch Intern Med* 1963;111(6):100–109.

58. Kid SM, Chasmar LR, Clapson JB. Frostbite in the prairies: a 12-year review. *Plast Reconstr Surg* 1993;92:633–641.

59. Urschel JD. Frostbite: Predisposing factors and predictors of poor outcome. *J Trauma* 1990; 30:340–342.

60. Sinks T. Hazards of working in cold weather include frostbite, hypothermia. *Occup Health Saf* 1988;57:20–25.

61. Antti-Poika I, Pohjolainen T, Alaranta H. Severe frostbite of the upper extremities—a psychosocial problem mostly associated with alcohol abuse. *Scand J Soc Med* 1990;18:59–61.

62. Urschel JD, Urschel JW, Mackenzie WC. The role of alcohol in frostbite injury [letter]. *Scand J Soc Med* 1990;18:273.

63. Kappes BM, Mills WJ. A sample of personality profiles on frostbite patients in Alaska 1980–86. *Arctic Med Res* 1988;47(Suppl. 1):243–245.

64. U.S. Public Health Service. *APHA-CDC recommended housing maintenance and occupancy ordinance*. Atlanta, Georgia: Centers for Disease Control, 1975.

65. Lloyd E. Hypothesis: temperature recommendations for elderly people: Are we wrong? *Age Ageing* 1990;19:264–267.

66. Collins KJ. Low indoor temperatures and morbidity in the elderly. *Age Ageing* 1986;15:212–220.

67. Bullard RW, Rapp GM. Problems of body heat loss in water immersion. *Aerospace Med* 1970;41:1269–1277.

14

Floods

JOSEPHINE MALILAY

Background and Nature of Floods

Of all natural hazards, floods occur most often and are the most widespread in scope and severity (*1, 2*). Among all natural disasters in the United States, floods are the main cause of death (*3*). Floods are defined as the overflow of areas that are not normally submerged with water or a stream that has broken its normal confines or has accumulated due to lack of drainage (*4*). When water levels rise above normal stages and overflow to the extent that surrounding communities become vulnerable to rapidly moving or rising water, flood events become hazardous.

Scope and Relative Importance of Floods

Like most natural hazards, flooding can lead to loss of life and property damage, with significant impact on public health that can extend far beyond recovery. From 1980 to 1985, there were approximately 160 flood-related events worldwide, in which at least 120,000 people were killed or injured and 20,000,000 were left homeless (*2*). In terms of physical losses, floods account for 40% of property damages from all natural disasters (*1*). In the United States, direct economic losses from floods amounted to $4 billion per year before the great midwestern floods of 1993 (*5*). In the Mississippi River Valley losses from this flood event alone are expected to surpass $10 billion (*6*), and long-term effects of contaminated water wells, mental health problems, and vector-borne diseases will require continued surveillance well beyond the response period.

Factors that Contribute to Flood Problem

Adequate weather forecasts, timely warning systems for hazardous flooding, and mitigative practices such as floodplain management have helped greatly to prevent or reduce the effects of floods on the health and well-being of communities in recent years (5, 7). Despite increased levels of preparedness, however, deaths, diseases, and injuries continue to occur in affected communities.

Several possible explanations for this predicament exist. First, the topographical makeup of some areas consistently presents a hazard to residents. For instance, inhabitants of Bangladesh, an alluvial plain delta created by three rivers, are subjected annually to inundation, a condition exacerbated during the rainy season with increased upland flow of rivers and high tides in the Bay of Bengal (8). In Puerto Rico, drainage basins differ in length and degree of steepness. Where drainage basins are long but not steep, deaths occur as motorists cross submerged bridges; people who are located near short and steep drainage basins experience unexpected surges of water and subsequently drown (9).

Floods may also accompany other natural disasters, such as coastal inundations, sea surges during hurricanes, or tsunamis related to earthquakes. Landslides occurring secondary to a flood disaster may exacerbate the previously described hazardous conditions.

Factors Affecting Flood Occurrence and Severity

Natural Factors

Various mechanisms may cause flooding, and different flood characteristics affect the occurrence and severity of the flood event. These characteristics, such as hydrometeorologic properties, geologic conditions, and seasonal variation, are largely inherent in the nature of flooding itself.

For example, heavy rainfall may result in flash flooding. Flash floods exhibit two characteristics. First, they follow a causative event, such as excessive rainfall in a catchment system or sudden release of water in a natural or human-made dam, within minutes or hours and with high-velocity flows and great volumes of water. Second, with flooding commonly lasting less than 24 hours (1), they are accompanied by an extremely short warning and response time, with potential for great loss of life (10). Furthermore, specific factors affecting flash flooding consist of the intensity, amount, and duration of rainfall; general topography of the land; soil conditions; and ground cover (10, 11).

On the other hand, riverine floods, which usually result from rainfall or meltdown of snow and ice, are slow-rising. Like flash floods, riverine floods are affected by climatic factors such as intensity and amount of rainfall. The size, track, and rate of movement of a storm are additional hydrometeorological factors affecting the occurrence and severity of riverine floods. Moreover, characteristics of natural or human-made drainage basins, including size, shape, drainage density, and permeability, must also be considered (*1*).

Human-Generated Factors

Human alterations of the environment may also compromise normal drainage patterns and therefore predispose some areas to flooding. These include urbanization, agricultural practices such as overgrazing, activities such as deforestation, and the use of improper construction techniques and materials in protective structures such as flood embankments and levees.

Public Health Impacts of Flood Disasters: Historical Perspective

Mortality

Flood-related health effects have been documented in the public health literature extensively throughout the world, particularly in the People's Republic of China, Bangladesh, Brazil, Great Britain, the Netherlands, Portugal, and the United States. The results of these studies, some of which date back to flood disasters in the 1950s, describe mortality in absolute numbers as well as focus on populations displaced as a result of flooding (*12*). These studies have shown that flood-specific mortality varies by country. For example, in flood-prone Bangladesh, approximately 15,000 people are killed each year due to flood disasters (*13*). In the United States, with more than 20,000 cities and communities subject to flash flooding alone, the average annual loss of life due to floods has been estimated at between 47.6 and 146 deaths (*1, 14*). In the People's Republic of China, where more than 40 million inhabitants are estimated to be affected yearly by floods (*13*), approximately 1,000 people perished in the summer floods of 1994 (*15*). Continuing differential levels of mortality associated with individual flood events in various areas of the world warrant investigation of the factors that contribute to flood-related deaths, illnesses, and injuries.

As mentioned above, mortality from most floods is caused by flash flooding and the circumstances that surround the flash-flood event (*2*). In a study of flash-flood-related deaths in the United States from 1969 to 1981, 1,185 deaths were attributed to 32 flash floods, with an average of 37 deaths occurring per flash flood (*16*). In these floods, due primarily from dam ruptures associated with heavy rains (*16*), drowning caused an estimated 93% of these deaths. In general, mortality due to drowning is frequently observed in flash-flood incidents, examples of which occurred in Nmes, France, in 1988,

Puerto Rico in 1992, Missouri in 1993, and Georgia in 1994, when heavy water runoff inundated communities with great immediacy and intensity (*9, 17–19*).

Finally, increased levels of physical and emotional stress, particularly related to increased exertion in evacuating a flooded area and in cleanup activities, are evident after almost all natural disasters. Many flood-related deaths have been attributed to such stress and overexertion, which increase the likelihood for myocardial infarction and even cardiac arrest among people with preexisting heart conditions (*17*).

Morbidity

Infectious Diseases

Concern by the public and health authorities about potential outbreaks of communicable diseases normally arises after natural disasters. It has been believed that disruption of water-purification and sewage-disposal systems puts the community at risk of greater susceptibility to infections from contaminated food and water (*20–22*). Studies have shown, however, that such outbreaks rarely occur and that mass immunization programs for typhoid fever and cholera, commonly anticipated in the past, are unnecessary (*23–26*).

Nevertheless, the potential for transmission of water-borne disease (e.g., enterotoxigenic *Escherichia coli*, *Shigella*, hepatitis A, leptospirosis, giardiasis) and for increased levels of endemic illnesses in flood-affected areas is possible (*27*).

Surveillance of water- and vector-borne diseases, endemic illnesses, and cleanup injuries has been recommended and implemented during response and recovery periods in flood-affected communities (*27–30*). Although no significant increases were noted in communicable diseases after several flood events worldwide (*19, 20*), isolated instances of increases in endemic disease have been noted in some cases. After flooding during a spring thaw in 1983, an outbreak of diarrheal disease related to giardiasis was detected in Utah (*27*). After the heavy and extensive flooding in Sudan in 1988, endemic levels of acute hepatitis E infection and chloroquine-resistant malaria rose and were expected to increase with time (*31–34*). Finally, epidemiologists attributed most deaths and illnesses in Bangladesh in 1988 to nonspecific diarrheal disease after extensive flooding (*35*).

Surveillance of arboviral diseases, such as St. Louis encephalitis and western equine encephalitis, was a topic of increasing concerning after floods in the midwestern and southern United States in 1993 and 1994, respectively (*30*). Standing water from heavy rains produced habitats for the proliferation of mosquito populations that could have rapidly transmitted arboviruses. In these cases, surveillance indicated that the risk for transmission was minimal and thus averted costly large-scale plans for mosquito-control measures.

Chronic Health Effects
Chronic health effects secondary to a flood disaster have been documented in the literature. After flooding of a river valley in western New York in 1972, a cluster of deaths attributed to leukemia and lymphoma and a cluster of abnormal reproductive outcomes were thought to be associated with high natural background radiation in indigenous surface rock deposits, radiation from a nearby nuclear processing plant, and suspected radiation from a new town water well. Although radiation samples were within limits set by federal guidelines, the study suggested that the flood may have been a possible etiologic event for leukemia and lymphoma deaths (*36*).

Injuries
In the aftermath of a flood disaster, injuries are likely to occur as residents return to dwellings to clean up damage and debris. Electrocutions have occurred from downed power lines, electrical wiring, and improper handling of wet appliances. Injuries from fire and explosions from gas leaks also occur when lit matches are used to inspect darkened structures for damage. Although minor in nature, lacerations and punctures are common sequelae because postflood debris often consists of broken glass and nails (*37*).

The natural habitat of many types of wild animals may be altered by floodwaters. As a result, animals such as snakes may be forced to seek refuge from rising floodwaters in areas that may be inhabited or used by humans. Animal bites are possible, although past public health surveillance after floods has not indicated that animal bites have been a major problem (*28, 29, 38*).

Health Effects of Toxic Substances
In a flood, the potential for exposure to hazardous chemical and biological agents exists. Underground pipelines may rupture, storage tanks may be dislodged, toxic-waste sites may overflow, and chemicals stored at ground level may be released (*35*). The hazards are further exacerbated when industrial and agricultural areas are submerged under floodwater. Although one study showed that toxic substances caused no adverse health effects in one instance of flash flooding in France (*35*), another study showed that toxic substances presented a major health concern after extensive flash flooding and riverine flooding flushed unusually high levels of industrial and agricultural chemicals into the Mississippi River, its tributaries, and the Gulf of Mexico in 1993. Although no emergent health effects were immediately noted, the long-term effects have yet to be fully evaluated (*39*).

Mental Health Effects of Flood Disasters
An extensive amount of psychosocial literature is devoted to the mental health of flood victims (*40–43*). Longitudinal studies have focused on the psychological consequences of flooding on individuals and communities. Studies show that severe psychological

distress is rare (*42, 43*), although mild transient emotional problems are common (*41*). Results of one study that controlled for predisaster emotional symptoms showed that floods precipitated significant psychological reactions to stress and strain (*43*). Subgroups such as the elderly and the very young are probably at greater risk for psychological reactions, for a number of reasons. Psychosocial factors are further discussed in Chapter 6, "Mental Health Consequences of Disasters."

Other Potential Health Concerns

Dislodged coffins in flooded cemeteries have also led to concern for public safety and for the emotional distress of relatives of the deceased whose remains were exposed by floodwaters.

Contaminated well water after extensive flooding has raised concerns regarding the safety of drinking water from privately owned wells. For example, after the midwestern U.S. floods of 1993, regional studies in nine flood-affected states were conducted by state and federal authorities to determine the prevalence of wells contaminated with atrazine, coliforms, and nitrates.

A potential problem arising from the 1993 floods in the midwestern United States concerned adverse health effects from molds and mildew. Studies are currently under way to determine whether these have had any detrimental respiratory health impacts.

Factors Influencing Flood Mortality and Morbidity

In recent years, results of epidemiologic studies have extended knowledge regarding risk factors for flood-related mortality and morbidity. These results have led to the development of strategies for reducing or preventing deaths, illnesses, or injuries in populations at risk.

Natural Factors

Characteristics of stream-flow velocity and the terrain of an area can predispose residents and passersby to risks for death and injury. The timing of deaths during a flood disaster in Puerto Rico in early 1992 indicated that most of the deaths occurred during a particularly violent surge of water that followed an initial premonitory smaller wave consisting of leaves and other debris (*9*). Moreover, topographical features of land in a flooded area can present significant hazards to motorists and passersby. For example, in Puerto Rico, drainage basins differ in length and degree of steepness. Where drainage basins are long but not steep, deaths have occurred as motorists crossed submerged bridges; likewise, deaths also took place near shorter, steeper drainage basins when unexpectedly violent waves of water surged through the area (*9*).

Landslides may occur secondary to a flood disaster and exacerbate hazardous conditions. After widespread flooding caused by a tropical storm in Puerto Rico in 1988, nearly half of the deaths were attributed to traumatic asphyxia from landslides (20).

Human-Generated Factors

Human settlement frequently occurs in flood-prone areas, thereby increasing a community's vulnerability to the effects of flooding. Although flood-control measures have been instituted through floodplain management in some areas of the world, lush river valleys and attractive coastal areas continue to attract large numbers of settlers for obvious economic and social reasons.

Lack of awareness of the dangers posed by fast-moving floodwaters has led to inappropriate behaviors by people encountering floodwaters. For instance, recreational activities such as wading, bicycling, or driving into floodwaters led to several deaths during the midwestern floods in the United States (17). Motorists in particular are at high risk for death when driving into swiftly moving water or when traffic is diverted by floodwater (9, 10, 17, 18, 37). In fact, of all flood-related deaths due to drowning, most occur among occupants of motor vehicles (9, 17, 18). These deaths may be attributed in part to a misconception that motor vehicles provide adequate protection from rising or swiftly moving waters. When people drive through water, their vehicles become more buoyant because the momentum of the water is transferred to the vehicle. For example, for each foot that water rises up the side of a car, an estimated 1,500 pounds of force are applied to the vehicle due to the displaced water. Thus, as little as 2 feet of water is capable of sweeping away most vehicles (11).

The use of alcohol and other intoxicants impairs judgment and thus increases risks for both flood-related mortality and morbidity. In the Puerto Rico flooding that occurred during a holiday evening in 1992, 12 of 16 (75%) adults who died and who had blood alcohol levels measured had concentrations greater than 0.01 percent. Of these people, 5 had blood alcohol levels that exceeded 0.1 percent (9).

Paradoxically, engineering flood controls may actually contribute to greater human losses and physical damages after a flood disaster (e.g., levee failure). In most strategic flood-mitigation programs, the overall planning of flood controls, including the design and construction of structures, is intended to reduce the effects of impending flooding. These controls include overtopping of embankments, protecting embankments from erosion, improving drainage systems, and promulgating dam safety regulations (44). During the Georgia floods in July 1994, half of the deaths that occurred in Sumter County were attributed by local authorities to the rupture of earthen dams whose unleashed waters then inundated surrounding creeks, causing widespread flooding (18).

Prevention and Control Measures

The severity of flood disasters is largely affected by the timing of phases in which a flood event takes place. Known as the disaster cycle, the temporal phases that make up a disaster event involve mitigation measures, warning and preparedness activities, response, and recovery, as outlined by Western and modified by Cuny (*45, 46*). Before, during, and after a flood event, activities may be undertaken by the population at risk and emergency responders at each phase to prevent or reduce the risk for injury, illness, or death.

Mitigation

Mitigation is defined as the reduction of the harmful effects of a disaster by limiting the disaster's impact on human health and economic infrastructure. In the past, mitigation measures have been used in the traditional fields of engineering and urban planning; currently, these measures refer to structural or policy-oriented modifications that can be made independent of a disaster event. Flood-related mitigative activities reduce deaths and injuries by ensuring structural safety through enforcing adequate building codes, promulgating legislation to relocate structures away from flood-prone areas, planning appropriate land use, and managing coasts and floodplains. Some mitigative actions involving engineering and administrative strategies are used to ensure public safety when flooding is imminent. Adequately designed and constructed flood-control structures such as levees and floodwalls offer protection; however, as the flooding in the American Midwest during the summer of 1993 showed, these fail from time to time. In an effort to promote population movement away from flood-prone areas, some flood-control policies call for initiating government buyout of homes and converting such areas along rivers to wetlands. Despite these attempts, however, human settlement in these areas continues to grow.

Warning and Preparedness

Early detection, warning, and appropriate citizen response to these warnings have proven to be effective in reducing disaster-related deaths. In the United States, weather forecasts and warnings of hazardous weather have enhanced public safety during flood events in recent years (*5*). Likewise, many countries have also implemented severe-weather watch and warning programs that allow local officials to take appropriate emergency management actions such as evacuation and sheltering.

In general, these systems consist of two components, both of which are based on the expected duration of the flood and the size of an affected area. Predicated on the use of large-scale weather patterns, *watches* are issued when meteorological conditions indicate that severe weather may affect a given area (*47*). When meteorologists determine that conditions create threats to human life and property, watches are upgraded to *warnings* (*47*). A crucial factor is the timing with which watches and warnings are issued to the public. During flash flooding in Puerto Rico in 1992, 20 of 23 deaths occurred before watches or warnings had been broadcast for specific municipalities (*9*).

Moreover, broadcasts should be issued with consideration to the timely receipt of warnings by the public. The Puerto Rico flash floods took place on Three Kings' Eve, an island-wide holiday when most residents were not home and probably did not have access to the broadcast media (9).

As discussed earlier, appropriate behavioral actions are critical in preventing deaths, injuries, and illnesses. Therefore, the design of effective messages to prompt desired behavioral outcomes is important. Special subgroups in the population may be at particular risk for the effects of flood events. These include the elderly, immigrants who do not speak the language of their new home, physically disabled people, and residents in remote areas for whom taking lifesaving actions may require special warnings or more lead time than usual before a flood to allow for safe evacuation.

Advances in science and technology (such as improved radar, satellite, and information-processing systems), sirens, and the use of dedicated weather channels by the public have increased lead time for watches and warnings for flood disasters. The effectiveness of detection and warning systems may now be evaluated, and recommendations for appropriate standards for such systems in assuring greater warning sensitivity and timeliness can be made (47).

Needs Assessment

After the impact of floods, rapid needs assessments should be conducted in order to determine the health and medical needs of a flood-affected community. These activities are especially important after sudden-impact flooding, during which the types, quantities, and delivery of services to meet needs vary daily during the emergency-relief period. A needs assessment typically consists of administering a standardized questionnaire that addresses the status of health, medical and pharmaceutical needs, the status of public health services, and the condition of utilities such as water supplies, sewage systems, and electricity. Individuals or households may be selected randomly to provide an overview of needs in their communities. Similarly, county health departments may be surveyed to determine the impact of the floods and requirements of local public health authorities (28, 48). Several surveys may be performed over the course of the emergency period (usually 1 week) to assess changes in the nature of the emergency.

Surveillance

A major postflood activity is public health surveillance of mortality and morbidity associated with the specific disaster. Mortality surveillance is performed to determine the nature and circumstances surrounding deaths caused by the flood so that appropriate preventive actions can be taken to reduce or prevent further mortality. Morbidity surveillance is conducted to determine (1) any increases in diseases that are endemic to the area, (2) any cases of infectious disease (waterborne or otherwise) that must be contained and controlled, and (3) any cases of injuries that may require public advisories or control of animal or insect populations. Flood-specific surveillance systems should also determine any increases in vector populations, such as mosquitoes, and laboratory-based surveillance of drinking-water sources, such as public and private wells.

A definition of flood-related deaths, illnesses, and injuries should be established before implementing the surveillance system. Local health authorities should also determine the length of time that the surveillance system will operate, usually for 1 month from the response through the recovery periods. During riverine flooding, however, this period may need to be lengthened, particularly when heavy rains and flash flooding persist throughout the rainy season. A comprehensive flood surveillance system should include reporting from different types of health and medical service providers (e.g., physicians, community health workers) and locations of these services (e.g., hospitals, private physicians' offices, field shelters). Moreover, decisions to include different sources of reporting in the surveillance system should be made early on, and every effort should be attempted to encourage or require outside organizations providing medical care (nongovernmental organizations, volunteers) to submit disease information to the local health department. Outcome status (e.g., treated or released, hospitalized, discharged, deceased) is important to include in programs that monitor diseases and injuries, particularly if follow-up epidemiologic studies are planned.

Results from the flood surveillance system should be compiled, analyzed, and disseminated to appropriate decision-makers periodically, usually on a weekly basis.

Further details of general disaster surveillance are presented in Chapter 3, "Surveillance and Epidemiology."

Response and Recovery

Several specific issues are germane to public health and safety in the aftermath of a flood event (*49*). These issues include (1) water quality; (2) food safety; (3) sanitation and hygiene; (4) precautions during cleanup activities upon returning to a flooded structure; (5) potential immunizations as determined by local health officials (e.g., administering tetanus vaccine to those with lacerations if indicated by the injured person's tetanus immunization history); (6) protective measures against potential disease vectors, such as mosquitoes, rodents, and other wild animals; (7) chemical hazards; and (8) mental health well-being measures such as stress reduction and counseling for both victims and responders. Taking personal protective and preventive measures during this period can significantly decrease the adverse public health consequences of a flood disaster.

When flooding occurs, local health departments will need to focus on obtaining information about emergency requirements, delivering services or supplies to communities in need, and controlling adverse health effects from the disaster. Local health authorities can also work with counterparts in public works and utilities to implement recommendations from past epidemiologic studies on hydrological disasters (e.g., controlling access to areas where many motor vehicle fatalities have commonly occurred during flash flooding). Recommendations from the investigation of circumstances of deaths after the Missouri floods of 1994 include identifying flooded roads to be blocked off from vehicular access, assuring the posting of warning signs at potential high-risk flooding locations, and issuing and reinforcing public media warnings (*37*).

Continuing Health Education to Public

Recommendations about sanitation and hygiene are determined by local health departments and cooperative extension units and vary from state to state. In general, encouraging the public to maintain proper sanitation and hygiene is paramount after hydrological disasters, and regular reinforcement of warning messages may be necessary. Details of prevention guidelines for individuals and households are found in the CDC pamphlet *Beyond the flood: a prevention guide for personal health and safety* (*49*).

Critical Knowledge Gaps

Although the risks for drowning while operating motor vehicles during flooding have been well elucidated, other important gaps in the present epidemiologic knowledge base have yet to be well studied. The following is a list of critical knowledge gaps related to the public health effects of floods:

- association between mortality and general topographic land features of surrounding areas where deaths have occurred
- association between mortality and type of mitigative measures taken (e.g., catchment systems or drainage basins, flood walls, and earthen dams)
- lack of knowledge about the relationship between risk factors in epidemiologic studies and risk factors from classic risk analysis (e.g., determination of predictors of deaths from dam bursts and flash floods) (*50*)
- adverse health effects from toxic biologic and chemical exposures due to flooding
- health outcomes associated with flooded blowholes, or huge underground caverns resulting from mining excavations
- the role of the health sector in overall intersectoral disaster preparedness and response (*51*)

Methodologic Problems of Epidemiologic Studies of Floods

In past flood-related studies the following methodologic problems have been identified:

- In case ascertainment of flood-related conditions, the criteria for determining whether a death, illness, or injury is flood-related have yet to be fully evaluated and standardized. Thus, when comparing various databases or studies on mortality and morbidity arising from a flood event, it is important to note the case definitions that were used in each investigation.

- Misclassification of disease, injury, or death related to a disaster event may happen when multiple types of disasters occur at the same time. Flooding, in particular, may result from the heavy rains that frequently accompany even minor hurricanes. A serious flood may cause mudslides that may actually be more hazardous than the flooding itself.

- The period following a flood disaster in which to count deaths, illnesses, and injuries in surveillance systems has yet to be established. In the past, determining the duration of surveillance (usually 1 month after the flood event) has been left to local authorities. Restricting surveillance activities to just 1 month may be inappropriate in flood disasters, since with continuing heavy rains, episodic flash flooding can occur repeatedly over the course of several weeks.

Research Recommendations

- Surveillance of flood-related morbidity, mortality, vector populations, and environmental health should continue throughout the response and recovery periods. Should any unusual conditions be noted, specialized investigations or surveys should be done so that appropriate interventions can be made.

- Based on the type(s) of data sources (e.g., hospitals, private physicians' offices, field clinics, etc.) for each system, systematic studies of the sensitivity, quality, and utility of information collected by various surveillance systems should be undertaken.

- Research should be conducted on the effectiveness of local watch and warning systems in eliciting evacuation. Both active and passive warning systems should be investigated.

- Studies should be conducted to further identify hydrologic and geologic risk factors for mortality, such as stream-flow velocity and topography of surrounding area.

- Investigations should be undertaken to examine the impact of mitigative structures and practices (e.g., flood walls, earthen dams, floodplain use) in increasing or decreasing mortality.

- Investigations should be conducted on the health effects of any toxic releases into floodwaters, particularly where industrial and agricultural chemicals are normally stored and transported.

- Systematic studies should be conducted to investigate any adverse health consequences due to community flood-preparedness activities (e.g., shoring embankments, building levees, etc.).

- Research should be undertaken to determine any adverse health outcomes associated with biological, chemical, and physical exposures during the recovery period.

Summary

Floods are the most frequently occurring of all types of natural disasters, accounting for an estimated 40% of damages. In the United States, they represent the leading cause of death from natural disasters.

Flood hazards are both natural and human-generated. Natural factors include topography and the natural makeup of catchment areas or drainage basins surrounding rivers and other waterways. Human-generated hazards include inadequate design and construction of flood-retention walls, nonsensitive flood watch and warning systems, inappropriate behaviors by people when they encounter floodwater, and increased human settlement in flood-prone regions such as coastal zones.

Public health issues specific for flood disasters include water quality, food safety, sanitation and hygiene, precautions during cleanup activities, potential immunizations as determined locally, protective measures against disease vectors, potential release of toxic substances, and adverse mental health consequences.

Effective flood watch and warning systems, especially for flash flooding, are absolutely critical for public safety. The timeliness, dissemination (through proper news media available to most people at a particular hour), and presentation of flood warnings in a manner that can be understood by most people in a given geographical area or culture are important factors that can reduce mortality and morbidity.

In response to health needs that are likely to arise, epidemiologic assessments to determine the need for certain health and medical services; continued public health surveillance; and monitoring of mortality, morbidity, vector populations, and water and sewage systems are recommended throughout the recovery period.

References

1. Alexander D. *Natural disasters*. New York: Chapman & Hall, Inc., 1993.
2. World Meteorological Organization. *The role of the World Meteorological Organization in the International Decade for Natural Disaster Reduction*. Report no. WMO-745. Geneva: World Meteorological Organization, 1990.
3. Frazier K. *The violent face of nature—severe phenomena and natural disasters*. New York: William Morrow & Company Inc., 1979.
4. Gunn SWA. *Multilingual dictionary of disaster medicine and international relief*. Dordrecht, the Netherlands: Kluwer Academic Publishers, 1990.
5. National Research Council. *The US national report. Facing the challenge*. Washington, D.C.: National Academy Press, 1994.
6. Parrett C, Melcher NB, James RW Jr. *Flood discharges in the upper Mississippi River Basin*. US Geological Survey Circular 1120-A. Denver (CO): U.S. Government Printing Office, 1993.
7. Organization of American States. *Primer on natural hazard management in integrated regional development planning*. Washington, D.C.: Organization of American States, 1991.
8. Seaman J. *Epidemiology of natural disasters*. Basel: S. Karger, 1984.

9. Staes C, Orengo JC, Malilay J, Noji E, Rullán J. Deaths due to flash floods in Puerto Rico, January 1992: implications for prevention. *Int J Epidemiol* 1994;23:968–975.

10. Gruntfest E, Huber CJ. Toward a comprehensive national assessment of flash flooding in the United States. *Episodes* 1991;14(1):26–35.

11. National Weather Service/American Red Cross/Federal Emergency Management Agency. *Flashfloods and floods . . . the awesome power!: a preparedness guide.* Report no. NOAA/ PA 92050, ARC 4493. Washington, D.C.: U.S. Department of Commerce, National Oceanic and Atmospheric Administration, National Weather Service, 1992.

12. French JG. Floods. In: Gregg MB, editor. *The public health consequences of disasters.* Atlanta: Centers for Disease Control, 1989:39–49.

13. International Federation of Red Cross and Red Crescent Societies. *World Disasters Report 1993.* Norwell, MA: Kluwer Academic Publishers, 1993.

14. National Weather Service (NWS). *Summary of natural hazard deaths for 1991 in the United States.* Rockville, MD: National Weather Service, 1992.

15. United Nations Disaster Assessment and Coordination Team. *Floods in southern China, 27 June to 11 July, 1994. Report.* Beijing, People's Republic of China: United Nations Disaster Assessment and Coordination Team, 1994.

16. French J, Ing R, Von Allmen S, Wood R. Mortality from flash floods: a review of the National Weather Service Reports, 1969–81. *Public Health Rep* 1983;98(6):584–588.

17. Centers for Disease Control and Prevention. Flood-related mortality—Missouri, 1993. *MMWR* 1993;42:941–943.

18. Centers for Disease Control and Prevention. Flood-related mortality—Georgia, July 1994. *MMWR* 1994;43:526–529.

19. Duclos P, Vidonne O, Beuf P, Perray P, Stoebner A. Flash flood Disaster—Nîmes, France, 1988. *Eur J Epidemiol* 1991;7(4):365–371.

20. Dietz VJ, Rigau-Perez JG, Sanderson LM, Diaz L, Gunn RA. Health assessment of the 1985 flood disaster in Puerto Rico. *Disasters* 1990;14(2):164–170.

21. Aghababian RV, Teuscher J. Infectious disease following major disasters. *Ann Emerg Med* 1992;21(4):362–367.

22. Toole MJ. Communicable disease epidemiology following disasters. *Ann Emerg Med* 1992; 21(4):418–420.

23. Western KA. *Epidemiologic surveillance after natural disaster.* Scientific Publication No. 420. Washington, D.C.: Pan American Health Organization, 1982.

24. Dai Z. No epidemics despite devastating floods. *Chin Med J* 1992;105(7):531–534.

25. Blake PA. Communicable Disease Control. In: Gregg MB, editor. *The public health consequences of disasters.* Atlanta: Centers for Disease Control, 1989:7–12.

26. Centers for Disease Control and Prevention. Current trends flood disasters and immunization— California. *MMWR* 1983;32:171–172,178.

27. Centers for Disease Control and Prevention. Outbreak of diarrheal illness associated with a natural disaster—Utah. *MMWR* 1983;32:662–664.

28. Centers for Disease Control and Prevention. Public health consequences of a flood disaster— Iowa, 1993. *MMWR* 1993;42:653–655.

29. Centers for Disease Control and Prevention. Morbidity surveillance following the Midwest flood—Missouri, 1993. *MMWR* 1993;42:797–798.

30. Centers for Disease Control and Prevention. Rapid assessment of vectorborne diseases during the Midwest flood, United States, 1993. *MMWR* 1994;43:481–483.

31. McCarthy MC, He J, Hyams KC, El-Tigani A, Khalid IO, Carl M. Acute hepatitis E infection during the 1988 floods in Khartoum, Sudan. *Transactions of the Royal Society of Tropical Medicine and Hygiene* 1994;88:177.

32. Homeida M, Ismail AA, El Tom I, Mahmoud B, Ali HM. Resistant malaria and the Sudan floods [letter]. *Lancet* 1988;2:912.

33. Novelli V, El Tohami TA, Osundwa VM, Ashong F. Floods and resistant malaria [letter]. *Lancet* 1988;2:1367.

34. Barclay AJG, Coulter JBS. Floods and resistant malaria [letter]. *Lancet* 1988;2:1367.

35. Siddique AK, Baqui AH, Eusof A, Zaman K. 1988 floods in Bangladesh: pattern of illness and causes of death. *J Diarrhoeal Dis Res* 1991;9(4):310–314.

36. Janerich DT, Stark AD, Greenwald P, Burnett WS, Jacobson HI, McCusker J. Increased leukemia, lymphoma, and spontaneous abortion in western New York following a flood disaster. *Public Health Rep* 1981;96(4):350–356.

37. Missouri Department of Health. *Flood mortality statistics, summer/fall 1993.* Jefferson City, MO: Missouri Department of Health, 1993.

38. American Red Cross/Federal Emergency Management Agency. *Repairing your flooded home.* Report no. ARC 4477/FEMA 234. Washington (DC): Federal Emergency Management Agency, 1992.

39. Goolsby DA, Battaglin WA, Thurman EM. *Occurrence and transport of agricultural chemicals in the Mississippi River Basin, July through August 1993.* United States Geological Survey Circular 1120-C. Denver, CO: U.S. Government Printing Office, 1993.

40. Kinston W and Rosser R. Disaster: effect on mental and physical state. *J Psychosomat Res* 1974;18:436–456.

41. Logue JN, Hansen H, Struening E. Emotional and physical distress following Hurricane Agnes in Wyoming Valley of Pennsylvania. *Public Health Rep* 1979;94(6):495–502.

42. Norris FH, Murrell SA. Prior experience as a moderator of disaster impact on anxiety symptoms in older adults. *Am J Community Psychol* 1988;16(5):665–683.

43. Phifer JF, Norris FH. Psychological symptoms in older adults following natural disaster: nature, timing, duration, and course. *J Gerontol* 1989;44(6):S207–217.

44. Watanabe M. Problems in flood disaster prevention. In: Starosolszky O and Melder OM, editors. *Hydrology of disasters. Proceedings of the World Meteorological Organization Technical Conference in Geneva, November 1988.* London: James & James, 1989:84–105.

45. Western K. *The epidemiology of natural and man-made disasters: the present state of the art* [dissertation]. London: Univ. of London, 1972.

46. Cuny FC. Introduction to disaster management, lesson 2—concepts and terms in disaster management. *Prehospital and Disaster Medicine* 1993;8(1):89–94.

47. Belville JD. The national weather service warning system. *Ann Emerg Med* 1987; 16(9):1078–1080.

48. Pan American Health Organization. *Assessing needs in the health sector after floods and hurricanes.* Technical paper no. 11. Washington, D.C.: Pan American Health Organization, 1987.

49. Centers for Disease Control and Prevention. *Beyond the flood. A prevention guide for personal health and safety.* Atlanta: Centers for Disease Control and Prevention, 1994.

50. DeKay ML, McClelland GH. Predicting loss of life in cases of dam failure and flash flood. *Risk Anal* 1993;13(2):193–205.

51. Shao XH. The role of health sectors in disaster preparedness: floods in southeastern China, 1991. *Prehospital and Disaster Medicine* 1993;8(2):173–175.

IV

HUMAN-GENERATED
PROBLEMS

15

Famine

RAY YIP

Background and Nature of Famines

Famine represents the most severe form of food insecurity, during which mass starvation and death take place within a relatively short span of time. Hence famine is often viewed as an acute and discrete event (*1*). There is compelling evidence, however, that a long-term process is responsible for the development of the underlying socioeconomic vulnerability that is required for famine to occur (*2*). In fact, famine represents failure to recognize or respond to increasing food insecurity over time. In times of famine, public health workers traditionally have participated in reactive relief efforts to control morbidity and mortality; potentially greater roles are available for public health workers in proactive efforts to prevent and mitigate famine (*3*). Although many of the underlying factors leading to increasing vulnerability are related to fundamental issues such as political stability and developmental policy—issues that may seem outside the reach of public health—it would be helpful, at least in the process of assessing vulnerability to famine, for public health workers to take some of the fundamental factors into consideration.

If famine is indeed the end result of a long-term process of increasing vulnerability, identifying opportunities for earlier intervention would be the best prevention strategy to consider. The focus of this chapter will not be on relief efforts or field management procedures during famine. Rather, this chapter will examine the underlying factors contributing to and the process leading to famine and will propose a broader role for public health workers in preventing and mitigating famine. Because there are wide

Table 15-1 Definitions of Major Terms Relevant to Famine

Food Security: Access by all people at all times to enough food for an active, healthy life. There are three dimensions in assessing food security—availability, accessibility, and adequacy.

Food Insecurity: Lack of access to enough food. There are two kinds of food insecurity: chronic and transitory.

Chronic food insecurity is a continuously inadequate diet caused by the inability to acquire food. It affects households that persistently lack the ability to buy enough food or to produce their own.

Transitory food insecurity is a temporary decline in a household's access to enough food. It is often the result of instability in food prices, food production, or household incomes.

Hunger: Recurrent and involuntary lack of access to food. Hunger may produce malnutrition over time.

Starvation: Severe deprivation of food where energy intake cannot sustain the basic need for long-term survival.

Malnutrition: Objective physical or laboratory findings of physical deterioration as a result of inadequate nutrient intake. *Primary malnutrition* is related to inadequate intake of nutrients including calories, or the result of starvation. *Secondary malnutrition* is related to disease processes leading to the inability either to consume or to utilize adequate nutrients for metabolic needs.

Famine: The most extreme form of food insecurity and often the result of transitory or acute deterioration of access to food. Increased malnutrition and mortality are the usual consequence of mass starvation during famine.

variations in some of the terms related to food insecurity, Table 15-1 lists definitions that are commonly used when discussing famine and food insecurity (*4, 5*).

Scope and Relative Importance of Famine

By nature, the dramatic images of mass starvation and mortality often associated with famine create the impression that it is a sudden disastrous event. This level of suffering commands media attention and, therefore, international relief efforts. In reality, famine contributes to only a small part of the overall suffering and mortality related to food insecurity. In many developing countries, large segments of the population suffer from milder forms of chronic food insecurity, with resulting malnutrition and mortality making up the bulk of human suffering related to food insecurity (*6*). Areas with long-term or recurrent food insecurity are most prone to famine when conditions worsen. In the past four decades there have been declining trends in the incidence and magnitude of famine. This decline has resulted from improving economic status, food security, and capacity to cope in famine-prone regions (*6*). Although the general trend is encouraging, famine related to armed conflict and political instability is still a common occurrence.

Factors that Contribute to Famine

Famine can be regarded as a form of disaster secondary to other disastrous events, such as drought and war, which often also result in another form of disaster: mass population displacements and refugee situations. To a large extent, these disaster events are closely linked. For example, mass population migration and concentration due to famine also create an environment of crowding and poor sanitation, leading to an increased prevalence of disease that further contributes to morbidity and mortality. The fundamental factors affecting the risk for famine are the stability of social, political, and economic conditions that are the determinants of food insecurity and that define the capacity to cope when the population is vulnerable, such as during a drought. Immediate risk factors of famine, such as drought or war, are closely linked to these fundamental factors; more vulnerable populations are less able to cope with a setback and are, therefore, more famine prone. Political instability in itself often results in armed conflict or civil strife, which can cause famine directly. In general, most incidences of famine can be attributed to either failure of food production or lack of food access due to conflict. Specific examples will be examined in this chapter.

Factors Affecting Famine Occurrence and Severity

Natural Factors

Natural disasters such as severe drought or flood resulting in widespread crop failure and food shortage are perhaps the best-known causes of famine. Other well-known natural factors are cyclones and destruction of crops by locust or plant disease. By far, severe and recurrent drought has been the most frequently observed immediate cause of famine affecting Africa. In recent years, Bangladesh has suffered several flood- and cyclone-related famines. The famous Irish potato famine in 1862 was the result of a viral disease called potato pilage. Over time, as the global capacity of food production and distribution has increased, famine due mainly to natural factors or agriculture failure has become less frequent (6). In recent times, famine due solely to natural disasters may have become the exception rather than the rule. It appears that a lack of capacity or willingness on the part of governments to manage food shortages competently is an essential ingredient for the occurrence of famine triggered by natural events. For this reason, there is also a strong man-made component of famine that results from natural disaster.

There are well-documented cases in which major food shortages, when properly managed, did not result in famine. Major famine was averted in India (1967), in Kenya (1984–1985), and in Botswana (1982–1987) (7, 8). The most recent example in which famine was averted was the severe drought in southern Africa in 1992, a drought that affected virtually all countries in the region. Crop-failure rates approached 80% in some of the most severely affected areas (9). Because of regional cooperation and external assistance in the form of grain shipments and distribution, however, famine was averted, even though there were significant economic consequences due to the crop failure and the purchase of some of the grain (*10*). In essence, famine related to natural disasters can be and often is mitigated, even when the level of food shortage is severe and the area affected is wide. When famine is attributed to a natural factor, it is more likely true that the natural event is simply the triggering event among many contributing factors, rather than the main cause of famine.

Human-Generated Factors

On the basis of an analysis of major famines that have occurred during this century, it appears that lack of access to food by the entire population or a segment of the population is a predominant factor leading to famine. The access problem—described by economists as failure of "entitlement"—can be regarded to a large extent as a human-generated problem (*11*). There are two aspects related to human-generated factors. One is that underlying factors lead to poverty and food insecurity, placing certain communities at an elevated risk for famine (*2*). The other aspect is that the sociopolitical situation often either directly creates famine or disables the capacity to cope with increasing food insecurity (*6*).

In the first case, underlying poverty creates certain areas that are chronically food insecure and constantly threatened with recurrent famine. The African Shale countries (Burkina, Chad, Mali, Mauritania, and Niger) are often cited as an example where the balance of population growth and food production is marginal even during good years and becomes disastrous when the region is faced with a natural calamity (*12*). A detailed review of factors related to economic or developmental policy leading to elevated vulnerability to food insecurity is beyond the scope of this chapter; in essence, however, poverty or underdevelopment is a major factor for chronic food insecurity and greater vulnerability to famine.

That human-generated factors often create barriers to food access is perhaps the most tragic aspect of famine. Unfortunately, this aspect appears to be the rule rather than the exception in all recent major famine situations. In the 1990s, all reported famines (in Angola, Ethiopia, Liberia, Mozambique, Somalia, and Sudan) had one thing in common: armed conflict (*6*). "War famine," as some have called it, not only can be the primary cause of the famine, but also can make relief efforts difficult, thereby worsening famine-related suffering and mortality. The recurrent famines in the horn of Africa (Ethiopia, Somalia, and Sudan) in recent years can be attributed to wars or civil strife in an area of chronic food insecurity often exacerbated by natural factors. Food blockades and the use of food as a weapon also create problems of access. Examples of this type of human-generated famine may be seen in the few famines that have occurred in Europe during this century, including the Leningrad siege of 1941 and the Dutch Famine of 1944. Disruption of agricultural production caused by war was the primary cause of famine in Kampuchea in 1979, in Mozambique throughout the 1980s, and in southern Sudan in the 1990s. The disruptive impact of war goes beyond agricultural production.

It also interferes with food distribution and other income-generating activities. Hence it reduces both food availability and access to food. Under such conditions, armed intervention is often necessary to achieve basic security for relief efforts. When war is the primary cause of famine, providing security through armed intervention may very well be the most effective means to halt the disastrous consequences of famine (*13*). Unfortunately, because of political constraint or lack of compelling national interest, it is often a difficult proposition to provide military intervention for humanitarian purposes. The delay or failure of intervention likely contributes the most to famine-related morbidity and mortality.

Even though food-production failure and lack of food availability are commonly cited as main causes of famine, hunger and starvation can occur, even though food is widely available, when a population lacks access to that food because they have no capacity to purchase or exchange food. A detailed analysis of major famines in recent history found that lack of access to food or uneven distribution of food were perhaps the most important cause of famine (*11*). In response to the recurrent famine and chronic food insecurity of the Sahel region of Africa, a detailed review by the Independent Commission on International Humanitarian Issues (ICIHI) concluded that human-generated mistakes far outweighed natural factors in recurrent famines (*12*). The severe famine in southern Somalia in 1993 is a case example where intense civil conflicts among local clans not only directly caused reduced food availability and access, but also paralyzed any famine-mitigation efforts, thereby turning a food shortage related to drought into a full-fledged famine. From the perspective of famine prevention and mitigation, some of the human-generated factors contributing to or causing famine, such as poverty and war, far outweigh natural factors. Because these factors involve economic, political, and sometimes military actions, they are far more complex than the management issues related to food-aid and relief operations during a famine.

Public Health Impacts of Famine: Historical Perspective

By definition, famine is characterized by increased morbidity and mortality related to starvation and disease. Next to mortality, malnutrition is the most commonly used indicator to measure the severity of famine. From an epidemiologic point of view, malnutrition and mortality are two indices that require different procedures for assessment. In reality, these two events are inseparable. Malnourished people are more likely to die because malnutrition increases susceptibility to disease; at the same time, physical signs of malnutrition are late indicators of starvation and disease (*14*). In general, there are severe disturbances of every aspect of society before and during famine; malnutrition and death are only part of the overall spectrum of disturbance. The major health-related events of the 1993 famine in southern Somalia were documented in a detailed analysis by the Refugee Policy Group (Fig. 15-1) (*15*). The chronology of events

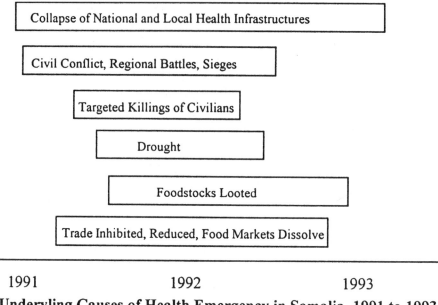

Collapse of National and Local Health Infrastructures

Civil Conflict, Regional Battles, Sieges

Targeted Killings of Civilians

Drought

Foodstocks Looted

Trade Inhibited, Reduced, Food Markets Dissolve

1991   1992   1993

Underyling Causes of Health Emergency in Somalia, 1991 to 1993

Figure 15-1. Chronology of health related events during the 1993 famine in southern Somalia. The onset of disturbances leading to severe food insecurity started in 1991, even though the famine did not gain international attention until near the end of 1992. (Courtesy of S. Hansch, Refugee Policy Group.)

showed that disturbances related to civil strife and food insecurity started in 1991; however, it was not until near the end of 1992 that the suffering and mortality reached a level that gained international attention.

Among health-based indicators, nutritional status is a useful indicator of efforts needed to manage relatively advanced food-insecurity situations, as well as to document full-fledged famine. The most commonly used indices to assess nutritional status for famine-related situations are weight-for-height of children and body-mass index (BMI) of adults. Low weight-for- height or low BMI is evidence of wasting or of recent and significant weight loss. The individual-based correlation between increased mortality and wasting state is well established (*16*). A review of multiple displaced populations by Pearson also demonstrated a strong association between the prevalence of wasting and mortality (Figure 15-2) (*3, 17*). For this reason, a recent World Health Organization (WHO) working group recommended the creation of a classification table to reflect the severity of the malnutrition problem on the basis of low weight-for-height (Table 15-2) (*18*). The purpose of this table is to bring attention to the fact that, since the worldwide prevalence of wasting for children younger than 5 years of age during nonemergency times is generally below 5%, prevalence levels even as low as 5%–10% indicate a

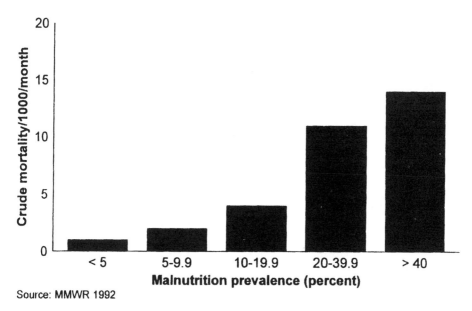

Source: MMWR 1992

Figure 15-2. Association of crude mortality rate with the prevalence of wasting (low weight-for-height) of children under the age of five based on information from 41 refugee camps *(3, 13)*.

serious problem. A prevalence of over 10% wasting can indicate an extremely severe situation. Even though severe wasting is a common observation during severe famines, epidemiologic assessment of the extent of severe malnutrition is not always feasible. In recent years, in the famine of southern Somalia, a wasting rate of 10%–35% was documented *(19)*, and a staggering rate of 75% was documented in southern Sudan in 1993 *(20)*. It is worth noting that a high rate of severe malnutrition or wasting is not unique to starvation; it can also be the consequence of a high rate of diarrheal disease among displaced populations. For example, in the Kurdish refugee crisis in 1991 and the Rwandan refugee situation in 1994, high rates of wasting and mortality were observed without apparent significant food shortages *(21, 22)*.

Table 15-2 A Decision Table to Define the Severity of Emergency Situations Based on the Prevalence of Low Weight-for-Height for Children Under the Age of 5

Classification of Severity	Prevalence of Wasting	Mean Weight-for-Height Z-Score
Acceptable	<5%	−0.35 or higher
Poor	5–9%	−0.36 to −0.65
Serious	10–14%	−0.66 to −0.90
Critical	≥15%	−0.91 or lower

Anthropometric measurements such as weight-for-height for children and BMI for adults do not provide specific information on the nature of the malnutrition. During famine, especially when there is mass population displacement, the cause of malnutrition could be primary (due to a lack of adequate food intake) or secondary (due to the disease process). For the most part, the relative contributions of these two major factors are difficult to separate, because malnourished people are more vulnerable than the well-nourished to disease, a situation that can further worsen nutritional status. From an intervention point of view, food distribution and disease control are equally important activities for reducing morbidity and mortality (*3*).

Energy deficit and weight loss or wasting are by far the most apparent signs of malnutrition and are routinely monitored by public health workers as measurements of the severity of advanced famine. Less apparent but often coexistent with energy deficit is micronutrient malnutrition due to the poor quality of the limited diet (*23, 24*). Vitamin A and iron deficiencies, common worldwide even during nondisaster times, often become exaggerated during disasters. Vitamin A deficiency has a strong influence on measles mortality if such an outbreak occurs (*25*), and severe anemia related to iron deficiency increases the risk for childhood and maternal mortality (*26*). Outbreaks of disease caused by other forms of micronutrient deficiencies (such as pellagra due to niacin deficiency, scurvy due to vitamin C deficiency, and beriberi due to thiamine deficiency) have occurred among famine-displaced populations in recent years (*24*). To a large extent, these outbreaks were related to nutrient deficiencies in the rations distributed (*23*).

Mortality

Historically, major famines were marked by the number of people who perished. In virtually all cases, mortality estimates were inexact for various reasons, including the influences of isolation and neglect that led to lack of access to food. These factors continue to make it impossible to assess properly the extent of famine-related mortality. The response to famine often results from media reports of excessive mortality rates (*6*). Although excess mortality is a late event of extreme food insecurity, recognizing this event is still critical for mounting national and international relief efforts. Unlike the assessment of nutritional status, which can be done by cross-sectional survey, mortality assessments are more difficult and require retrospective interviews or the establishment of a system to count deaths on an ongoing basis. Boss *et al.* (*19*) recently reviewed issues and critiques related to the need for a more standardized approach to mortality and nutritional assessment on the basis of the experience of the 1993 famine in southern Somalia.

A review of recent famines conducted by Hansch estimates that, even though famine-related death has been declining in the past several decades, at least 250,000 deaths due to starvation are still occurring annually in the 1990s (*27*). Historically, the single most severe famine of this century was the 1959–1962 famine in China. This catastrophe, which cost an estimated 26 million lives, was related to a disastrous farming and social policy called the Great Leap Forward (*28*).

Public Health Implications and Prevention Strategies in Famine

Primary prevention of famine should take place on global and regional levels, as well as within national political and economic systems. Secondary prevention—in order to avert the high morbidity and mortality that characterize famine—takes the form of managing vulnerable situations when there are circumstances of increased risk, such as population migration or significant shortfalls in food production. The last phase of a public health famine-prevention effort is damage control in the form of field-relief operations for food aid and public health services.

Unfortunately, the first phase of prevention must be carried out at a policy level that is not in the common operational domain of public health. Public health workers can best influence policy by providing credible information to policymakers and by advocating reform and action that can lead to a reduction in the occurrence of famine-prone situations. Perhaps the most effective role for public health workers is in enhancing famine-mitigation capacity by contributing to early warning and timely intervention. The traditional public health emphasis on field management of famine-affected and displaced populations is "too little and too late." Famine is a grim reality that will continue to occur, and more timely and adequate response as well as coordinated field operations are needed.

Prevention and Control Measures

Famine mitigation—the recognition of prefamine conditions and adoption of actions to prevent the onset of full-blown famine—is perhaps the most appropriate and feasible activity. Recognizing an area's increasing vulnerability to famine requires developing adequate warning systems similar to other public health surveillance systems. Such a system is technically feasible. The challenges facing famine mitigation are the willingness and ability to respond to the warning signals for appropriate action; such action is greatly dependent on the political and economic structure of the countries affected. A recent review of 46 incidences of famine during the twentieth century found that the common denominator is the lack of stable democratic government. This finding strongly suggests that long-term food security and short-term worsening of a situation leading to famine are closely tied to political and economic factors rather than to weather conditions or the quantity of food produced (*29*). The issues related to international developmental policy, economic structure adjustment, and the need for government systems that are more accountable to citizens are beyond the scope of public health approaches to enhance food security. For the discussion on famine warning and recognition here, one assumption is that there is some national and international capacity to respond to an urgent situation based on information from the warning system.

Efforts to mitigate famine will succeed only if both public health workers and policymakers accept the fact that commonly used famine-assessment indicators (e.g., elevated malnutrition and mortality rates) are actually late indicators and should not be relied upon as primary warning indicators. Elevated malnutrition and mortality basically indicate that the warning system and mitigation efforts have failed. Population migration, a sign widely regarded as an intermediate warning sign of famine, is actually a late sign of famine (30). Careful review of the process of famine development indicates that by the time people have left their homes or communities to seek food, there is already extensive suffering. Any congregation of displaced populations almost assures high morbidity and mortality related to infectious diseases and reduced host resistance. An ability to respond to the earliest warning indicators presents a chance for effective mitigation of a potential famine. Hence, the reorientation from late indicators to early indicators is the first step toward successful famine prevention.

Much of the assessment and surveillance of early warning signs relies on nontraditional public health indicators such as weather patterns, crop failures, and market food prices. There is a need to switch the role of public health from famine identification and management to famine mitigation. Much of the monitoring responsibility for early warning signs falls outside of the health sector (e.g., agricultural or economic sectors). Better intersectoral coordination is essential for the proper functioning of famine warning systems and for response to adverse warning signals.

Monitoring and Early Warning Systems

Currently, there are no standardized approaches for the assessment or surveillance of food-security situations for early warning signs of famine. In some countries, such as in India and Ethiopia, there are institutionalized long-term surveillance activities for famine warning (11). In many other countries, the warning is based on short-term cross-sectional assessments to define famine vulnerability when there is evidence of deteriorating conditions. Whether for long-term surveillance or one-time assessment, the general principle is similar: one must monitor different aspects of the chain of events that can lead to food insecurity. Table 15-3 shows a proposed common framework for a food-security surveillance system that can be implemented by the public health sector for famine warning. The major components or indicators defined for the assessment of food security (e.g., food availability, food accessibility, food and nutrition adequacy, and nutritional and health status) need to be measured and interpreted together to properly define vulnerability. To a great extent, the order of these major components can be viewed as the sequence of events leading to famine. Even though the specific indicators are obtained from multiple sectors, including health, it is quite feasible for a

Table 15-3 Common Framework for Food Security Surveillance or Famine Warning System*

Major Components	Food Availability	Food Accessibility	Food and Nutrition Adequacy	Health and Nutrition Status
General Contents	Food production; food distribution	Food price; purchasing power	Food quantity and quality; consumption pattern	Anthropometry; morbidity; mortality
Specific Indicators	Weather; early crop condition; harvest; food balance sheet; policy affecting production	Local food price; price of common staples; household incomes; price to income ratio; food stock; policy affecting rations and subsidies	Food frequency of key items; perception of adequacy (hunger)	Weight-for-height/BMI or weight loss of children and adults; incidence of measles, diarrhea; mortality

*Inputs from multiple components permit the formulation of vulnerability. The "proximal" components of food availability and accessibility are of greater warning value than "distal" events, which signal the presence of famine.

public health agency to be the coordinating point for summarizing and interpreting information. It is unlikely that a single overriding indicator among the many required can provide an accurate assessment or forecast. Part of the art of early warning is to assess the situation by synthesizing information from multiple components of the system. However, some events or indicators, such as weather failure, that affect harvest and potential food availability in the earlier part of this framework have greater value in early warning for action, whereas other events, such as morbidity and mortality, in the later part are late indicators for assessing the severity of the famine. Some useful information for assessing famine vulnerability can actually be qualitative information (e.g., national policy on food subsidies or evidence of population migration or food rioting). In the case of long-term monitoring-based systems, the relative change of the indicators is far more useful than the absolute value of the indicator at a given time, in part because some of the surveillance indicators for hunger and food insecurity—although they can be expressed as a quantitative index—lack adequate means to define their validity at a specified level without reference to some baseline value. For this reason, long-term monitoring is far more useful than one-time cross-sectional surveys in assessing famine vulnerability. Examples of information sources for the major components of an early warning system are detailed below.

Major Sources of Indicators for Events Affecting Food Availability

Both natural and human-generated factors known to affect food production can be incorporated as part of a systematic information-collection system to determine general food availability. Major factors affecting political and economic stability can be captured from the media or government information sources that routinely monitor economic indicators. In the case of naturally triggered reductions in food production, since drought is the most common cause, the earliest warning can be provided by weather- or rainfall-based assessments, early estimates of crop failure, and later, harvest-yield information.

Weather-Based Surveillance for Early Warning of Famine

Severe weather conditions, especially drought, are the most common cause of crop failures and food shortages that can trigger famine. In most parts of the world, the relationship between rainfall and food production is a predictable one. Because there are several months of lead time between severe drought and severe shortages of food, initiating response efforts on the basis of reliable information about weather and early crop failure will provide a much greater margin of safety than the usual response does. Generally, response efforts do not begin until after the harvest, when there is actual food scarcity and significant changes in food price are already evident.

On-the-ground rainfall monitoring is a time-honored method for collecting infor- mation as part of an early warning system for drought and famine. However, the ability to collect and use this information consistently as part of the famine warning system within a given area varies. Currently, well-developed aerial-sensing technologies rou- tinely monitor worldwide weather patterns and measure rainfall over a specific period for both large and smaller regions. The best-known weather sensing system uses the METROSAT satellite (*31*). Using an infrared radiometer, the satellite estimates current rainfall on the basis of cold cloud duration. Satellite information is calculated every 10 days by the Department of Meteorology at the University of Reading in the United Kingdom. Aerial-determined cold-cloud duration has been well correlated with actual thunderstorm-generated rainfall, as well as with ultimate crop yield.

The major food shortage related to the 1992 drought in southern Africa can be well demonstrated by an image collected by the Food and Agriculture Organization/Southern Africa Development Coordinating Committee (FAO/SADCC) project (Fig. 15-3) (*32*). This image shows the difference in rainfall amounts between the 1991 and 1992 planting seasons (January and February). Except for the western part of Angola, the entire region had much less rainfall in 1992, giving clear evidence of widespread drought across the entire region. Later, in May 1992, it was confirmed that drought-affected areas sustained crop failures ranging from 40% to 100%. If response efforts had been started in Feb- ruary, the massive food-procurement and distribution efforts subsequently undertaken would have been more manageable than they were at the start of actual food shortage. One advantage of the aerial-sensing method is that coverage of a large area is possible; another is that it is an activity that can be carried out even when a given country lacks the willingness or capacity to conduct famine-warning activities.

Agriculture-Based Early Monitoring for Food Availability

Compared with using weather information to predict severe food shortages, monitoring crop progress and early signs of crop failure before harvest season provides an early to

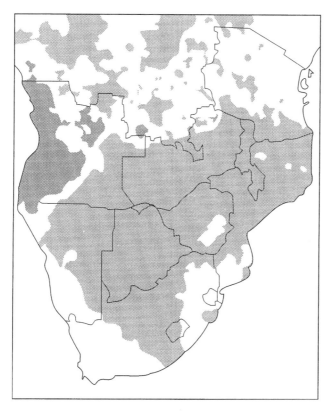

Figure 15-3. An example of rainfall estimation based on satellite images of cold cloud coverage for the month of January, 1993 for southern Africa (light shade: less rain, dark shade: more rain, no shade: no change). This image demonstrated widespread rain failure during the critical planting season in southern Africa except for Angola. Thus, this image provided an accurate estimate of the drought and forecasted the severe crop failure that followed.

intermediate warning signal of impending famine. Like weather-based surveillance, crop monitoring can be done on the ground, by systematically collecting information on crop growth and destruction, and through the use of aerial-sensing technology. In most countries, there are well-established systems within the agricultural sector for monitoring planting, progress (e.g., preharvest assessment), and crop yield (e.g., harvest assessment). Generally, the ministry of agriculture and local and regional offices of the Food and Agriculture Organization (FAO) are the best centralized sources for food-production-based information, and they are often part of national famine warning systems. In addition, information on food and grain importation that can affect a country's food balance can be obtained from the office in charge of agriculture and economic statistics.

Predictions of future food availability made on the basis of agricultural information are useful for famine early-warning purposes, but they are often underutilized as mechanisms to trigger early interventions to combat increasing food insecurity. Aerial-sensing technology can monitor crop coverage and growth conditions for wide geographic areas. The current global system for aerial crop-based surveillance is a series of polar-orbiting satellites administered by the U.S. National Oceanic and Atmospheric Administration (NOAA), which collects data daily using a high-resolution radiometer. Data are transformed and disseminated in the form of the Normalized Difference Vegetation Index (NDVI), with a 7-kilometer resolution (*31, 33*). The NDVI is a measure of greenness and vegetative vigor that has been well correlated with other weather-based information, as well as with on-the-ground assessments of crop growth and yield. NDVI data are used by comparing local current-month NDVI information with historic monthly-average NDVI data from multiple past years.

For assessments of harvest and food production in smaller areas, locally based harvest estimation through the agricultural system is the best approach and is institutionalized in many countries. During emergency situations, or when there is a need to obtain information independently, household-based assessments to determine yields of recent harvests, food stock on hand, and coping mechanisms for food shortages can be conducted. Such summary information from these assessments can often adequately characterize the larger area that the sample household represents.

Major Sources of Indicators for Events Affecting Food Accessibility

One of the principle reasons for reduced food accessibility is lack of food availability, particularly for rural subsistence farmers. However, for various sociopolitical reasons, famine is often the result of lack of access by poor populations—often when food is readily available (*11*). One way to assess food accessibility, regardless of whether or not there is reduced food availability, is to measure the cost of food relative to purchasing power. There are many ways to measure relative food costs and family incomes. A simplified approach that can be implemented within the framework of a public-health-based surveillance system is described here.

Market-Based Food-Price Monitoring

Overall food availability in a given area is usually reflected by market price. Market price is a good indicator of food accessibility because increasing food prices will make it more difficult for people not engaged in subsistence farming to meet their basic needs. Food price, of course, can go up with increasing shortages or production failures (reduced availability). It can also go up as a result of increased demand or broader market pressures. For example, in the 1943 Bengal famine there was little reduction in crop yield, but the combination of increased cereal prices because of wartime demand and the loss of cheaper imported cereals from Burma because of Japanese occupation resulted in mass starvation among the landless rural poor (*11*). On the other hand, there are also clear examples where severe food shortages have not resulted in food-price increases. In the 1973–1974 famine in Ethiopia, cereal prices in markets surrounding the hardest-hit region, Wollo, did not increase throughout the period of the famine because the level of poverty and destitution was so great at Wollo (*11*). Most people had little purchasing power to command the market; hence there was no food price increase. These opposing case studies point out one of the pitfalls of interpreting information from a single source or single system. It is imperative to utilize multiple parameters to make an overall assessment of famine vulnerability.

In general, cereal markets of major staples such as maize, rice, and wheat are the best indicators for broad scale market-based monitoring. Increasing cereal prices are usually a reliable signal of decreasing food accessibility. On the other hand, in countries where livestock is a major part of agricultural production, livestock price is a helpful signal of diminished resources due to drought or other conditions. As conditions make it more difficult to raise livestock, stress sales of less healthy animals usually occur; hence the market reflects a lower livestock price.

At the community level, one simple low-cost monitoring approach is to conduct periodic market-basket surveys to assess household vulnerability. Market-basket surveys define a ''basket'' as a fixed number and quantity of commonly consumed items. The unit price of each item can then be periodically obtained from a fixed number of markets to calculate the overall cost of the basket defined. The content of the market basket can be based on the basic nutritional need of an average family, say for 1 month. Food cost can then be more meaningfully compared with income information as an additional index for food accessibility. Monitoring the trends of cost of food items in a food basket from multiple locations in itself is a useful index. A model of this approach has been used as part of the emergency public health surveillance system for Armenia since 1992 (*34*). Figure 15-4 details the changes in basket price (using local currency and then converting that currency to its value in U.S. dollars as a guide) over a 2-year period as economic conditions continued to deteriorate with relatively little increase in family income.

Income or Purchasing-Power Monitoring

If feasible, monitoring of household income or purchasing power is helpful in assessing food accessibility relative to the cost of food. For urban populations, one could use a fixed-income value, such as average teacher salary or pensioner entitlement as defined by the government, average income based on surveys of clinic attendees, and household-based surveys as part of the hunger-monitoring activities described below. The ratio of food cost and estimated household income is likely the best quantitative expression for income-based monitoring.

Food Consumption or Hunger-Based Monitoring for Food Adequacy

The net outcome of reduced food accessibility is consumption of an inadequate quantity and quality of food. The degree and the acuity of the deterioration of food-consumption

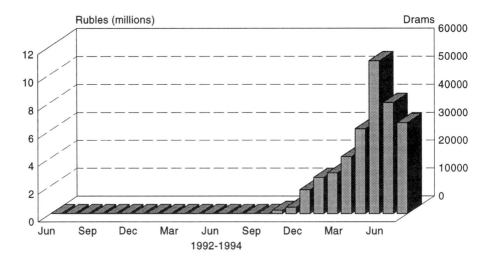

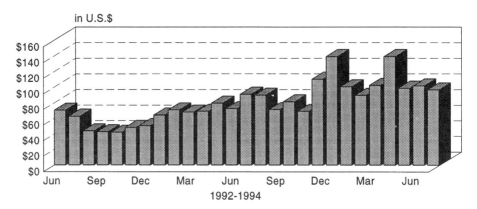

Figure 15-4. An example of monthly market-basket food prices based on a defined amount of fixed food items (''market basket'') as part of the Emergency Public Health Surveillance System of Armenia. The unit price of each food item was obtained monthly at the same markets for the computation of the cost of the entire basket. The upper panel is based on Russian rubles or Armenian drams, and the lower panel is based on U.S. dollars to illustrate the impact of local currency devaluation. Income based on local currency clearly did not keep pace with the rapidly escalating prices of food as reflected in the top panel.

patterns (as concurrent indicators of food insecurity) are likely the most direct indicators of famine vulnerability. Even though there are many well-developed dietary assessment methods that can provide good estimates of individual energy and nutrient-intake and consumption patterns (e.g., 24-hour dietary recall and detailed frequency of food-consumption survey), for practical purposes, these methods are unsuitable as part of a famine-warning system. In recent years, simplified frequency-of-food-consumption questionnaires have been developed, and hunger-related questions have been used for purposes of food-security monitoring. In settings where it is feasible either to conduct periodic rapid surveys or to administer questionnaires on a continuous basis in primary health care settings as part of nutritional surveillance activities, trends on degree of food consumption can potentially be assessed. The strategy is to ask a few food-consumption-related questions and to monitor the relative change in responses from the same population over time. Selected food-frequency items could be either food items that are more costly and, therefore, likely to be consumed less frequently with increasing shortages, or items known as "famine food" that are undesirable in general but consumption of which tends to increase with growing food shortages. In essence, this system uses a few selected food items as indicators for broader consumption patterns. Other types of questions, such as "Did your family have enough food to eat this past month?", are known as hunger-related. They test subjective perception of adequacy of food intake. On the surface, such questions may seem simplistic and lack the means to assess the accuracy of the response. However, as a surveillance index for food security, the change in response rate over time provides significant clues for changing vulnerability. One component of the Emergency Public Health Surveillance System of Armenia was the repeated survey of pensioners (*34, 35*). The response to such hunger-related questions showed sensitivity to the seasonal variation of food supply (i.e., reduction in positive responses in summer as food becomes more abundant, and increase in positive responses during winter as food becomes scarce). Instead of repeated surveys, it is feasible to obtain such information on a continuous basis from selected sentinel sites if the primary health care system is intact.

Health-Indicator-Based Warning Systems

Nutritional Status

The monitoring of nutritional status based on anthropometry is one of the most widely used tools to define the severity or the consequences of significant food insecurity. The main advantage of nutritional surveys or ongoing surveillance is that the information is relatively easy to obtain on a consistent basis and is objective in nature. However, one major disadvantage of nutritional status as an indicator is that it is a relatively late indicator of significant food insecurity, reflecting the consequence of significant energy deficit or disease. Further, the absence of elevated rates of malnutrition does not necessarily imply that the situation is secure. Unfortunately, this latter point is not commonly appreciated and may result in overreliance on nutritional surveys as the main assessment tool for famine vulnerability (e.g., interpreting the situation as secure on the basis of the absence of elevated prevalence of severe malnutrition). Most nutritional surveys take the form of one-time cross-sectional surveys that require a significantly elevated prevalence to be regarded as definite evidence of food-crisis problems (*18*). In places where there is ongoing nutritional surveillance, the nutritional status of the population can be compared across time. Small changes in nutritional status over time are far more sensitive indicators of increasing food insecurity. Kelly reported that a continuous nutrition-monitoring system in the Wollo region of Ethiopia showed that mean weight-for-height changes took place earlier than changes in livestock market trends and migration patterns (*36*).

The most readily used index of malnutrition is the relative weight-for-height ratio, which is reflective of recent weight loss and indicates protein-energy malnutrition. For children, the weight-for-height index is based on the international or WHO growth reference, developed by the National Center for Health Statistics at the Centers for Disease Control and Prevention (*37*). A weight-for-height value below -2 standard deviations of the reference mean is commonly used as the case definition of wasting or evidence of "acute malnutrition" for population-based assessments. The usefulness of this indicator for assessing famine severity is related to the fact that, during nondisaster times, the worldwide baseline variation of low weight-for-height is relatively stable at 3%–6%. Thus, even in the absence of predisaster or baseline information, any significant elevation from this level of weight-for-height indicates an increased level of malnutrition. In fact, studies from multiple displaced populations have found that low weight-for-height prevalence of as little as 5%–10% is associated with increased mortality (*18*). Increased prevalence of low weight-for-height (or wasting) is a useful indicator of the severity of a famine. For the purposes of food aid and nutritional supplementation, prevalence of low weight-for-height is also often used as a direct measurement of the proportion of children, or of the population, that requires food or nutritional supplementation. Unfortunately, this may not be an appropriate application of the wasting indicator, because good evidence exists to suggest that when the prevalence of wasting increases, the entire weight-for-height distribution in the population is shifted downward, indicating that the whole population is affected or has lost weight, not just those who meet the cutoff criteria of weight-for-height < -2 SD of the reference (*21*). However, in emergency situations, individual measurements of low weight-for-height can be used as a screening tool to find severely wasted children ($\sim$weight-for-height < -3 SD of the reference) who are at high risk for dying; this group would then be eligible for immediate therapeutic intervention. Even though an elevated rate of wasting is indicative of severe crisis, the lack of elevated rates of wasting cannot be equated with low population vulnerability to famine, because wasting is a late and severe indicator of suffering and may not reflect severe food shortage until it has already reached an advanced stage. It is also possible, when conditions are very severe, that the most malnourished people will have already died. This situation will give the false appearance of a relatively low prevalence of wasting in the population (*21, 38*). Other height- and weight-based anthropometric indices, such as height-for-age or weight-for-age, which have little bearing on disaster situations, usually have much higher prevalence in developing countries.

The nutritional status of children is commonly used as an index for the entire population, because children are the most vulnerable to the effects of food insecurity and disease. However, in times of severe food shortage, no part of the population is spared. Documentation of severe undernutrition among adults can be just as helpful in characterizing the extent of suffering. For adults, the commonly used quantitative measure for nutritional status is body-mass index (BMI: weight (kg)/ height (M)^2). A BMI value of 16 has been defined as indicative of severe wasting for population-based assessments (*18*).

Because measuring height and weight during emergency situations is not always feasible, there has recently been an increase in the use of mid-upper-arm-circumference (MUAC) as a substitute for determining weight-for-height. MUAC can be simply measured by using a short measuring tape. Low MUAC consistent with malnutrition is defined on the basis of a fixed cutoff circumference of 12.5 or 13 cm. However, there is good evidence that MUAC based on a fixed cutoff as described above is not a suitable substitute for the screening of children suffering from wasting based on low weight-for-height (*18*). This is because low MUAC measurements often detect younger children who happen to have smaller arms and are not suffering from wasting. For this reason, the application of MUAC will require the use of age- or height-based references in order to assess wasting conditions properly (*18*).

Morbidity and Mortality

The collection of morbidity information is particularly useful among displaced populations, which usually suffer from high rates of disease due to the stress leading to migration and the crowding and unsanitary conditions of relocation sites. Quantitative information can be obtained from disease surveillance systems if they exist, or data can be obtained through household surveys as part of nutrition or food-security surveys. Information concerning diarrheal disease is commonly collected in this manner. Because elevated morbidity and mortality are late warning indicators (or trailing indicators) of famine, the detection of elevated morbidity and mortality would indicate need for urgent actions to manage the situation. Generally, baseline mortality is considered to be one death per 10,000 per day. Mortality exceeding this rate is of great concern. Table 15-4 summarizes key recommendations related to field assessment of public health indicators during famine based on a review of the famine experience in southern Somalia in 1993 (*19*).

Assessing Famine Vulnerability on the Basis of Multiple Sources of Information

The determination of famine vulnerability is based on analyzing various indicators of the major components for food security assessment: food availability, food accessibility, consumption pattern, and health and nutritional status. As described above, multiple indicators can be used for each of the major components. The assessment of vulnerability can be based on large geographic areas (i.e., entire countries or regions), local communities, or households. Because there is no standard set of indicators used for the warning system or for food security assessment, there is no common procedure to define a population's vulnerability to famine. In part, this lack of a standardized approach for

Table 15-4 Recommendations for Surveys of Health Indicators in Emergency Situations

---

A. General Recommendations

- Work with relevant decision-makers to define specific objectives for the study.
- Utilize scientifically appropriate survey methodology.
- Document all deviations from the planned methodology.
- Discuss the results with relevant decision-makers.
- Prepare a written report:
  State objectives;
  Detail methodology;
  Provide case definitions;
  Describe training of interviewers;
  Define time periods, study subjects, and age groups;
  Present and discuss results;
  Append copy of questionnaire, survey tools, or assessment forms.
- Disseminate study results in a timely manner.

B. Specific Recommendations

Nutritional Data

- Use weights and heights for measurement of acute malnutrition.
- Present low weight-for-height data as percentage of children less than -2 SD (z-score) of the reference median and mean z-scores with a written interpretation of the findings.
- Count children with edema as being severely malnourished.

Mortality Data

- Report as the proportion of the population at the beginning of the recall period who died during that period.
- Calculate an average daily death rate (deaths per 10,000 per day) for the recall period.
- Determine the cause of death.

Morbidity Data

- In general, these are less useful than mortality and nutritional data.
- Immunization coverage data may be helpful, especially if vaccination record cards have been distributed.

Source: Adapted from Boss *et al* (*15*).

assessment is due to the need for adapting methods under different circumstances. For example, indicators that are useful for monitoring trends in subsistence farming communities may not be useful in urban areas. Even though specific indicators and procedures cannot be standardized, a more unified framework or general approach in assessing famine vulnerability is certainly indicated in order to facilitate comparison over time and across populations and to promote consistent decision-making and action. Currently, there are several assessment models used by different organizations. The design and methodology of assessment models depends on the level at which the vulnerability assessment is to be carried out—at the household, local community, subregional, regional, or country level.

Some of the components of a food-security assessment, such as the systematic collection of information on household food-consumption patterns and health and nutritional status, can be collected by using structured survey methods or from routine health data from primary health care settings. The collection of such information can be regarded as part of the traditional public health approach for monitoring. However, for the food-availability and accessibility components of the monitoring system (including the assessment of coping strategies), most of the information sources are not part of traditional public health surveillance systems. These components of the food-security monitoring system often rely more on qualitative or anthropological approaches to define the nature of the problem. As the overall public health effort shifts toward efforts to prevent the worsening of milder forms of food insecurity, rather than toward reactive efforts to respond to full-fledged famine, proper assessment and action will require integrating traditional and nontraditional public health approaches.

A large-area food-security assessment was conducted in Mali in the early 1990s. The system was administered by the USAID Famine Early Warning System (FEWS) (39). In this assessment, the household income model for understanding food security was used to determine vulnerability to famine. This model used a total of 23 indicators divided into two components—chronic or structural indicators and current or short-term indicators. The 10 indicators of chronic vulnerability were grouped into the following 4 categories: the economic importance of livestock and cereals, the quality of the agro-pastoral season (food availability), other sources of income, and physical access to markets and the urban infrastructure (food accessibility). The 13 current indicators were grouped into the following 3 categories: quality of the past 3 agro-pastoral seasons, observed market responses, and civil unrest or insecurity. Because of civil strife in northern Mali and a poor 1993 harvest for a large area, the food-security situation was determined to be highly to extremely vulnerable for a good part of the country.

Even though multiple models are employed by the FEWS to assess vulnerability at country and regional levels, a common framework is used to summarize each assessment into a level of vulnerability. Table 15-5 presents the FEWS vulnerability index with corresponding coping strategies and interventions to consider (39). This framework helps point out that famine is the severe end of the food-insecurity spectrum and that the objective of assessment is to define appropriate coping strategies and early interventions.

Another approach better suited for assessing the vulnerability of smaller areas or communities has been developed by Young. This approach is suitable for field application by public health workers. It is detailed in an Oxfam monograph on assessment and response for food scarcity and famine (40). This particular model outlines three general methods for data collection. First, an initial assessment is conducted by reviewing existing information. Then rapid assessment at a few sites is performed to gather new information based on qualitative approaches. Finally, structured surveys, focusing on objective measurements of household food, income, property assets, and nutritional status of younger children, are carried out.

In summary, famine prevention requires both recognition and action during the earlier stages of food insecurity. Recognition of early food insecurity requires an adequate

Table 15-5 FEWS Vulnerability Index of Food Security

Level of Vulnerability	Conditions of Vulnerability	Typical Coping Strategies and/or Behaviors	Interventions to Consider
Slightly Vulnerable	**Maintaining or Accumulating Assets and Maintaining Preferred Production Strategy**	**Assets/resources/wealth:** Either accumulating additional assets/resources/wealth or only minimal net change in assets, resources or wealth over a season/year, i.e., coping to minimize risk (normal "belt-tightening" or seasonal variations). **Production Strategy:** Any changes in production strategy are largely volitional for perceived gain, and not stress related.	**Developmental Programs**
Moderately Vulnerable	**Drawing-down Assets and Maintaining Preferred Production Strategy**	**Assets/resources/wealth:** Coping measures include drawing down or liquidating less important assets, husbanding resources, minimizing rate of expenditure of wealth, unseasonable "belt-tightening" (e.g., drawing down food stores, reducing amount of food consumed, sale of goats or sheep). **Production Strategy:** Only minor stress-related change in overall production/income strategy (e.g., minor changes in cropping/planting practices, modest gathering of wild foods, interhousehold transfers and loans, etc.)	**Mitigation and/or Development: Asset Support** (release food price stabilization stocks, sell animal fodder at "social prices," community grain bank, etc.)

		Mitigation and/or Relief: Income and Asset Support (food-for-work, cash-for work, etc.)
Highly Vulnerable	**Depleting Assets** and **Disrupting Preferred Production Strategy**	
	Assets/resources/wealth: Liquidating more important investments, but not yet "production" assets (e.g., sales of cattle, bicycles, and possessions such as jewelry). **Production Strategy**: Coping measures being used have a significantly costly or disruptive character to the usual/preferred household and individual lifestyles, to the environment, etc. (e.g., time-consuming wage labor, selling firewood, farming marginal land, labor migration of young adults, borrowing from merchants at high interest rates).	
		Relief and/or Mitigation: Nutrition, Income and Asset Support (food relief, seed packs, etc.)
Extremely Vulnerable or At-risk	**Liquidating Means of Production and Abandoning Preferred Production Strategy**	
	Assets/resources/wealth: liquidating "production" resources (e.g., sale of planting seeds, hoes, oxen, land, prime breeding animals, whole herds). **Production Strategy**: seeking nontraditional sources of income, employment, or production that preclude continuing with preferred/usual ones (e.g., migration of whole families).	
		Emergency Relief (food, shelter, medicine)
Famine	**Destitute**	
	Coping Strategies Exhausted: no significant assets, resources, or wealth; no income/ production.	

warning system that involves monitoring activities in multiple sectors. The monitoring system must be functional, with adequate political support to respond effectively to the warning signals. The greatest challenge appears to be that often only late or trailing indicators are taken seriously, and by the time these late indicators appear, famine is already occurring. The public health challenge is to reorient famine-mitigation efforts to focus on true early-warning indicators, which become evident prior to the onset of mass starvation and suffering.

Mitigation and Control Measures

Famine prevention is far more desirable than efforts to control and manage famine once it is under way. Unfortunately, famine control and management are the rule rather than the exception for public health workers who traditionally have become involved when the food-insecurity situation has already reached famine stage. Public health workers have become expert at on-site management of health and nutrition programs as part of emergency relief efforts. Many of the issues and procedures of emergency relief programs are related to providing support to large, concentrated displaced populations. (This is also the case for refugees displaced because of war or civil conflict. The chapter ''Complex Emergencies'' [Chapter 20] details many of these operations. Another good source of information dealing with issues relevant to morbidity and mortality control measures during famine is the CDC publication ''Famine-affected, refugee, and displaced populations: recommendations for public health issues'' (*3*). For a very detailed step-by-step field manual, Appleton of Save the Children compiled a practical guide on the planning and management of feeding programs based on drought-relief programs in Ethiopia (*41*). These two publications are useful as field manuals for staff participating in the field management of famines).

A number of common and recurrent problems are encountered in every large-scale emergency relief operation (*3, 42*). From a broader public health management perspective, if some of these operational constraints can be dealt with, better control of the situation, with decreased morbidity and mortality, will result. Proposals to deal with these common problems can be summarized as follows (*3, 13, 42*):

- Strong overall leadership and coordination for field operations are needed. Often, dozens of different organizations with workers are present in the field without adequate coordination.
- Long-term logistical capacity to respond with large-scale emergency relief efforts should be developed.
- Measures to ensure safe water, sanitation, and disease control should be emphasized in addition to the staffing of health services for curative measures. Much of the morbidity and mortality is a result of the high concentration of the population living together in a relatively small area without an adequate basic sanitary infra-

structure. In essence, there is the need for implementation of traditional basic public health measures (*21*).

- To ensure equity of food distribution, food distribution and nutrition programs should be based on the needs of the entire population, not solely on the needs of those with evidence of severe malnutrition (*43*).

Specific programs or components that are relevant to famine control are reviewed below.

Food-Aid Programs

Food-aid programs can be implemented at several levels, depending on the severity of the food-insecurity problem. Generally, a displaced population in a camp setting has little capacity to provide for itself and must depend on relief distributions. In such a setting, there are three ways to provide food:

- General food distribution or the provision of dry rations. Allocated food is based on 2100 kcal per person per day and is often provided as cereal, oil, and milk powder (*44*).
- Mass feeding with cooked meals. This approach is sometimes necessary in extreme emergency conditions when there is no capacity for the displaced households to cook for themselves. This approach can also be used to control maldistribution or illicit selling of dry rations.
- Supplementary feeding of an additional ration for the more nutritionally vulnerable subpopulations, such as children younger than age 5, pregnant and lactating women, children selected on the basis of anthropometric deficit, and those who are ill. This supplementary ration can be provided either as dry rations or as on-the-spot wet feedings to ensure that the food is consumed by the targeted groups. Often supplementary feedings are provided only for children meeting certain anthropometry-based criteria for malnutrition. There is no good evidence that such practice is sound; in a stressed population, children who do not meet the strict anthropometry criteria for malnourishment are equally vulnerable and affected as those who actually meet the criteria (*43*). A more reasonable approach would be to provide supplementation to all children within a community. Such a selection strategy is based on evidence that the community as a whole is at greater risk for being worse off (e.g., higher rates of malnutrition or disease). However, if there are insufficient resources to feed all children under the age of 5, priority should be given to the younger children because they are more vulnerable to the consequences of energy malnutrition.
- Therapeutic (intensive) feeding programs intended for medical treatment for severely wasted children and adults, such as those with weight-for-height scores below -3 standard deviations or 70% of the reference median. This practice targets the most malnourished children and adults. Extremely wasted individuals, regard-

less of whether the primary cause is starvation or diarrheal disease, are at high risk of dying; therapeutic feeding is definitely a needed clinical intervention for those in such life-threatening situations. It is worth noting that because of the intense resources required for therapeutic feedings, it is not a feasible practice in time of widespread famine.

For nondisplaced populations during urgent situations, free-food distribution based on the same principle of general food distribution is often the only option. It is feasible to provide both supplementary feedings and therapeutic feeding programs during more stable situations. In less acute situations, there are several options other than free-food distribution, the most common of which is implementing a food-for-work program. The advantage of this type of program is that it is self-targeting; only those individuals who truly need the food will take part in the program because of the significant work output required to exchange for food. Activities that can help reduce food-aid requirements include (1) supplying provisions such as seeds and tools to reestablish farming activities; (2) providing income-generating opportunities among the displaced population; and (3) providing opportunities for trading. Useful guides and operational manuals for food-aid-related activities include the UNHCR Food Aid Briefing kit (45), "The Drought Relief in Ethiopia" by Save the Children (41), and the summary article titled "Management of Nutrition Relief for Famine Affected and Displaced Populations" by Seaman (46).

Two difficult issues faced by food-aid programs are (1) how to avoid the creation of long-term dependency and (2) how to avert any potential adverse impacts on agricultural production when food security improves. In a number of cases relief supply kept food prices too low for farmers to obtain equitable returns from the market. Management of food-aid programs requires careful consideration of the long-term impact so as to preclude the creation of greater states of vulnerability in the future.

Management After Acute Phase of Famine

Despite relief efforts, after the most extreme phase of food insecurity, the affected population and community are still in a vulnerable condition. Regardless of the triggering event or underlying cause, the stress of famine undermines future capacity for food production and development related to the economic depression that is associated with famine. For this reason, the same affected population may become more vulnerable for future famines. The transition from the acute to the postacute phase of famine requires the effective transformation of relief activities to longer-term developmental activities. For example, free-food distribution can be replaced by food-for-work programs. Such a substitution can also help to rehabilitate the community's economic infrastructure. Emergency health programs using medical volunteers can be transformed to programs to rebuild primary health care capacity of the local community. Long-term support for the proper transition to postfamine rehabilitation likely will reduce future vulnerability for recurrent famine.

Critical Knowledge Gaps

Current abilities and technology to assess famine vulnerability are only partially developed. The greatest area for improvement lies in developing a more standardized framework or approach to assessing various aspects of the food-security situation so that decisions can be based on a more uniform system or criteria. The process of assessment can be accomplished by public health workers who are not necessarily food-security experts.

Perhaps the largest knowledge gap in famine-mitigation activity involves knowing what action to take to halt imminent situations after vulnerability assessment. To some extent this problem is the result of the compartmentalization of the monitoring unit apart from the complex national and international infrastructure that is needed to respond to famine. Historically, intervention for famine has not become a issue until the level of devastation has become evident and the extent of suffering in terms of morbidity and mortality is already high. In this respect, the knowledge gap that impedes famine prevention and control takes the form of common misconceptions about famine. The following points may be important for public health workers, as well as policymakers, to appreciate:

- Famine is not a discreet event. It results from the worsening of chronic or deteriorating socioeconomic conditions and food security. Effective monitoring and warning systems must cover various levels and various aspects of the support system for food security. It is essential that prefamine stages be recognized and defined when mitigation efforts are still possible.
- Famine is preventable. This is especially the case when food insecurity is triggered by natural factors. There are a number of examples of major famines averted through timely interventions. The proper documentation of such positive lessons is more important than the more popular approach—analyses of lessons learned after a major famine occurs.
- Early indicators must be used for famine warning. In assessing food insecurity and famine vulnerability, a number of early indicators can be used to trigger action; these early signals of impending famine should be relied on more than late indicators, such as malnutrition and mortality.
- Nutritional status must be appropriately interpreted. The absence of elevated rates of malnutrition and mortality cannot be equated to the absence of food insecurity or famine vulnerability. But the presence of elevated malnutrition and mortality rates indicates unequivocally that famine is already taking place.

- Action and response must be linked to information provided by the warning system. Like any other public health surveillance system, for a famine early-warning system to be effective, a built-in system of action and response components is essential. In the case of food security, surveillance requires the involvement of nonhealth sectors such as agriculture, transportation, and finance.

Methodological Problems of Epidemiologic Studies

The focus of epidemiologic approaches in famine-related activities, as suggested in the previous section, should be on the development of more useful and more widely comparable famine early-warning systems. Because the assessment of famine vulnerability requires the analysis of a complex set of indicators collected from different sources and from different population organization levels, a more uniform approach to the collection and interpretation of various indicators will help direct efforts to monitor and simplify comparisons. To the extent possible, different components of the assessment can be standardized to facilitate field operation.

Epidemiology is a useful tool, but not the only tool, because traditional epidemiologic studies are based on the collection and analysis of strictly public-health-related, quantitatively variable information. Nonhealth early-warning indicators, such as factors affecting food availability and accessibility, can also be put into an epidemiologic framework to achieve greater comparability or standardization, thereby facilitating interpretation and hence decision-making. A number of indicators that are nonquantitative in nature provide complementary information or detect problems that do not lend themselves to traditional quantitative methods. Since it is unlikely that all useful food-security indicators can be obtained efficiently using traditional epidemiologic approaches, an understanding of both the usefulness and limitations of various qualitative research methods will be helpful for the collection of data as well as for the interpretation of information related to nonhealth famine indicators.

Research Recommendations

A review of various issues related to famine indicates that much is known about the nature and background of famine and food insecurity among a small circle of technicians who are preoccupied with this issue. Among policymakers who are in a position to prevent or mitigate famine, and among public health workers in general, however, there appears to be a knowledge gap regarding the nature of famine. Rather than more research, greater promotion of knowledge about the preventability of famine and the nature of chronic food insecurity is indicated. Improvement of early-warning systems from a technical perspective may not increase the effectiveness of famine mitigation if the linkage to action is weak. It appears that there is greater urgency for policy reform than for applied research.

Several potential research activities can help to improve our capacity to prevent and mitigate famine: For advocacy purposes, we need

- better documentation of major natural disasters, such as drought, that through active intervention did not result in famine. Case example demonstration of the fact that famine is preventable likely will create greater willingness to consider the merits of early implementation of intervention activities.
- better analyses to show that long-term underlying factors, such as inappropriate economic and developmental policies, poverty, and chronic food insecurity, are major contributory factors to the onset of famine in famine-prone region of the world. Such information may help to turn attention from short-term management during crisis situations toward longer-term developmental activities that can reduce famine vulnerability.

For monitoring and early-warning purposes, we must develop

- definition of a series of indicators for different aspects of food-security assessment that have some predictive value for famine occurrence and are relatively easy to collect;
- definition of standardized approaches for the collection and interpretation of various indicators that can be used for food-security monitoring;
- a simple conceptual framework that summarizes various indicators for the assessment of famine vulnerability.

For field operations and management purposes:

- We should create a standardized monitoring system for food distribution and disease surveillance, and develop measurements to monitor increases in malnutrition and mortality.
- We should expand the definition and content of public health operations beyond food aid and basic health care to include such issues as water and sanitation for mass displaced populations.
- We need to define an emergency program content that is appropriate for the particular stage of famine and that allows for the efficient transformation from relief to rehabilitation when the acute emergency phase has passed.

References

1. Currey B. Is famine a discrete event? *Disasters* 1992;16:138–144.
2. D'Souza F. Famine: Social security and an analysis of vulnerability. In: Harrison GA, editor. *Famine*. New York: Oxford University Press, 1988.

3. Toole MJ, Malkki RM. Famine-affected, refugee, and displaced populations: recommendations for public health issues. *MMWR* 1992;41(RR-13):1–76.

4. Leidenfrost N. *Definitions concerned with food security, hunger, undernutrition, and poverty.* Washington, D.C.: U.S. Dept of Agriculture, 1993.

5. Reutilinger S, van Holst Pellekaan J. *Poverty and hunger: issues and options for food security in developing countries.* Washington, D.C.: The World Bank, 1986.

6. Kates RW. Ending deaths from famine: the opportunity in Somalia. *N Engl J Med* 1993; 328:1055–1057.

7. Downing TE. Monitoring and responding to famine: lessons from the 1984–85 food crisis in Kenya. *Disasters* 1990;14:204–229.

8. Teklu T. The prevention and mitigation of famine: policy lessons from Botswana and Sudan. *Disasters* 1994;18:35–47.

9. Office of U.S. Foreign Disaster Assistance. *Southern Africa drought assessment.* Washington, D.C.: Office of U.S. Foreign Disaster Assistance, 1992.

10. Collins C. Famine defeated: Southern Africa, UN wins battle against drought. *Africa Recovery* August 9, 1993:1–13.

11. Sen AK. *Poverty and famine: an essay on entitlement and depravation.* Oxford, England: Clarendon Press, 1981.

12. The Independent Commissions on International Humanitarian Issues. *Famine: a man-made disaster?* New York: Random House, 1985.

13. Sharp TW, Yip R, Malone J. The role of military forces for emergency international humanitarian assistance: observations and recommendations from three recent missions. *JAMA* 1994;272:286–290.

14. Pinsturp-Andersen P, Burger S, Habicht JP, Peterson K. *World Bank health priorities review: protein energy malnutrition.* Washington, D.C.: The World Bank, 1992.

15. Hansch S, Lillibridge S, Egeland G, Teller C, Toole M. *Excess mortality and the impact of health interventions in the Somalia humanitarian emergency.* Washington, D.C.: Refugee Policy Group, 1994.

16. Pelletier D, Frongillo A, Habicht JP. Epidemiologic evidence for a potentiating effect of malnutrition on child mortality. *Am J Public Health* 1993;83:1130–1133.

17. Pearson-Karell B. *The relationship between childhood malnutrition and crude mortality among 42 refugee populations* [thesis]. Atlanta, GA: Emory University, 1989.

18. World Health Organization. *Report of the WHO expert committee on physical status: the use and interpretation of anthropometry.* Geneva: World Health Organization, 1995.

19. Boss LP, Toole MJ, Yip R. Health and nutrition assessments in Somalia during the 1991–92 famine: recommendations for standardization of methods. *JAMA* 1994;272:371–376.

20. Herwaldt BL, Bassett DC, Yip R, Alonso CR, Toole MJ. Crisis in southern Sudan: where is the world? *Lancet* 1993;342:119–120.

21. Yip R, Sharp TW. Acute malnutrition and high childhood mortality related to diarrhea: lessons from the 1991 Kurdish refugee crisis. *JAMA* 1993;270:587–590.

22. Paquet, van Soest. Mortality and malnutrition among Rwandan refugee in Zaire. *Lancet* 1994; 344:823–824.

23. Toole MJ. Micronutrient deficiency disease in refugee populations. *Lancet* 1992;333:1214–1216.

24. Tomkins A. Nutritional deficiencies during famine. *Trop Doct* 1991;21(Suppl. 1):43–46.

25. Nieburg P, Waldman RJ, Leavell R, *et al.* Vitamin A supplementation for refugee and famine victims. *Bull World Health Organ* 1988;66:689–697.

26. Yip R. Iron deficiency: contemporary scientific issues and international programmatic approaches. *J Nutr* 1994;124:1479S–1490S.

27. Hansch S. *How many people die of starvation in famine-related humanitarian emergencies?* Washington, D.C.: Refugee Policy Group, 1994.

28. Riskin C. Food, poverty, and development strategy in the People's Republic of China. In: Newman LF, editor. *Hunger in history: food shortage, poverty, and depravation.* Oxford, England: Basil Blackwell, 1990.

29. Johnson S. *A comparative analysis of failure to prevent famine in the twentieth century* [thesis]. Atlanta, GA: Emory University, 1995.

30. Harrison GA. *Famine.* New York: Oxford University Press, 1988.

31. Tulane University Famine Early Warning System (FEWS) Project (Tulane/Pragma Group). *Vulnerability assessment—July 1994: Mauritania, Mali, Burkina Faso, Niger, Chad, Ethiopia.* New Orleans: Tulane University, 1994.

32. Southern Africa Development Coordinating Committee (SADCC) Regional Early Warning Unit. *Food security special update—9th March 1992.* Harare, Zimbabwe: SADCC, 1992.

33. Idso SB, Jackson RD, Reginato RJ. Remote-sensing of crop yields. *Science* 1977;196:19–25.

34. Centers for Disease Control and Prevention: Emergency public health surveillance in response to food and energy shortage—Armenia, 1992. *MMWR* 1993;42:69–71.

35. McNabb S, Welch K, Laumark S, Peterson DE, Ratard RC, Toole MJ, et al. Population-based nutritional risk survey of pensioners in Yerevan, Armenia. *Am J Prev Med* 1994; 10:65–70.

36. Kelley M. Entitlement, coping mechanisms and indicators of access to food: Wollo region, Ethiopia, 1987–88. *Disasters* 1992;16:322–328.

37. Hamill PVV, Drizid TA, Johnson CL, Reed RB, Roche AF, Moore WM. Physical growth: National Center for Health Statistics percentiles. *Am J Clin Nutr* 1979;32:607–629.

38. Nieburg P, Berry A, Steketee R, Binkin N, Dondero T, Aziz N. Limitations of anthropometry during acute food shortage: high mortality can mask refugee's deteriorating nutritional status. *Disasters* 1988;12:253–258.

39. May CA. *Vulnerability and food security in the Famine Early Warning System (FEWS) project: guidelines for implementation.* FEWS Working Paper 2.2. Arlington, VA: U.S. Agency for International Development FEWS Project, 1990.

40. Young H. *Food scarcity and famine: assessment and response.* Oxfam practical health guide no. 7. Oxford, England: Oxfam Publications, 1992.

41. Appleton J. *Drought relief in Ethiopia: a practical guide for planning and management of feeding programs.* London: Save the Children UK, 1987.

42. Toole MJ, Waldman RJ. Prevention of excess mortality in refugee and displaced populations in developing countries. *JAMA* 1990;293:3296–3302.

43. Yip R, Scanlon K. The burden of malnutrition: a population perspective. *J Nutr* 1994; 124:2043s–2046s.

44. Allen L, Hobson CP. *Estimated mean per capita energy requirements for planning emergency food aid rations.* Institute of Medicine Report. Washington, D.C.: National Academy Press, 1995.

45. United Nations High Commission for Refugees (UNHCR). *Food aid briefing kit.* Geneva: UNHCR, 1992.

46. Seaman J. Management of nutrition relief for famine affected and displaced populations. *Trop Doct* 1991;21 (Suppl. 1):38–42.

16

Air Pollution

RUTH A. ETZEL
JEAN G. FRENCH

Background and Nature of Acute Episodes of Air Pollution

Sources of Air Pollutants

Pollutants may enter the air from natural or synthetic sources. Air always carries natural pollutants such as pollens, spores, molds, yeast, fungi, and bacteria; and forest fires, windstorms, volcanic eruptions, and droughts cause smoke, dust, and other pollutants to enter the air. Yet all the pollution wrought by nature counts for little when compared with the effects of pollutants associated with human activity (*112*). The major sources of synthetic air pollutants include the burning of fossil fuels, particularly coal; emissions from smelters, steel plants, and other heavy manufacturing facilities; and emissions from mobile sources such as automobiles, trucks, and airplanes. The primary pollutants from these major sources are sulfur dioxide (SO_2), nitrogen dioxide (NO_2), carbon monoxide (CO), suspended particulates, ozone, hydrocarbons, acid aerosols of sulfates and nitrates, and heavy metals. Although emissions from chemical manufacturing may affect the area immediately surrounding the source, they do not have the same impact on regional air pollution as the aforementioned pollutants.

336

Factors Contributing to a Buildup of Concentrations of Air Pollution

Natural Factors

Adverse meteorologic conditions cause air pollutants to accumulate. One such condition is stagnation in which low wind speeds (<4 km/hour [7 mph]) do not allow air pollutants to disperse. Another adverse condition is a thermal inversion at or not far above the earth's surface whereby ground-level air is cooler (rather than warmer) than the air layer above. The most common cause of a thermal inversion is nighttime cooling of a stratum near the ground (caused by clear skies that permit surface heat to escape) in conjunction with light winds that do not disperse the pollutants. However, an inversion can also be caused by complicated large-scale meteorologic events usually associated with high atmospheric pressure. Within an inversion layer, vertical atmospheric motions that normally might disperse pollutants are minimized. Sometimes an inversion layer hovering over a city acts as a lid, keeping pollutants from escaping upward, the only direction for them to go when wind speed is insufficient to disperse them horizontally.

The greatest potential for a buildup of air-pollution concentrations occurs in areas with a high frequency of both low wind speeds and thermal inversions. The problem is intensified in areas in which air movement is restricted by surrounding hills or mountains.

Human-Generated Factors

Humans have been exposed to synthetic sources of air pollution since they lit their first fire. The air of many of the earliest towns was rife with smoke and noxious odors emanating from trades such as tanning. Only with the general use of coal, however, did air pollution begin to be a major problem. Until the early Middle Ages, wood was the prime source of heat throughout Europe. By the 1200s, however, forests near settlements were depleted, and people needed a new fuel. Increasingly, Europe followed the example of Asia, whose coal-burning technology had been described by travelers such as Marco Polo.

The use of coal fouled the air so badly that in 1273 England's King Edward I passed a law prohibiting the burning of at least one type of coal, and in the early 1400s Henry V formed a commission to oversee the use of coal in London. In 1661, Charles II ordered scientist John Evelyn to survey the effects of the increasing air pollution over the city. Evelyn recognized the relationship between the ''dismal cloud'' over London and a number of fatal diseases, but his warnings about the need for air-pollution controls were ignored.

After the introduction of coal, buildups of air pollution sporadically afflicted towns, but urban centers still had fairly small populations, industry operated on a small scale, and the outpourings of industrial contaminants were not yet the norm. Thus the effects of early episodes of air pollution were relatively minor. By the late 1800s, however, industry was booming, larger and larger populations were concentrating in cities, and increasing amounts of chemical pollution were entering the air. As a result, in December 1873, when particularly adverse weather conditions occurred, a thick cloud of pollution gathered over London. This episode resulted in 1,150 deaths, making it one of the earliest air-pollution disasters (*3*).

Since 1873, in the industrialized world there have been at least 40 episodes in which sudden buildups of air pollution have caused widespread casualties. London experienced such episodes in January 1880, February 1882, December 1891, and December 1892. During the autumn of 1909, Glasgow, Scotland, suffered an acute episode, resulting in 1,063 deaths. In 1911 in a report on the Glasgow episode, Dr. Harold Antoine Des Vouex coined the word "smog" as a contraction of smoke-fog (*4*).

In 1911, the highly industrialized valley of the Meuse River in Belgium experienced a thermal inversion that trapped all pollutants along its 15-mile length. The resultant buildup of pollution caused scores of casualties. Virtually the same weather conditions recurred in December 1930. Few air-pollution controls had been established in the interim, and by 1930 the valley had become even more industrialized. The 1930 thermal inversion caused 63 deaths, and 6,000 people became ill (*5*).

The first reported air pollution disaster in the United States occurred in Donora, Pennsylvania, in October 1948. Donora is situated in a horseshoe-shaped valley of the Monongahela River, and the city contained large plants that produced steel, wire, zinc, and sulfuric acid. Fog closed in on the area, accompanied by a pollutant-trapping thermal inversion. Twenty deaths were attributed to the resultant buildup of air pollutants, and 1,190 people became sick (*6*).

In December 1952, London experienced another air-pollution episode, which resulted in 4,000–8,000 deaths (*7*). Although other acute air-pollution episodes have occurred since 1952 in such places as New York City; Los Angeles, California; Birmingham, Alabama; and Pittsburgh, Pennsylvania, none was of the magnitude of the episodes mentioned above. These latter episodes resulted in few deaths and relatively mild symptoms in a small subset of the population (*8–10*).

Since the United States Congress passed the Clean Air Act in 1963 and the Clean Air Act Amendments in 1970 and 1990, air quality in the United States has greatly improved, and the number of acute episodes of air pollution has decreased substantially.

Factors Influencing Morbidity and Mortality During the Early Disasters

Several studies conducted after these early air-pollution disasters provided some information on the types of adverse effects experienced during the episodes, the population segments at highest risk for experiencing adverse effects, and the nature of the air pollutants responsible for the effects observed. Although these studies varied in depth and design, their findings were consistent.

Meuse Valley, Belgium, 1930

The results of an investigation launched shortly after the Meuse Valley episode in 1930 indicated that most of the 63 deaths occurred among elderly persons and people who were not necessarily in poor health (although no age-specific rates were determined). Also among the dead were relatively young people who had preexisting diseases of the heart and lungs. Although people from these two groups were among the first to die, as the episode continued, thousands of otherwise healthy people became ill, and some of them died. No single pollutant could be blamed, and no pollutant ever reached the dose determined in laboratory settings to be lethal. Rather, it was thought that pollutants acting in combination intensified one another's effects. Probably the worst offender was the combination of sulfur dioxide and sulfuric acid mist. The investigators also judged that nitrogen oxides from fuel combustion and industrial processes contributed to the casualties and that particles of metallic oxides made the polluted air more hazardous (*11*).

Donora, Pennsylvania, 1948

The most thorough investigation of an episode of air pollution was carried out by the U.S. Public Health Service and the Pennsylvania Department of Health after the 1948 episode in Donora, Pennsylvania. In these studies, researchers determined that 5,190 Donorans—almost 43% of the people in the area—were made ill to some degree by the smog. The principal health effect was an acute irritation of the respiratory tract and, to a lesser extent, of the digestive tract and eyes. During the smog, 33% of the people in Donora developed cough, the most common single symptom. Other reported symptoms, in descending order, were sore throat, constriction of the chest, shortness of breath and difficulty in breathing, headaches, nausea and vomiting, smarting of the eyes, tears, and nasal discharge. Relatively few of the people affected by the smog escaped with an illness considered mild. Of every 100 people who became ill, at least 24 suffered severe symptoms and 39 experienced symptoms of moderate severity (as determined by how disabling the symptoms were, how much medical care was required, and how long symptoms lingered after the smog).

The morbidity rate rose with age; 31% of people age 20–24 years of age, 55% of those 40–44 years of age, and 63% of those 60–65 years of age became ill. The severity of illness also rose with age.

Preexisting disease of the heart or lungs was a major factor in many of the deaths from the smog, but not all of the deceased had histories of chronic disease. In four instances, the decedents had been in excellent health until they were affected by the smog. Autopsy reports for two of the victims listed bronchitis, pulmonary edema, and hemorrhage as the cause of one death and cor pulmonale as the cause of the other. The decedents ranged in age from 52 to 84 years (*12*).

A decade after the disaster, investigators reassessed the impact of the acute episode on the health status of the population of Donora and found that people who had become ill during the smog subsequently died younger and were ill more often than those who had not been affected during the episode. For those who had suffered severe complaints during the smog, death rates were particularly high. Even people who had no history of heart disease but who developed symptoms during the smog continued to suffer impaired health.

The investigators reported that a combination of pollutants had probably caused the disastrous effects. Sulfur oxides combined with airborne particles of metals and metallic compounds were the likely cause of the injuries incurred during the episode of smog (*12*).

London, England, 1952

Although no in-depth study was done immediately after the London smog episode, an analysis of death certificates and reports from several physicians who attended the ill during this episode revealed findings similar to those reported in the study in Donora, Pennsylvania.

The first evidence of illness and death associated with the smog was found among livestock. The opening of the Smithfield Club Show, one of Britain's most important livestock exhibitions, coincided with the onset of the air-pollution episode. The livestock—prize cattle brought from the best herds in the United Kingdom—were young, fat, and in prime condition. Despite the animals' good health, some 160 became ill soon after the onset of the smog. At first, the breathing of a cow or bull increased slightly, causing the animal to keep its mouth open. As the smog worsened, the animal's breathing became faster and more labored. Many animals in marked distress hung out their tongues and panted like dogs. Many grew feverish and refused to eat. Sixty developed severe symptoms and required major veterinary treatment. A dozen of the cattle—in pain and beyond hope—were slaughtered, and another animal died. Detailed examination of the carcasses indicated that the animals had suffered extreme respiratory irritation resulting in emphysema, pneumonia, and pulmonary edema.

Among humans, the most common symptoms were respiratory disorders, chiefly an extremely irritating cough sometimes accompanied by gray phlegm. Patients were debilitated by shortness of breath, convulsive coughing, and painful gasping for air. Many developed cyanosis and wheezing. The most severely ill patients were those with histories of heart or respiratory disease. At the Emergency Bed Service, requests on behalf of patients with heart problems were more than three times normal, and those on behalf of patients with respiratory disorders were nearly four times normal. Among patients with both heart and respiratory problems, the demand was even greater, and these people were the first to die. Typically, those ill from the smog took from 4 to 9 days to recover.

During the smog period, the number of deaths exceeded the norm by 2,851. In the following week, more than 1,224 other deaths were attributed almost exclusively to the smog. A study of death certificates for the months after the smog showed evidence of excess deaths occurring up to 12 weeks after the episode, bringing the estimated total deaths attributed to the episode to 8,000. People 65 years of age or older had a death rate 2.7 times the normal rate for their age group, and those age 45–64 had rates 2.8 times higher. Infants under 1 year of age had rates 2 times normal. No human autopsy reports were provided.

The coroner's statistics showed that during the episode, deaths occurred both inside and outside the home. Twenty-eight cardiac patients died suddenly while at their place of work or elsewhere outside their homes. One hundred five people suffered heart attacks while engaged in sedentary activities inside their homes.

The harmful agents in the London episode were thought to be a combination of irritant pollutants—principally smoke and sulfur dioxide. Smoke concentrations during the smog were measured at 5 times London's normal level. Particles of soot showed up universally in the residents' sputum. The general level of sulfur dioxide throughout the smog was about 6 times normal; in some areas, the sulfur dioxide concentration rose to 12 times the norm. An estimated 60% of the total pollution in the smog originated from domestic fires in which soft coal was burned. The remainder of the pollution came from commercial sources and motor vehicles (*7, 13*). Stronger air-pollution-control measures were instituted after the acute episode, with particular attention given to the control of smoke and suspended particulates.

New York City, 1953

A statistical study of emergency room visits and death certificates after an acute episode of air pollution in New York City in 1953 established that during the smog, a substantial number of people suffered cardiac and respiratory distress. Moreover, results of the final study indicated that 175–260 people died because of the smog (*8*).

Summary of Findings

Information from these early disasters shows that the population at greatest risk of morbidity and mortality is the group with preexisting respiratory and cardiac conditions. These people are the first to develop symptoms and among the first to die. As the episode continues, other segments of the population—particularly the old and the very young—become symptomatic, and many die. The primary symptom is respiratory irritation manifested by cough, but gastrointestinal symptoms such as nausea and vomiting may also occur. Cardiopulmonary complications are the major cause of death, and the limited information available from autopsy reports suggests that infection, pulmonary edema, and hemorrhage may contribute to death. The only study giving the location and activity of the decedents before they died was a report on the London episode of

1952, and that information showed that remaining indoors had no protective effect. However, because a major source of pollution in that episode was domestic coal fires, the indoor environment may also have been heavily polluted.

The follow-up study in Donora, Pennsylvania, suggests that people who experience symptoms during an acute episode of air pollution may have an elevated risk for subsequent illness and early death. The more severe the symptoms during the episode, the more severe the residual effect.

Although the technology for measuring pollutants at the time of these earlier disasters was quite crude by today's standards, there was some consistency in the assessment that a combination of pollutants rather than a very high level of a single pollutant was probably responsible and that the principal hazard was sulfur dioxide in combination with metallic particles.

Studies of Subsequent Moderate Air-Pollution Episodes

In the United States, air-pollution disasters resulting in very high morbidity and mortality have been averted since the institution of air-pollution regulations. However, moderate air-pollution episodes continue to occur under adverse weather conditions. These episodes have provided air-pollution investigators the opportunity to apply newer techniques and to understand better the contribution of lower levels of air pollution to morbidity and mortality. These newer studies have addressed the association between air pollution and mortality, between air pollution and specific types of morbidity, between air pollution and hospital and emergency room admissions, as well as pollution dispersion patterns and the indoor/outdoor ratio during air-pollution episodes.

Mortality

In a meta-analysis of seven United States studies examining the relationship between gravimetrically measured airborne particles and mortality, Schwartz suggested that a 100 microgram/m^3 increase in daily total suspended particle (TSP) concentrations is associated with about a 6% increase in mortality. This correlation is independent of SO$_2$ levels. The same TSP coefficient also explains the more than 2-fold increase in mortality in London in 1952 (*14*). In another study, by examining the death certificates from Philadelphia for the 5% of days with the highest particulate air pollution and the 5% of days with the lowest particulate air pollution during 1973–1980, Schwartz assessed whether the pattern of deaths at lower concentrations appeared similar to the pattern seen in the 1952 London air-pollution disaster. There was little difference in weather between the high- and low-pollution days, but total suspended particulate matter concentrations averaged 141 micrograms/m^3 on the high-pollution days versus 47 micrograms/m^3 on the low-pollution days. The highest numbers of deaths on the high-pollution days were from chronic obstructive pulmonary disease (COPD) and pneumonia, but the numbers of deaths for heart disease and stroke with respiratory factors listed as underlying contributory causes of death were also elevated. These observations parallel those of London in 1952 as well as the age pattern of the relative risk of death (*15*).

Spix et al. assessed the health effects associated with high ambient pollution due to unfavorable geography and emissions from coal burning in Erfurt, Germany, during 1980–1989. They used a multivariate model including corrections for long-term fluctuations, influenza epidemics, and meteorologic conditions. Daily mortality rates increased by 10% when SO_2 levels increased from 23 to 929 micrograms/m^3 and by 22% when particulate levels increased from 15 to 331 micrograms/m^3 (*16*).

Krzyzanowski and Wojtyniak studied the association between daily mortality and daily concentrations of suspended particulates and sulfur dioxide during the winters of 1977–1989 in Cracow, Poland. Suspended particulate levels exceeded 300 micrograms/m^3 on 21% of the days, and SO_2 levels exceeded 200 micrograms/m^3 on 19% of those days. Krzyzanowski and Wojtyniak estimated that the daily number of deaths due to respiratory system disease increased by 19% and that the number due to circulatory system disease increased by 10%, with an SO_2 concentration increase of 100 microgram/m^3. After adjusting for SO_2 levels, they found that suspended particulates had no additional effect (*17*).

Hospital Admissions and Emergency Room Use

Lipfert conducted a critical review of studies of the association between air pollution and the demands for hospital admissions and emergency room use, including studies of air-pollution episodes, time series analyses, and cross-sectional studies. Almost all of the studies reviewed found statistically significant associations between hospital use and air pollution; overall, a 100% increase in air pollution was associated with a 20% increase in hospital use. Respiratory diagnoses were emphasized in most studies, and cardiac diagnoses were included in five of the studies. The air pollutants most often associated with changes in hospital use were particulate matter, sulfur oxides, and oxidants. The link between air-pollution level and hospital use was limited to major air-pollution episodes (*18*).

From 1985 to 1987, in Barcelona, Spain, Sunyer *et al.* studied the relationship between emergency room admissions for chronic obstructive pulmonary disease and levels of SO_2 and black smoke, taking into consideration winter and summer periods as well as influenza epidemics. They found that an increase of 25 micrograms/m^3 in sulfur dioxide (24-hour average) produced adjusted changes of 6% and 9% in emergency room admissions for chronic obstructive pulmonary disease during winter and summer, respectively. A similar change was found for black smoke, although the change was smaller in summer. The association of each pollutant with chronic obstructive pulmonary disease admissions remained significant after researchers controlled for the other pollutant (*19*).

In the Ruhr District of West Germany, Wichman *et al.* studied hospital admissions, outpatient services, ambulance transports, and consultations in doctors' offices that occurred during a 5-day smog episode in 1985 and for 6 weeks following that episode;

they compared the frequency of these occurrences in the impacted area with their frequency in a control community. During the episode period, mortality and morbidity increased in the smog area, but there was no substantial increase in the control area. The total number of deaths was 8% in the smog area but 2% in the control area. Hospital admissions were 15% in the affected area vs. 3% in the control community, and outpatient visits were 12% in the smog area vs. 5% in the control community. The effects were more pronounced for cardiovascular disease than for respiratory disease. The maximum ambient concentrations exerted effects on the same days, whereas the daily averages were more pronounced after a delay of 2 days (20).

Smoke from bush fires has been linked to increases in emergency room visits for asthma in Sydney, Australia (21), and smoke from forest fires has been linked to increases in emergency room visits for asthma in California (22). These and other studies indicate that localized air-pollution episodes may play an important role in emergency room visits for asthma exacerbations (23).

Analysis of Dispersion Patterns During Air-Pollution Episode

A recent air-pollution situation that attracted worldwide attention was caused by the Kuwait oil fires. On February 23, 1991, more than 700 oil wells were set on fire throughout Kuwait. Careful monitoring showed that the levels of four major air pollutants (sulfur dioxide, nitrogen dioxide, carbon monoxide, ozone) did not reach harmful levels in residential areas. The average level of particulate matter measuring less than 10 microns (PM_{10}) during the period of the oil fires occasionally reached 500 micrograms/m^3. However, Kuwait has frequent sand and dust storms, and the average level of PM_{10} in Kuwait is 600 micrograms/m^3, the highest in the world.

Hazards posed by the smoke were less severe than had been anticipated because the plume of the fires rose up to 3,000 to 5,000 feet, mixed with the air, and then dispersed for several thousand miles over several weeks. As the plume traveled, it became more widely dispersed and also more diluted. The highest concentrations occurred in the areas nearest the affected oil fields and the areas immediately downwind. Luckily, few people except the firefighters were in this area.

Data collection from polyclinics and hospital emergency rooms in Kuwait began in January 1991. Preliminary analyses of emergency room surveillance conducted at two hospitals in Kuwait City from January 1 to April 30 showed no documented increase in the proportion of visits for acute upper- and lower-respiratory infections or asthma during the period after the oil wells were ignited. While few major acute health effects were attributable to the pollution from the oil well fires in Kuwait, it is not known whether people will have long-term health problems as a result of exposure to the oil well fires.

Protective Effect of Houses on Air Pollution Episodes

Danish investigators looked at the relationship between indoor and outdoor pollutants in 17 dwellings under varying conditions during an air-pollution episode. They found that staying indoors in a normal living room with closed windows and doors reduces the aerosol inhalation dose by a factor of 3. Operating a vacuum cleaner while staying indoors increases this reduction factor to about 9. Airing out the house 1 hour after the passage of a plume of 3 hours' duration raises these two factors to 6 and 12, respectively (*24*).

Single Pollutant or Combination?

These recent studies of less serious pollution episodes have provided more definitive information on the magnitude of change in air-pollution levels that will contribute to morbidity and mortality. Because patterns of morbidity and mortality seen at lower pollution levels are comparable to those observed at higher levels, these studies have reconfirmed the relationship between air pollution and serious health effects. However, results of these studies contain many inconsistencies in the specific pollutants reported to be associated with these effects. In some instances, total suspended particulates alone were incriminated; in other situations, SO_2 independent of total suspended particulates was associated with effects; and in some cases, fine particulates, particularly sulfates, were the associated pollutants. In most instances, a combination of TSP, SO_2, and black smoke was involved. These inconsistencies are not surprising given the fact that particulate air pollution is a mixture of solid particles and liquid droplets that vary in size, composition, and origin. Fine particulate pollution also contains acid sulfate and nitrate particles. The concentration of this combination of mixtures can change in varying settings and under varying conditions.

An alternative explanation for the association between pollution levels and health effects is that these complex mixtures may serve as surrogates for the specific agents associated with adverse effects. Because some of these studies did not monitor air pollution on a daily basis or use more than one monitoring station in a community, some study results may inaccurately reflect actual exposures in the study population. Peak concentrations in the rural regions may be as high as or even higher than levels in the urban/industrialized areas, and, depending on prevailing winds, an area may be affected either by emissions in the immediate area or by transported regional pollutants. Under these circumstances, the measured pollutant level may reflect conditions on the day and in the area where measurements were taken rather than the actual exposure of the population during the entire pollution episode.

The amount of time that people spent indoors during the air-pollution episode was often not considered in these studies and could be an important factor in assessing exposures.

Prevention and Control Measures

The principal steps to follow to prevent injury and death associated with acute air-pollution episodes are as follows:

- Recognize meteorologic conditions such as low wind speed and thermal inversions that might lead to a buildup of air pollutants. Meteorologists with the National Oceanic and Atmospheric Administration (NOAA) have an ongoing monitoring program for recognizing the presence of such adverse conditions in the United States. The NOAA meteorologists alert the U.S. Environmental Protection Agency (EPA) when such conditions are identified.
- Measure air-pollution levels during adverse meteorological conditions and prevent the buildup of hazardous levels of pollutants.
  - (a) EPA, in conjunction with state and local air-pollution agencies, has an ongoing air-monitoring network that covers many large industrial regions of the United States. Thus, a system is in place to monitor the ambient air in these areas during adverse meteorologic conditions. If a thermal inversion or air stagnation occurs outside the monitoring network, air-monitoring resources from federal, state, or local government agencies may be used.
  - (b) When air-pollution levels exceed the short-term standard, the EPA or the responsible state agency issues an air-pollution alert. EPA has the authority to shut down factories if it judges that continuing emissions from such sources during the adverse meteorologic conditions would pose a hazardous air pollution situation (25).

- Ensure that all personnel stationed or working in the immediate vicinity of dangerous air pollution levels be medically evaluated prior to their assignment for preexisting cardiac and pulmonary diseases and issued appropriate personal protective equipment. Ensure also that they receive sufficient training in the use of this equipment and in appropriate safety precautions.
- Alert susceptible segments of the population to take appropriate action and minimize their exposure to hazardous levels of pollution. The EPA, as well as some state health departments, has developed guidelines to be issued during air-pollution alerts. These guidelines contain precautions that susceptible members of the population should take under various conditions of air-pollution buildup (26). The Pollution Standard Index developed by the EPA is shown in Table 16-1. This index is used by many state and local health departments in the United States.
- Advise people residing in areas with significant air-pollution levels about measures they can take to reduce their exposures. These include limiting outdoor activities, keeping windows shut, and monitoring changes in their own health status. People should be educated as to early warning signs and symptoms of potentially serious exposure: runny nose, sore throat, watery eyes, chest pain, headache, nausea, dizziness, cough, and shortness of breath. Those people experiencing symptoms should be instructed to seek medical attention.
- Advise medical personnel of the potential health hazards posed by air pollution, and ensure that they are prepared to recognize possibly related health problems within the populations they serve. Medical personnel should be especially vigilant

in looking for the often subtle clinical presentations of the toxic effects of substances such as hydrogen sulfide and carbon monoxide, and they should know how to treat patients manifesting these effects. Both of these toxic inhalants have specific antidotal treatment with which medical personnel should be familiar.

- Disseminate information. Often an air pollution episode has gone unrecognized by a major portion of the population in the area involved. During the episodes in London and New York, many of the illnesses and deaths were not reported as being associated with the poor air quality. The media, particularly television and radio, can play a vital role in informing the public of potential adverse health effects of an air-pollution episode and of the precautions that should be taken. These precautions should include simple voluntary measures such as not smoking, maintaining an adequate diet, and learning to recognize symptoms of potential adverse effects and knowing steps to follow if such symptoms appear. It is important to have a communication network whereby people identifying adverse meteorologic conditions and a buildup of air pollution can convey this information through appropriate channels to the media for broad dissemination.
- Conduct surveillance. Through its air-monitoring network, the EPA conducts an ongoing surveillance program of ambient air quality in the United States. The resulting data permit potential problem areas to be identified in the event of adverse meteorologic conditions. Due to passage and enforcement of the Clean Air Act and its amendments, air quality in the United States has improved considerably, and the number of air pollution alerts has decreased dramatically.
- Provide further assessment of an acute air pollution situation.
  (a) Experts in the fields of environmental monitoring, air pollution, pulmonary medicine, clinical and laboratory toxicology, and public health should make site visits to the affected area.
  (b) Experts in emergency medicine should evaluate the medical facilities in the affected areas in terms of their capabilities to both diagnose and treat medical conditions that may occur as a result of exposure to air pollution. These facilities should have adequate cardiac and respiratory monitoring equipment, oxygen-delivery systems, chest X ray machines, airway-management equipment (e.g., endotracheal tubes), medications (e.g., beta-adrenergic agents) and supplies of antidotes for hydrogen sulfide poisoning (e.g., cyanide antidote kits).
  (c) Air monitoring should be conducted in major residential areas. Specific pollutants to be measured will depend on the individual circumstances but may include respirable particulates, sulfur dioxides, ions of hydrogen, hydrogen sulfide, and nitrogen oxides.
  (d) Surveillance systems for adverse health effects should be expanded in order to monitor the health status of people exposed to the air pollution. In addition, the availability of medical records for long-term follow-up of highly exposed people should be assessed by public health officials.

Table 16-1 Comparison of PSI* Values with Pollutant Concentrations, Descriptor Words, Generalized Health Effects, and Cautionary Statements

Index Value	Air Quality Level	Pollutant Levels					Health Effect Description	General Health Effects	Cautionary Statements
		TSP (24-hour) µg/m³	SO₂ (24-hour) µg/m³	CO (8 hour) mg/m³	O₃ (1-hour) pmm	NO₂ (1-hour) pmm			
500	Significant	600	2,620	50	0.6	2.0		Premature death of ill and elderly. Healthy people will experience adverse symptoms that affect their normal activity.	All persons should remain indoors, keeping windows and doors closed. All persons should minimize physical exertion and avoid traffic.
400	Emergency	500	2,100	40	0.5	1.6	Hazardous	Premature onset of certain diseases in addition to significant aggravation of symptoms and decreased exercise tolerance in healthy persons.	Elderly and persons with existing diseases should stay indoors and avoid physical exertion. General population should avoid outdoor activity.

300	Warning	420	1,600	30	0.4	1.2	Very unhealthful	Significant aggravation of symptoms and decreased exercise tolerance in persons with heart or lung disease, with widespread symptoms in the healthy population.	Elderly person with existing heart or lung disease should stay indoors and reduce physical activity.
200	Alert	350	800	15	0.2§	0.6	Unhealthful	Mild aggravation of symptoms in susceptible persons with irritation symptoms in the healthy population.	Persons with existing heart or respiratory ailments should reduce physical exertion and outdoor activity.
100	NAAQS	150	365	9	0.12	†	Moderate		
50	50% of NAAQS	50‡	80‡	4.5	0.06	†	Good		
0		0	0	0		†			

*Pollution Standard Index.

†No index values reported at concentration levels below those specified by "Alert Level" criteria.

‡Annual primary NAAQS.

§400 pg/m3 was used instead of the O3 Alert Level of 200 pg/m3 (see text).

Critical Knowledge Gaps

- The protective effect of staying indoors to prevent the acute health effects associated with an air-pollution episode has never been adequately evaluated.
- The protective effect of using specialized filters for home heating and air-conditioning systems during air-pollution episodes needs to be evaluated.
- The protective effect of a diet rich in antioxidants to prevent the adverse health effects of air pollutants needs to be evaluated.
- The effectiveness of public warning systems needs to be evaluated.

Methodologic Problems of Epidemiologic Studies

A common study design for assessing the health impacts of air pollution is the *hybrid ecologic study*. In hybrid ecologic studies of population health outcomes, researchers use time-series analyses to investigate relationships between air-quality data and population health outcomes. These studies differ from traditional ecologic studies in that they involve the use of community measures of air quality from air-monitoring stations and the analysis of the number of events (such as hospitalizations or emergency room visits) over time and evaluate how these numbers vary with variations in air quality. These studies have several limitations. First, they use crude measures of people's exposure to air pollution. Second, they assume uniform exposure to air pollution, a situation that is unlikely because of variations in people's activities. Third, the quality of the outcome data is questionable because of inherent problems of using hospitalization and emergency room data. For example, ill people who do not seek care at a hospital or emergency room are not included in the study, and there may be observer bias in assigning International Classification of Diseases (ICD) codes.

Research Recommendations

Although research studies have greatly augmented our understanding of risk factors associated with acute episodes of air pollution, the following research issues should be addressed in the event of future air-pollution episodes:

- During an air-pollution episode and for a period of time following the episode, ongoing air-pollution measurements of a broad spectrum of agents should be taken daily to determine the specific pollutants that might be associated with death and disease. More attention should be given to assessing the actual exposure of the study population, more widely distributed monitoring stations throughout the study community should be used, and the amount of time people spend indoors during the episode should be noted.

- During an episode, a reporting system should be established to assess more accurately the number of illnesses and deaths associated with the episode as well as the nature and severity of the illnesses. Reports should include information provided by private physicians, hospital inpatient and outpatient admissions, household sampling, and medical examiners and coroners.
- Case control studies should be conducted to determine whether limiting exercise and remaining indoors provide protection from illness or death.
- A cohort of affected individuals should be followed over time to determine whether they are at higher risk of having chronic health problems than are unaffected members of the exposed population.

Summary

Acute episodes of air pollution are caused by a buildup of pollutants during periods of low wind speed (<4 km/hour) or during thermal inversions. Increased industrial emissions coupled with increased aggregation of people in urban areas during the latter part of the nineteenth century created circumstances wherein large numbers of people were exposed to hazardous air pollution during adverse meteorologic conditions. Since 1870, at least 40 episodes of air pollution have been accompanied by deaths and illnesses. The largest number of deaths reported from an episode occurred in London, England, in 1952 when an estimated 8,000 people died from the effects of air pollution. People at greatest risk of morbidity and mortality from such episodes are those with preexisting respiratory and cardiac conditions. They are among the first to have symptoms and among the first to die. The old and the very young are also at increased risk of becoming ill and dying. The primary effect of air pollution is respiratory irritation manifested by cough and chest discomfort, but gastrointestinal symptoms such as nausea and vomiting may also occur. Cardiopulmonary complications are the major cause of death, and information available from a limited number of autopsy reports suggests that pulmonary edema, infection, and hemorrhage may contribute to death.

Findings from one study suggest that people who experience symptoms during the episode may be at higher risk for subsequent illness and premature death than those who experience no symptoms during the episode. The more severe the symptoms during the episode, the more severe the residual effect.

Although the technology for measuring pollutants at the time of these earlier episodes was quite crude by today's standards, studies of these episodes have been fairly consistent in showing that a combination of pollutants rather than a very high level of a single pollutant was responsible for the health effects and that the principal hazard was sulfur dioxide in combination with metallic particles.

Subsequent studies of episodes of moderate air-pollution levels have corroborated earlier findings from studies of more severe episodes concerning the populations most at risk and the types of illness and deaths associated with such episodes. They have also shed some light on the magnitude of change in pollution levels associated with illness and death. However, findings relating to the specific pollutants associated with morbidity and mortality are inconsistent. These inconsistencies may be attributed, in part, to the limitations of some of these studies as well as to the ever-changing complex mixture of pollutants involved in these episodes.

Death and injury from episodes of air pollution can be prevented by rapidly identifying instances of low wind speed and thermal inversions, by monitoring air pollutants during the period of adverse meteorologic conditions, by limiting pollution emissions when necessary, and by advising susceptible segments of the population to take preventive measures appropriate under specific air-pollution conditions. The Clean Air Act and its amendments have led to improved air quality in the United States, and the number of episodes of air pollution has decreased substantially.

References

1. Jacobson A. Natural sources of air pollution. In: Stern A, editor. *Air pollution*. New York: Academic Press, 1962: 175–208.
2. Smith KR. *Biofuels, air pollution and health: a global review*. New York: Plenum Press, 1987.
3. Halliday EC. A historical review of air pollution. In: *Air pollution*. Geneva: World Health Organization, 1961.
4. Lewis H. *With every breath you take*. New York: Crown Publishers Inc., 1965.
5. Ashe W, Kehoe R. *Proceedings of the National Conference on Air Pollution*. Public Health Service document no. 654, 1958.
6. Miller NR. Donora. *New Medical Materia* 1963;February: 23–24.
7. Smithard EHR. The 1952 fog in a metropolitan borough. *Monthly Bull Ministry of Health* 1954;February:26–35.
8. Greenburg L, Jacobs MB, Drolette BM, Field F, Braverman MM. Report of an air pollution incident in New York City, November 1953. *Public Health Rep* 1962;77:7–16.
9. Stebbings JH, Fogelman DG. Identifying a susceptible subgroup: effects of the Pittsburgh air pollution episode upon schoolchildren. *Am J Epidemiol* 1979;110:27–40.
10. Nelson CJ, Shy CM, English T, *et al*. Family surveys of irritation symptoms during acute air pollution exposures: 1970 summer and 1971 spring studies. *Journal of the Air Pollution Control Association* 1973;23(2):81–90.
11. Firket M. Sur les causes des accidents servenus dans la vallee de la Meuse, lors des brouillards de december 1930. *Bull Belgian Roy Acad Med* 1931;11:683–741.
12. Public Health Service. Air pollution in Donora, Pennsylvania: epidemiology of unusual smog episode of October 1948. *Public Health Bull* 1949;306:173.
13. Ministry of Health, United Kingdom: Morbidity and mortality during the London fog of December 1952. Report No. 95. London: *Ministry of Health Reports on Public Health and Medical Subjects,* 1954.
14. Schwartz J. Particulate air pollution and daily mortality: a synthesis. *Public Health Rev* 1991/1992;19:39–60.
15. Schwartz J. What are people dying of on high pollution days? *Environ Res* 1994;64:26–35.

16. Spix C, Heinrich J, Dockery D, *et al.* Air pollution and daily mortality in Erfurt, East Germany, 1980–1989. *Environ Health Perspect* 1993;101:518–526.

17. Krzyzanowski M, Wojtyniak B. Air pollution and daily mortality in Cracow. *Public Health Rev* 1991;19:73–81.

18. Lipfert F. A critical review of studies of the association between demand for hospital services and air pollution. *Environ Health Perspect* 1993;101:229–268.

19. Sunyer J, Saiz M, Murillo C, Castellsague J, Martinez F, Anto J. Air pollution and emergency room admissions for chronic obstructive pulmonary disease. *Am J Epidemiol* 1993; 137:701–705.

20. Wichman H, Mueller W, Allhoff P, *et al.* Health effects during a smog episode in West Germany in 1985. *Environ Health Perspect* 1989;81:129–130.

21. Churches T, Corbett S. Asthma and air pollution in Sydney. *NSW Public Health Bulletin* 1991;2:72–73.

22. Duclos P, Sanderson LM, Lipsett M. The 1987 forest fire disaster in California: assessment of emergency room visits. *Arch Environ Health* 1990;45:53–58.

23. Wheaton EE. Prairie dust storms—a neglected hazard. *Natural Hazards* 1992;5:53–63.

24. Roed J, Gjoerup H, Prip H. Protective effect of houses on air pollution episodes. *Denmark Government Reports, Announcements, and Index (GRA&I)* 1987;11:1–30.

25. Environmental Protection Agency. *Guide for air pollution episode avoidance.* SN5503–0014. Research Triangle Park, NC: Environmental Protection Agency Office of Air Programs, 1971.

26. Environmental Protection Agency. *Measuring air quality: the pollutant standards index.* EPA 451/k-94–001. Research Triangle Park, NC: Environmental Protection Agency Office of Air Quality Planning & Standards, 1994.

17

Industrial Disasters

SCOTT R. LILLIBRIDGE

Background and Nature of Industrial Disasters

Disasters that result from a society's technological activities are termed industrial or human-made. Such disaster events threaten the health of populations and are often associated with the release of hazardous substances or their by-products into the environment. Most catastrophic chemical releases or spills occur in the transportation phase of the industrial process (1). Because many manufacturing processes involve petroleum products, explosions and fires often occur in these disasters and may result in blast, burn, or inhalation injuries (2–5). Environmental consequences of industrial disasters may include chemical contamination of the water table, the soil, the food chain, or common household products (6, 7), and the resulting adverse health effects may be delayed for years and then appear as subtle impairments to the neurologic or immune systems (8, 9).

Mitigation of industrial disasters requires a multidisciplinary approach to protect the health of the public. Public health officials must communicate with various critical emergency personnel (e.g., law-enforcement officials, safety engineers) whose professions lie outside the traditional health field. At a minimum, industrial-disaster planning for health care professionals involves coordinating prehospital emergency-response procedures and ensuring that health professionals are able to access toxicologic information rapidly and that medical personnel have adequate training to provide emergency care in a chemically contaminated environment (10). Unfortunately, few public health professionals have received sufficient training in toxicology, environmental health, epidemiology, or occupational medicine to protect communities that might be endangered by an industrial disaster *(11, 12)*. This chapter addresses emergency public health issues associated with non-nuclear industrial disasters. (See Chapter 19, "Nuclear Reactor Incidents.")

Scope of the Problem

Industrial disasters and their public health consequences are increasing, particularly as societies with limited experience in occupational safety undergo rapid industrialization (Table 17-1) *(13)*. Recurrent problems related to industrial safety in developing countries include the inability to ensure the proper use of new technology, the lack of prehospital emergency medical services, and the underdevelopment of occupational health as a medical specialty *(14)*. Incidents such as warehouse fires in Bangkok, Thailand, in 1991 and the methyl isocyanate release in Bhopal, India, in 1984 highlight the risk to surrounding populations when heavily industrialized areas are located near residential communities *(8, 15, 6)*. In addition, low socioeconomic status may place the most vulnerable segment of the population at greatest risk from industrial disasters because these people have limited access to emergency services and live near hazardous industrial sites *(17, 18)*. The lack of effective urban zoning regulations that separate residential communities from industrial sites also contributes to this problem *(19)*. Occupational groups at risk for injury from industrial disasters include plant workers, emergency responders, the media, and law-enforcement officials *(1)*. Medical personnel who treat chemically contaminated people during an industrial disaster may also be injured unless they follow proper decontamination procedures and have access to and use appropriate personal protective equipment (PPE) *(20, 21)*.

The vulnerability of developed nations to industrial disasters is enhanced by their dependence on an increasing number of vital "lifeline" services such as electrical power, telecommunications, and natural gas that must be supported by a high level of sustained industrialization. From 1988 to 1992, more than 34, 000 chemical accidents occurred in the United States *(22)*. Most (85%) releases or spills in the United States

Table 17-1 Major Industrial Disasters Worldwide from 1945 through 1986

Time Period	Number of Events	Number of Deaths	Deaths per Year
1945–1951	20	1,407	201
1952–1958	20	558	80
1959–1965	36	598	85
1966–1972	52	993	142
1973–1979	99	2,038	291
1980–1986	66	9,382	1,340

Source: Glickman TS, Golding D, Silversman ED. *Acts of God and acts of man—recent trends in natural disasters and major industrial accidents.* Washington, D.C.: Center for Risk Management, Resources for the Future, 1992. *(13)*

Table 17-2 Hazardous Substances Emergency Events Surveillance, 1990–1992 (substances released during all hazardous-substance emergency events and during all such events resulting in personal injury,* by chemical category in selected states)

Substance Category	During All Events		During Events Resulting in Personal Injury	
	No.	%[†] Percentage	No.	%[‡] Percentage
Volatile organic compounds	727	(18)	93	(12)
Herbicides	588	(15)	126	(16)
Acids	553	(14)	148	(19)
Ammonias	448	(11)	103	(13)
Metals	261	(7)	21	(3)
Insecticides	217	(5)	80	(10)
Polychlorinated biphenyls	212	(5)	6	(1)
Bases	152	(4)	40	(5)
Chlorine	157	(4)	43	(6)
Cyanides	21	(1)	9	(1)
Unclassified	698	(17)	108	(14)
Total	4,034	(100)	777	(100)

*Refers to injuries and all other adverse health effects.

[†]Percentage of all substances released.

[‡]Percentage of all substances released during events that resulted in personal injury.

Source: Centers for Disease Control and Prevention. Surveillance for emergency events involving hazardous substances—United States. Surveillance summaries. *MMWR* 1994;43(SS-2):1–6. *(23)*

involve a single chemical agent, usually a volatile hydrocarbon compound (Table 17-2) *(23)*. Other substances that are commonly associated with industrial disasters include herbicides, ammonia, and chlorine *(23)*. In addition to fixed-site industrial hazards (e.g., manufacturing plants, storage tanks) throughout the United States, more than 4 billion tons of hazardous materials are moved each year on the nation's transportation routes *(24)*. Because such massive quantities of hazardous materials are moved on the nation's highway, rail, and pipeline systems each day, communities that apparently are not at risk for an industrial disaster may suddenly be required to respond to a major hazardous-materials emergency *(25)*.

Although less dramatic than a major explosion, environmental contamination from the toxic residue of industrialization has resulted in health and environmental problems of immense proportions. For example, more than 10, 000 sites in the United States have been identified as United States Government–managed environmental cleanup sites (or Superfund sites) because of lingering toxic effects at the sites and the concern for public safety *(25)*. Proper restitution of the environment will require expensive reclamation projects to correct contamination caused by chemical substances ranging from heavy metals to polychlorinated-biphenyls. Worldwide, problems involving the industrial contamination of food substances have raised interest in the importance of being able to investigate and identify rapidly such offending agents in the future *(7)*. Unfortunately, more than 600 new chemical substances enter the marketplace each month *(1)*. Such explosive growth in the rate of introduction of new chemical substances into the economy increases the likelihood that new agents will find their way into the food and water supply unless health professionals maintain proper concern for environmental health.

Two common emergency-response problems have surfaced in previous disasters. First, medical professionals with public health and emergency medical skills have not been included in community industrial disaster planning. This exclusion results in a lack of coordination between the public health and other critical emergency-response personnel (e.g., law enforcement, fire-safety officials, rescue personnel, regulatory agencies, disaster-management officials) during the actual disaster response. Second, public health officials usually do not view emergency preparedness for industrial disasters as an extension of their duties to protect the health of their communities. Consequently, communities near industrial sites may not benefit from effective industrial safety programs that include preparedness activities ranging from emergency response training to disaster planning for the needs of special populations.

Factors Affecting the Severity and Occurrence of Industrial Disasters

Natural Factors

The location of industrial sites in regions subject to natural disasters can substantially increase a nearby community's risk for industrial disasters *(26)*. Floods, earthquakes, and hurricanes not only destroy a community's civil infrastructure but also devastate its industrial base. Because natural disasters often affect a vast geographic area and disrupt communications and transportation systems, reports detailing secondary industrial emergencies may be delayed. In addition, limited emergency response resources may have been allocated to more readily apparent problems such as dealing with displaced people, fighting fires, and locating people who are trapped in collapsed buildings. Natural disasters also disrupt critical industrial safety systems, such as refrigeration systems, that may depend on electricity or on a sustained water supply to remain operational. The abrupt cessation of these services may result in the loss of industrial cooling processes vital to keeping hazardous chemicals in an inert liquid state and preventing them from converting to unstable volatile gases. Such a change in chemical state may result in sudden volume expansion of the contents of a storage vessel and cause leakage or explosions.

Human Factors

Human factors also contribute to industrial disasters. Human error from fatigue or inadequate training may increase the risk associated with industrial disasters *(27, 28)*.

Recent industrial disasters abroad raise serious questions about safely implementing potentially dangerous industrial technology in developing countries that lack strong occupational and industrial health expertise or functioning emergency medical systems. Social or cultural impediments in some regions limit the acceptance of realistic industrial-disaster training. As a result of lack of awareness and the paucity of effective industrial-disaster preparedness and mitigation measures, the threat of technological catastrophes will increase throughout the world. In the future, industrial terrorism may become a more common way to achieve political and military objectives. For example, in Kuwait after the Persian Gulf War, hundreds of oil wells were set ablaze and the resultant fires caused significant air pollution *(3)*. Other wells were left to discharge oil onto the desert floor and into Persian Gulf waters. Unfortunately, the environmental consequences of warfare directed against a nation's industrial base do not stop at that country's borders.

Public Health Impacts: Historical Perspective

On December 3, 1984, the world's deadliest industrial disaster occurred in Bhopal, India, when methyl isocyanate (MIC) vapor was vented into the atmosphere as the result of an operator error and malfunctioning safety systems within a Union Carbide plant in Bhopal. MIC is an intermediate product in the manufacture of carbamate pesticides (boiling point 39C, freezing point -80C) and has a vapor density that is heavier than air *(29, 30)*. Weather conditions at the time of the chemical release resulted in an atmospheric inversion. This inversion caused the plume of MIC to move slowly across the ground, spreading throughout residential neighborhoods and public gathering places. Because the release occurred at night and because warnings of the release were either delayed or not issued, many victims became aware of the dangers only when they were awakened by the irritating effects of MIC to their eyes and throats. In the darkness, victims suffering from the effects of MIC were unable to determine the precise source of the toxic plume; unfortunately, some moved toward the source of MIC rather then toward areas of relative safety. More than 2,500 people in the adjacent community may have died, and 200,000 persons were affected by the chemical release *(31, 32)*. Thousands of victims, seeking urgent medical assistance, overwhelmed local medical facilities. At the time of the disaster, many community officials and residents had no knowledge about the types of hazardous materials produced and contained within the Union Carbide plant. Consequently, emergency-response authorities were initially unclear about the nature and toxicity of the offending chemical agent, the type of medical treatment needed, and the extent of decontamination victims had to undergo before they could be treated.

The chemical release of MIC in Bhopal involved many deficiencies in common industrial safety measures and practices. For example, normal plant operation allowed long-term storage of MIC in large 40-ton tanks *(33)*. Typical industrial safety recom-mendations call for hazardous materials to be stored in smaller (e.g., 1–2-ton) containers to limit the chemical threat to workers and nearby communities in the event the integrity of a vessel is breached. Another design flaw included a protective water spray system that was intended to reduce gaseous discharges that reached a height of 12–15 meters. Tragically, the plant's flare tower was constructed to release toxic gases at a height of 33 meters, far above the level of the "protective" water spray *(33)*. Other factors associated with the Bhopal disaster included multiple failed or inoperative safety sys-tems at the industrial site. For example, nonfunctioning emergency systems included a ventilation scrubber that was designed to reduce the concentration of an agent involved during a chemical release *(34)*. Human factors also played a role. For example, at the time of the disaster, the number of people who worked the night shift was limited, and the training of plant staff in managing chemical releases may not have been adequate. Safety manuals were printed only in English. In addition, plant managers had limited knowledge of the toxic nature of MIC, and the plant had no emergency plans in the event of a major chemical release *(33)*.

The Bhopal disaster mirrors the situation that is found in many developing countries. In Bhopal, emergency preparedness and basic industrial safety for technological dis-asters were inadequate, and the marginal prehospital emergency medical system was not able to address rapidly the urgent health needs of the affected population. Subse-quent clinical studies, ongoing litigation, and the magnitude of the human impact as-sociated with the Bhopal disaster have highlighted the importance of ensuring adequate industrial safeguards in developing countries. However, incomplete epidemiologic stud-ies, laboratory sampling, and initial documentation of the clinical status of patients during the emergency response phase of the disaster at Bhopal limit the full evaluation of the public health impact of this disaster *(32, 35)*. Unfortunately, such deficiencies in emergency preparedness for, and response to, industrial disasters have been the norm.

Factors Influencing Morbidity and Mortality

Natural Factors

Proper industrial-site selection includes not only a consideration of nearby residential populations but also an appreciation for regional natural hazards such as earthquakes and floodplains. Other natural forces also influence the morbidity and mortality asso-ciated with an industrial disaster. For example, local weather conditions at the time of the Bhopal disaster resulted in an atmospheric inversion. This inversion increased the concentration of MIC near the ground and delayed the dispersion of this hazardous substance. Certain natural phenomena may resemble a catastrophic industrial chemical release. For example, Lake Nyos, in Cameroon, Africa, is located within the craterlike depression of an active volcanic field *(36)*. A massive amount of carbon dioxide gas released from beneath the lake bed of this volcano in 1986 is believed to have asphyxiated more than 1,700 people while they slept.

Human Factors

Although human error is an important factor associated with industrial disasters, the most important single factor that contributes to a population's risk from industrial disasters is allowing communities (whose residents are often impoverished, undocumented workers and families of workers) to settle immediately adjacent to hazardous industrial complexes. Throughout the developing world, the lack of effective residential zoning laws has resulted in the location of many communities near such complexes. In addition, many communities lack a coordinated emergency-response system that links the industrial site with local public safety agencies. Delayed notification of the appropriate authorities during a chemical release or spill reduces the time available for coordinating an appropriate emergency response and delays the evacuation of people at risk. In addition to concerns about warning and evacuation, preexisting medical conditions, such as lung or heart disease, may increase a person's risk for injury or death from the unintended release of toxic substances *(37)*.

Other human factors associated with plant operations that may increase rates of morbidity or mortality associated with an industrial disaster result from using highly toxic substances in industrial processes when less dangerous chemicals are available. In addition, poorly designed or maintained industrial plants and other factors such as worker fatigue due to poor shift planning or to overly long work periods may also increase morbidity and mortality rates *(27)*. Inadequate training for both routine and emergency plant operations and the lack of worker and employer participation in occupational safety programs increase the likelihood that such a disaster will occur and have severe effects on the population.

Prevention and Control Measures

Hazard Identification

The initial public health step in mitigating the effects of industrial disasters is determining the extent of the adverse consequences likely to result from a potential spill or release. This process, called hazard identification, requires identifying all chemical products that are stored, manufactured, or transported by local industry and that might affect the community in the event of an industrial disaster. In the United States, Material Safety Data Sheets (MSDS) provide a standardized way to communicate information about chemicals that are used or stored at industrial sites or that are being transported.

MSDSs detail the physical characteristics of the chemical agent and the expected health effects associated with human exposure. This information must be made available to health and safety officials who are responsible for planning for and responding to industrial emergencies. MSDSs also include information on chemical reactions and hazard-neutralization strategies. Using these data, officials can evaluate the range of potential hazardous-materials emergencies and their potential adverse health effects as part of local emergency-preparedness activities *(24)*. Worldwide, the United Nations' Substance Identification Number and the United Nations' Hazard Classification are found on International Chemical Safety Cards (ICSC) and contain information similar to that contained on MSDSs but have the added feature of providing more emergency medical-response data *(38)*.

Vulnerability Analysis and Risk Assessment

Another major industrial-disaster-mitigation activity is *vulnerability analysis (39, 40)*. This activity attempts to identify vulnerable populations and the adverse public health consequences associated with a potential chemical release, industrial fire, explosion, or other industrial processes. Vulnerable populations may be people with disabilities, children attending school, or patients and medical personnel working in nearby hospitals. Once vulnerable populations are identified, good disaster planning requires that officials determine the likelihood that a specific chemical substance will achieve toxic concentrations in the vicinity of that vulnerable population. This determination is known as *risk assessment*. Vulnerability analysis and risk assessment help disaster planners focus limited resources on plant sites or vulnerable populations that have the greatest potential for experiencing adverse consequences as a result of an industrial disaster. Ideally, such planning would focus on chemical substances discovered in the community through the hazard-identification process described above.

Emergency Preparedness

As part of their responsibility to protect communities from the effects of industrial disasters, public health professionals should facilitate communication between the local clinical community (e.g., hospitals, ambulance services) and occupational health professionals at the industrial site. Other industrial-disaster-mitigation activities for public health officials may include coordinating these activities: (1) arranging the medical care and proper referral destinations for patients exposed to hazardous materials, (2) establishing warning systems to alert nearby communities of a chemical release, and (3) determining minimal threshold concentrations of toxic chemicals that would require the community to evacuate in the event of a chemical release *(1)*. The initial epidemiologic activity required to protect public health during the emergency response phase of an industrial disaster is to conduct an initial disaster damage assessment *(34, 41)*. Proper epidemiologic assessment should try to determine the extent of the immediate chemical risk to the population, to prioritize critical response actions and resources, and to lay the groundwork for measuring chemical exposures and health outcomes in the future. In addition, epidemiologic assessment should determine if additional lifesaving or environmental health services will be required immediately at the disaster site.

Accurate and timely information concerning the physical properties of chemical agents and their clinical effects is an important requirement of industrial disaster preparedness and routine occupational health. Information on proper chemical neutralization, plume-dispersion estimation models, and appropriate antidotes for victims are vital elements of disaster management. For example, Table 17-3 contains a partial list of chemical agents and their associated antidotes that might be required by hospitals located near industrial sites. Information on hazardous material or chemical data bases is available on a variety of compact disc, read-only memory (CD-ROM) databases or accessible via on-line services (e.g., dial-in using a personal computer modem). These systems can help public health workers rapidly obtain detailed information about a hazardous substance *(24)*. Written reference material has the obvious advantage of being easy to use and is potentially less expensive. In addition, obtaining critical toxicologic information from books or manuals does not depend on functioning utilities (e.g., electricity, telephone lines) during a disaster. Regional poison-control centers provide 24-hour assistance in many countries. During an industrial disaster, a poison-control center can provide clinical information to medical responders *(42)*. These centers can give disaster-response personnel toxicologic information about both the nature of the offending agent and appropriate therapy, thereby limiting further exposure or injury. Table 17-4 lists federal organizations and resources that distribute information on hazardous materials and emergency management *(24)*. In addition to federal information resources, private companies and industrial consortia such as CHEMTREC offer this type of information or service.

During the emergency-response phase of the disaster, poison-control centers can give information on the selection of antidotes and their proper administration to victims. In many locations, these centers offer ongoing public health surveillance for acute and chronic environmental exposures and can coordinate the rapid distribution of antidotes during an industrial disaster. Most chemical spills involve one agent whose toxicity and medical treatment are known. However, since very few chemical agents have specific

Table 17-3 Toxins or Chemical Agents that Have Specific Antidotes

Toxin or Chemical Agent	Antidote
Cyanide	Sodium thiosulfate
Arsenic, Mercury	Penicillamine
Organophosphates	Atropine
Hydrogen Fluoride	Calcium gluconate
Aniline	Methylene blue

Table 17-4 Examples of U.S. Government Hazardous Materials and Toxicologic Information Sources

National Library of Medicine (NLM)
  NLM offers many electronic data bases such as MEDLINE and TOXLINE, which provide literature references, and CHEMLINE and TOXLIT, which provide information from books, and journals and information on other hazardous-materials databases.

NIOSH Pocket Guide to Chemical Hazards
  This text offers key information and data on 398 chemicals or substance groupings that are commonly found in the workplace.

National Response Center (NRC)
  The NRC provides 24-hour assistance and hazardous-materials information to people responding to major industrial accidents.

Agency for Toxic Substances and Disease Registry (ATSDR)
  ATSDR provides 24-hour assistance to emergency responders who require assistance in managing hazardous-materials emergencies. Such assistance includes information on treatment protocols, laboratory support, and emergency consultation related to assessment and decontamination.

Centers for Disease Control and Prevention (CDC)
  CDC provides the same level of services as ATSDR during hazardous-materials emergencies and also is capable of dealing with industrial disasters involving biologic agents.

National Pesticide Telecommunications Network (NPTN)
  This network provides information for dealing with pesticide exposures to medical personnel and emergency responders.

Source: Borak J, Callan M, Abbot W. *Hazardous materials exposure: emergency response and patient care.* Englewood Cliffs, NJ: Prentice-Hall, Inc., 1991. *(24)*

antidotes, proper patient decontamination remains one of the few effective medical remedies for treating patients who have been exposed to most hazardous substances.

Medical preparedness for an industrial disaster should include training medical personnel to care for patients in a contaminated environment and to treat chemically contaminated patients. A reasonable strategy for local public health officials would be to begin by training medical personnel at the industrial site and by training emergency medical personnel in the nearby community. Personal protective equipment (PPE) and a respirator to protect the airway from the effects of harmful chemicals are required to protect industrial workers and hazardous-materials emergency responders who may be required to work in hazardous environments *(43, 44)*. Other protective measures may be required to protect the skin and the eyes. Although increasing the levels (levels A–D) of personnel protective equipment has been recommended by the Environmental Protection Agency (EPA), depending on the magnitude of the hazard, level B is the generally recommended level of personal protection for entering an environment where the extent of the chemical hazard is not fully known. Level B protection consists of: (1) chemical-resistant clothing, boots, and hood; (2) double-layered chemical-resistant gloves; and (3) positive-pressure self-contained breathing apparatus. Clearly, performance impediments imposed by this level of equipment limit the effectiveness of emergency-response personnel in the field.

Generally, providing protective gear (e.g., gas masks) is impractical and potentially dangerous to the general population *(45, 46)*. The training needed by laypeople to use PPE effectively and the level of ongoing PPE maintenance and refresher courses required have generally been prohibitive when balanced against the relatively low probability of hazardous-materials disasters. Resources are often better spent on developing other industrial-disaster-mitigation strategies, such as evacuating people from the site of chemical exposure *(47, 48)*.

Planning for mass decontamination generally requires that the decontamination occur outdoors. Ensuring that chemically contaminated patients do not enter treatment facilities or emergency vehicles without first undergoing decontamination is vital if emergency medical operations are to be sustained during an industrial disaster. Specific equipment needs for decontamination include a water source, brushes, and mild soaps and detergents *(43, 44)*. Managing the effluent properly after patient decontamination is also part of hazardous-materials medical preparedness. Effective patient decontamination requires training and should be part of routine industrial-disaster drills *(49, 50)*. Medical planning for industrial disasters must include mechanisms to refer disaster victims from primary care sites to other medical facilities where critical specialty services (e.g., burn care) are available. Before an industrial disaster occurs, referral arrangements should be made with hospitals that have the capability of providing burn-care services and hyperbaric oxygen and surgical subspecialty (e.g., plastic surgery) services to potential victims. Patients may sustain burns and inhalation damage from fires in addition to the full range of traumatic injuries associated with explosions *(51)*. For instance, primary-blast injuries resulting from the direct effects of blast shock waves may threaten the lives of patients who may not show external signs of life-threatening injury *(52)*.

To assist states and local governments with the health component of hazardous-materials emergency-preparedness and -response activities, several resources are available within various federal agencies or departments (Table 17-5). Increasing emphasis on proper industrial disaster planning at the local level through such federal initiatives as Title III of the Superfund Amendments and Reauthorization Act (SARA) of 1986 has made planning and cooperation among emergency response organizations, local industry, and the community critical steps in industrial-disaster preparedness *(25)*. As a result of these legislative developments, industrial-site hazard-disclosure and com-

Table 17-5 Examples of U.S. Government Agencies and Departments that Provide Health and Environmental Emergency Technical Assistance during Industrial Disasters

Centers for Disease Control and Prevention
Agency for Toxic Substances and Disease Registry
Department of Defense
Environmental Protection Agency
United States Coast Guard

Table 17-6 United Nations Organizations or Joint Agencies that Provide Technical Consultation with Land-Based Industrial Disasters

United Nations Environment Programme (UNEP)
International Programme for Chemical Safety (IPCS)
World Health Organization (WHO)
World Meteorological Organization (WMO)
International Labour Organization (ILO)
Food and Agricultural Organization (FAO)
Industrial Development Organization (INIDO)

Source: United Nations Centre for Urgent Environmental Assistance (UNCUEA). *UNCUEA update* No. 3. Geneva, Switzerland: United Nations Centre for Urgent Environmental Assistance (UNCUEA), February 1994. *(16)*

munity-preparedness activities for industrial disasters are increasingly common in the United States. Worldwide, intergovernmental resources available through the United Nations' system provide technical assistance to countries with emergencies or with an interest in improving their industrial-disaster-prevention and -mitigation capacity (Table 17-6) *(53)*.

Emergency Response

Many disaster-management tools are available to assist public health officials in managing the health and medical aspects of an industrial disaster. Such tools include Computer-Aided Management of Emergency Operations (CAMEO), which was developed by the National Oceanic and Atmospheric Administration (NOAA) *(24)*. CAMEO is a personal computer (PC)–operated software program that allows disaster planners to create a database of industrial chemicals present at a local industrial site and to estimate rapidly the plume-dispersion patterns associated with a given chemical release. Such geographical-based information systems allow health officials to relate health and medical data to specific locations where vulnerable populations might be concentrated *(54)*. Such information can also assist local emergency managers in evacuating the affected community. In addition to United States Government (USG) information systems, many commercial vendors can assist health officials in establishing a community-specific geographical-based emergency information system that focuses on local hazardous materials. These systems can be used to enhance emergency medical response related to specific chemical risks within the community.

Assessment of Exposure

Urgent public health responsibilities associated with industrial disasters include measuring the chemical exposure of the affected population, characterizing injuries and the causes of death among victims, and evaluating the efficacy of the emergency medical response. These investigations may require skills from many allied health fields (e.g., pathology, laboratory science, toxicology, and environmental and occupational health). Measuring a person's or population's level of exposure to a particular chemical agent as a result of an industrial disaster includes considering the exposure time to a particular chemical agent; the route of chemical exposure (e.g., inhalation versus skin contact); and, perhaps, the distance from the source of chemical release *(55, 56)*. In the long term, it is appropriate to consider risk factors for chemical exposure by focusing on especially vulnerable groups and risky patterns of behavior *(10)*. Collecting this type of data often requires a detailed epidemiologic investigation. Specialized laboratory resources to analyze environmental samples (e.g., air, water, soil) or to measure physiologic changes associated with chemical exposure are often critical components of such epidemiologic investigations *(57)*. Since there are few biomarkers available to measure the level of human exposure to chemical agents, complex analytic models may be needed to accurately determine the degree of chemical exposure and the adverse health effects in the affected population. To determine a population's biological effect from exposure to a particular hazardous substance, detailed medical evaluations may be required in order to document associated clinical signs or symptoms *(29)*.

Surveillance

Surveillance is the logical continuum of the initial epidemiologic task of disaster assessment. Usually, surveillance activities begin as soon as life-threatening situations, such as a chemical plume, fire, or spill, is controlled and after contaminated patients have received appropriate emergency medical care *(10)*. Proper surveillance may involve obtaining medical information from workers or from members of the community, abstracting data from treatment facilities, or evaluating medical examiner reports for cause-of-death information *(58–60)*. In addition, information describing denominator data, incidence rates, the relative severity of injury, and the range of clinical presentations will serve as the basis for future population-based studies. Registries to track victims over time may be required for both medical and legal reasons.

Critical Knowledge Gaps

Many additional information resources must be developed to support public health officials in their efforts to prevent industrial disasters. The optimum flow of new chemical-product health information from the manufacturer to the health community has yet to be determined. Currently, no single comprehensive information source exists to keep public health officials apprised of the hundreds of new chemicals that enter the global market each year. Few state health departments are able to perform advanced laboratory analysis to support environmental health investigations of the myriad substances found in the industrial sector. Inexpensive direct laboratory tests and equipment that can be used rapidly in disaster settings to measure human exposure to chemical substances must be developed. In addition, the lack of a comprehensive nationwide surveillance program for chemical spills, releases, and subsequent adverse health effects has yet to be developed. Consequently, it is impossible to measure accurately the national impact of hazardous-material events. Other limitations in our knowledge concerning industrial disasters include difficulties in modeling the chemical exposure of populations, the lack of biomarkers, and the fact that many chemicals have not been fully studied.

Methodologic Problems of Epidemiologic Studies

Because manufacturer liability may be associated with technological disasters, all parties involved in litigation may demand rigorous scientific investigations to measure a person's exposure to a specific chemical substance and to link that event to a subsequent adverse health effect. When evaluating people who have been potentially exposed to harmful chemical substances, such factors as the length of exposure, a person's occupation, the severity of the exposure, the route of exposure (e.g., cutaneous versus ingestion) must be considered (56). Measuring human exposure to chemical substances through laboratory sampling has its limitations, because few chemicals have specific and quantifiable biomarkers. Because industrial disasters may affect many people and overwhelm medical facilities, accurate medical documentation describing injury and treatment may be lacking.

In addition, the health effects from a chemical exposure resulting from an industrial disaster may be delayed, and patients may need to be followed up medically for years or even decades. Table 17-7 depicts examples of chemical exposures that have known long-term health effects (61). Unfortunately, researchers estimate that the toxicity of only 7% of all known chemical substances has been fully investigated (31). Epidemi-

Table 17-7 Examples of the Medical Consequences of Chemical Accidents

Category	Example	Agent
Carcinogenic	Primary liver cancer	Polychlorinated biphenyls
Teratogenic	Cerebral palsy syndrome	Organic mercury
Immunological	Abnormal lymphocyte function	Polybrominated biphenyls
Neurological	Distal motor neuropathy	Tri-o-cresyl phosphate
Pulmonary	Parenchymal damage	Methyl isocyanate
Hepatic	Porphyria cutanea tarda	Hexachlorobenzene
Dermatological	Sicca syndrome	Toxic oil syndrome

Source: Baxter PJ. Review of major chemical incidents and their medical management. In: Murray V, editor. *Major chemical disasters—medical aspects of management.* London: Royal Society of Medicine Services Limited, 1990:7–20. *(61)*

ologic and toxicologic research often relies on animal models to establish the biological plausibility of an association of a particular toxic substance with a specific adverse health effect. Unfortunately, animals models may not accurately reflect the toxic effects that occur in humans. Proper epidemiologic study design for investigating the adverse health effects in a population affected by chemical exposure requires careful consideration of the common methodologic problems that arise. For example, even when registries accurately follow up patients longitudinally, finding suitable control subjects for case-control environmental exposure studies may be difficult, particularly if many years have passed since the initial exposure or if confounding influences that affect human health, such as increasing age and smoking, also have been in effect. Cross-sectional studies are useful in estimating prevalence, but the incidence of a developing medical condition resulting from exposure to a hazardous substance cannot be determined. Case-series reports may suffer from limited representativeness to the population being studied. Consequently, it is difficult to present convincing causal evidence that a specific chemical exposure is associated with a particular adverse health outcome. Cohort studies have limited value when the adverse health outcome under investigation is relatively rare. However, this study methodology may be extremely helpful when focused on high-risk populations (e.g., victims, emergency responders) *(62)*.

Research Recommendations

- Research to determine specific biomarkers for each hazardous chemical should be pursued vigorously because accurate assessment of chemical exposures is critical to managing industrial disasters appropriately. Currently, exposures to hazardous materials are difficult to measure, because many of the adverse health effects are associated with nonspecific signs and symptoms in the affected population. The science of determining specific biomarkers for each chemical is still in its infancy but offers hope for accurately assessing chemical exposures in the future.
- Applied research must be conducted to assist disaster managers in adapting new technologies to reduce the adverse health effects associated with industrial disasters. For example, the ineffectiveness of outdoor warning systems could be overcome through indoor electronic warning systems. The confusing array of new technologies that can be applied to mitigate the adverse health effects of industrial disasters has not yet been fully integrated into medical planning and emergency response.
- Disaster-preparedness and emergency-response standards for communities located near industrial sites need to be better developed. Currently, no universal professional consensus exists to guide local communities in developing such plans.
- Additional research is needed to clarify the criteria used for evacuating a com-

munity or sequestering its residents within their homes until a chemical plume has passed.

- Research is needed in order to understand how chemical substances degrade and how their disposal is best managed, because the ultimate fate of many chemical substances discharged into the environment is unknown.
- Research to standardize the assessment and tracking of health effects associated with industrial disasters is urgently needed. Currently, there is no consensus on the proper method to objectively measure an industrial disaster's severity and its subsequent environmental impact. Consensus will greatly facilitate the development of international data bases on industrial disasters. Such information would be valuable for future industrial-disaster-preparedness and mitigation and prevention activities.

Summary

Worldwide, industrial disasters are increasingly common and have profound implications for public health. Industrialized countries have become dependent on a wider array of chemical processes to manage their increasingly complex societies. Many developing countries are undergoing rapid industrialization without enough attention to industrial safety or occupational health. Prevention and mitigation of industrial disasters requires appropriate training of health professionals in emergency preparedness associated with hazardous materials and the proper application of new technologies to reduce adverse public health consequences. Recent trends in countries with strong worker safety and industrial safeguards indicate that deaths and injuries from industrial disasters are decreasing. These trends suggest that, when effective preparedness and mitigation programs are applied to the industrial sector, adverse health effects associated with these disasters can be prevented.

References

1. Doyle CJ, Upfal MJ, Little NE. Disaster management of massive toxic exposure. In: Haddad LM, Winchester JF, editors. *Clinical management of poisoning and drug overdose*. Philadelphia, PA: W. B. Saunders Company, 1990: 483–500.
2. Centers for Disease Control. *Health effects: the Exxon Valdez oil spill. A report to the President*. Washington, D.C.: National Response Team, 1989:32–33.
3. Etzel R. *Environmental impact: Kuwait oil fires. Report of the EPA/CDC assessment team*. Atlanta: Centers for Disease Control, 1991.
4. Etzel R. *Oil well fire/release, Uzbekistan, March–April, 1992. Report of the EPA/CDC assessment team*. Atlanta: Centers for Disease Control, 1992.
5. Phillips YY. Primary blast injury. *Ann Emerg Med* 1986;15:1446.
6. Centers for Disease Control. Preliminary Report: 2,3, 7, 8-tetrachlorodibenzo-p-dioxin exposure to humans—Seveso, Italy. *MMWR* 1988;37:733–736.

7. Centers for Disease Control. Followup on toxic pneumonia—Spain. *MMWR* 1981;30:436–438.

8. Andersson N. Technological disasters: towards a preventive strategy: a review. *Trop Doct* 1991;21(Suppl. 1):70–81.

9. Straight MJ, Kipen HM, Vogt RF, Maler RW. *Immune function test batteries for use in environmental health field studies.* Atlanta, GA: Agency for Toxic Substances and Disease Registry, 1994.

10. Falk H. Industrial/chemical disasters: medical care, public health and epidemiology in the acute phase. In: Bourdeau P, Green G, editors. *Methods for assessing and reducing injury from chemical accidents.* Chichester, England: John Wiley and Sons, 1989:105–114.

11. Waeckerle JW, Lillibridge SL, Burkle FM, Noji EK. Disaster medicine: challenge for today. *Ann Emerg Med* 1994;23:715–718.

12. Binder S, Sanderson LM. The role of the epidemiologist in natural disasters. *Ann Emerg Med* 1987;16:1081–1084.

13. Glickman TS, Golding D, Silversman ED. *Acts of God and acts of man—recent trends in natural disasters and major industrial accidents.* Washington, D.C.: Center for Risk Management, Resources for the Future, 1992.

14. Lillibridge SR, Noji EK. *Trip report: industrial preparedness Bombay, India. World Environmental Center—Centers for Disease Control and Prevention emergency preparedness visit of March 1993.* Atlanta, GA: Centers for Disease Control and Prevention, 1993.

15. Brenner SA, Miller L, Noji EK. *Chemical fire explosion disaster in Bangkok, Thailand.* Atlanta: Centers for Disease Control and Prevention, 1992. EPI-AID 91-34-2.

16. United Nations Centre for Urgent Environmental Assistance (UNCUEA). *UNCUEA update No.3.* Geneva, Switzerland: United Nations Centre for Urgent Environmental Assistance (UNCUEA), February 1994.

17. Le Claire G. *Environmental emergencies—a review of emergencies and disasters involving hazardous substances over the past 10 years. Vol. 1 Report.* Geneva: United Nations Centre for Urgent Environmental Assistance (UNCUEA), 1993.

18. International Federation of Red Cross and Red Crescent Societies. *World disaster report 1993.* Norwell, MA: Kluwer Academic Publishers, 1993.

19. Noji EK. Public health challenges in technological disaster situations. *Arch Public Health* 1992;50:99–104.

20. Nadig R. Hazardous materials releases and decontamination. In: Goldfrank LR, editor. *Toxicologic emergencies*, 5th ed. Norwalk, CT: Appleton & Lange, 1994:1265–1276.

21. Centers for Disease Control and Prevention. Recommendations for civilian communities near chemical weapons depots: guidelines for medical preparedness. *Federal Register* 1994; 59(143):1–34.

22. National Environmental Law Center and the U.S. Public Research Interest Group. *Chemical releases statistics.* Washington, D.C.: Associated Press International (API), 1994.

23. Centers for Disease Control and Prevention. Surveillance for emergency events involving hazardous substances—United States. Surveillance summaries. *MMWR* 1994;43(SS-2):1–6.

24. Borak J, Callan M, Abbot W. *Hazardous materials exposure: emergency response and patient care.* Englewood Cliffs, NJ: Prentice-Hall, Inc., 1991.

25. Melius J, Binder S. Industrial disasters. In: Gregg M, editor. *The public health consequences of disasters.* Atlanta: Centers for Disease Control, 1989:97–102.

26. Office of U.S. Foreign Disaster Assistance. *Egypt—Disaster assessment response team report of the November 1994 flood/fire disaster.* Washington, D.C.: Office of U.S. Foreign Disaster Assistance, 1994.

27. Krieger GR. Shift work studies provide clues to industrial accidents. *Occup Health Saf* 1987; January-1987:21–34.

28. Yechiam Y. Preventive safety measures in industrial plants with chemical hazards: Intel's experience. *Public Health Rev* 1993;20:324–325.

29. Dhara R. Health effects of the Bhopal gas leak: a review. *Epidemiologia e Prevenzione* 1992; 52:22–31.

30. Lorin HG, Kulling PEJ. The Bhopal tragedy—what has Swedish disaster medicine planning learned from it. *J Emerg Med* 1986;4:311–316.

31. Mehta PS, Anant AS, Mehta SJ, *et al.* Bhopal tragedy's health effects: a review of methyl isocyanate toxicity. *JAMA* 1990;264:2781–2787.

32. Anderson Neil. Disaster epidemiology: lessons from Bhopal. In: Murray V, editor. *Major chemical disasters—medical aspects of management.* London: Royal Society of Medicine Services Limited, 1990:183–195.

33. Shrivastava P. *Bhopal: anatomy of a crisis.* Cambridge, MA: Ballinger Publishing Co., 1987.

34. Sanderson LM. Toxicologic disasters: natural and technologic. In: Sullivan JB, Krieger GR, editors. *Hazardous materials toxicology—clinical principles of environmental health.* Baltimore, MD: Williams and Wilkins, 1992:326–331.

35. Koplan JP, Falk H, Green G. Public health lessons from the Bhopal chemical disaster. *JAMA* 1990;264:2795–2796.

36. Baxter PJ. Volcanoes. In: Gregg M, editor. *The public health consequences of disasters.* Atlanta: Centers for Disease Control, 1989:25–32.

37. Baxter PJ, Ing RT, Falk H, *et al.* Mount St. Helens eruptions, May 18 to June 12, 1980: an overview of the acute health impact. *JAMA* 1981;246(22):2585–2589.

38. Organization for Economic Cooperation and Development (OECD). *Health aspects of chemical accidents: guidance on chemical accident awareness, preparedness and response for health professionals and emergency responders.* Paris: Organization for Economic Cooperation and Development (OECD), 1994.

39. National Response Team. *Hazardous materials emergency planning guide.* Washington, D.C.: National Response Team, 1987.

40. Noji EK. Chemical hazard assessment and vulnerability analysis. In: Holopainen M, Kurttio P, Tuomisto J, editors. *Proceedings of the African workshop on health sector management in technological disasters. 1990 Nov 26–30; Addis Ababa, Ethiopia.* Kuopio, Finland: National Public Health Institute, 1991:56–62.

41. Lillibridge SR, Noji EK, Burkle FM. Disaster assessment: the emergency health evaluation of a population affected by a disaster. *Ann Emerg Med* 1993;22:1715–1720.

42. Tong TG. Risk assessment of major chemical disasters and the role of poison centres. In: Murray V, editor. *Major chemical disasters—medical aspects of management.* London: Royal Society of Medicine Services Limited, 1990:141–148.

43. Agency for Toxic Substances and Disease Registry (ATSDR). *Hospital guidelines for medical management of chemically contaminated patients.* Atlanta: Agency for Toxic Substances and Disease Registry (ATSDR), 1992.

44. Agency for Toxic Substances and Disease Registry (ATSDR). *Prehospital guidelines for medical management of chemically contaminated patients.* Atlanta: Agency for Toxic Substances and Disease Registry (ATSDR), 1992.

45. Bleich A, Dycian A, Koslowsky M, Solomon Z, Wiener M. Psychiatric implications of missile attacks on a civilian population. *JAMA* 1992;268:613–632

46. Golan E, Shemer J, Arad M, Nehama H, Atsmon J. Medical limitations of gas masks for civilian populations: the 1991 experience. *Mil Med* 1992;157:444–446.

47. Duclos P, Sanderson L, Thompson FE, Brackin B, Binder S. Community evacuation following a chlorine release, Mississippi. *Disasters* 1988;11:286–289.

48. Duclos P, Binder S, Riester R. Community evacuation following the Spenser metal processing plant fire, Nanticoke, Pennsylvania. *J Hazardous Materials* 1989;22:1–11.

49. Federal Emergency Management Agency and the Department of the Army. *Planning guidance for the chemical stockpile emergency preparedness program*. Washington, D.C.: Federal Emergency Management Agency, 1992.

50. United States Army Medical Research Institute of Chemical Defense. *Medical management of chemical casualties*. Aberdeen Proving Ground, MD: Chemical Casualty Office of the United States Army Medical Research Institute of Chemical Defense, 1992.

51. Department of Defense. Blast injuries. In: Bowen TE, Bellany RR, editors. *Emergency War Surgery*. Washington, D.C.: U.S. Government Printing Office, 1988:74–82.

52. Waeckerle JF. Disaster planning and response. *N Eng J Med* 1991;324:815–821.

53. Yeater M, Ockwell R. *International emergency response capabilities—a review of existing arrangements both within and outside the UN system*. Geneva: United Nations Environment Programme (UNEP), United Nations Centre for Urgent Environmental Assistance (UNCUEA), 1993.

54. Stockwell JR, Sorensen JW, Eckert JW. The U.S. EPA geographic information system for mapping environmental releases of toxic chemicals. Toxic chemical release inventory (TRI). *Risk Anal* 1993;13:155–164.

55. Centers for Disease Control. Dermatitis among workers cleaning the Sacramento river after a chemical spill—California. *MMWR* 1991;40:825.

56. Agency for Toxic Substances and Disease Registry (ATSDR). *ATSDR public health assessment guidance manual*. Chelsea, MI: Lewis Publishers, 1992.

57. Dhara RV, Kriebel D. The Bhopal gas disaster: it's not too late for sound epidemiology. *Arch Environ Health* 1993;48:436–437.

58. Glass RI, Noji EK. Epidemiologic surveillance following disasters. In: Halperin WE, Baker E, editors. *Textbook of public health surveillance*. New York: Van Nostrand Reinhold, 1992:195–205.

59. Baron RC, Etzel RA, Sanderson LM. Surveillance for adverse health effects following a chemical release in West Virginia. *Disasters* 1988;12:356–365.

60. Parrish RG, Falk H, Melius JM. Industrial disasters: classification, investigation and prevention. *Recent Advances in Occupational Health* 1987;3:155–168.

61. Baxter PJ. Review of major chemical incidents and their medical management. In: Murray V, editor. *Major chemical disasters—medical aspects of management*. London: Royal Society of Medicine Services Limited, 1990:7–20.

62. Piantadosi S. Epidemiology and principles of surveillance regarding toxic hazards in the environment. In: Sullivan JB, Krieger GR, editors. *Hazardous materials toxicology. Clinical principles of environmental health*. Baltimore, MD: Williams and Wilkins, 1992:61–64.

18

Fires

LEE M. SANDERSON

Background and Nature of Fire Disasters

Since ancient times, fires have had an adverse impact on public health. With time, that impact has changed. The scientific literature suggests many criteria for defining disasters, including cause, duration, extent of damage, and number of casualties. Organizations such as the Metropolitan Life Insurance Company (MLIC) and the Occupational Safety and Health Administration (OSHA) consider a catastrophe (disaster) to be an event that causes at least 5 casualties—five people must die, according to MLIC; 5 people must either die or be hospitalized, according to OSHA. The National Fire Protection Agency (NFPA) currently defines catastrophic fires as residential fires that result in 5 or more deaths and nonresidential fires that result in 3 or more deaths. Causal patterns vary with time, and the risks that contemporary America faces are quite different from those faced 30, 50, or 100 years ago. A basic understanding of how these risks have changed assists us in identifying prevention measures that were efficacious in the past or that may be useful in the future.

In the United States, fire disasters that resulted in tens or hundreds of deaths used to be relatively rare. Today, it is clear from statistical evidence that the major adverse public health effect of fires is the total mortality and morbidity that results from fires in one- and two-family residences.

Scope and Relative Importance of Fire Disasters

According to a Metropolitan Life Insurance Company study (1), fires accounted for 31.2% of all disasters in the United States from 1941 through 1975 (Table 18-1). Fur-

Table 18-1 Civilian Disasters and Associated Deaths, by Type of Disaster, United States, 1941–1975

Type of Disaster	Number of Incidents	Number of Deaths
Fire and Explosion	1,369	12,128
Houses, apartments	935	5,716
Hotels, boarding houses	101	1,072
Hospitals, nursing homes	59	861
Public places	12	835
Other	262	3,644
Motor vehicle	1,659	10,516
Air transportation	451	7,756
Water transportation	225	2,226
Railroad	78	1,342
Weather phenomenon	335	8,279
Mines and quarries	94	1,612
All other	162	1,252
TOTAL	**4,393**	**45,117**

Source: Metropolitan Life Insurance Company. Catastrophic accidents, a 35-year review. *Stat Bull Metrop Insur Co* 1977;58:1–4. *(1)*

thermore, fires accounted for 26.9% of all disaster-associated mortality. Fully 68.3% of the fires and 47.1% of the associated deaths occurred in houses or apartments. Only 7.4% occurred in temporary public residences (hotels and boardinghouses), 4.3% in treatment centers (nursing homes and hospitals), and 0.9% in public places.

Burn injuries continue to be a common problem, both in the United States and throughout the world *(2)*. Each year in the United States, fires result in 5,000 to 6,000 deaths and more than 1 million injuries that require medical attention. Of these injuries, 90, 000 result in admissions to hospitals and 300, 000 involve visits to emergency rooms *(3)*. Fatal burns represent a disproportionate loss of person-years of life compared to mortality resulting from chronic disease. Nonfatal burns often have severe consequences for the victim, for his or her family, and for society, including costly medical care, permanent or temporary unemployment, and physical or mental sequelae *(2)*.

Factors that Contribute to Fire Disasters

The relative importance of types of fire disasters has changed over time. Historically, the occurrence of citywide conflagrations or natural firestorms were of primary public health importance. In contemporary times, the greatest public health risks of fire in the United States occur in single-family homes or duplexes.

Data from NFPA show that in the United States from 1980 through 1984, 87.5% of all fire disasters and 83.5% of all associated deaths occurred in residential properties *(4)*. For 1984, 67.2% of all residential fire disasters occurred in one- or two-family dwellings (excluding mobile homes), 16.3% occurred in apartments, 10.9% occurred in mobile homes, and 6.6% occurred in rooming or lodging facilities. Therefore, from a public health perspective, any focus on fires should emphasize occurrences involving single-family residences or duplexes.

Factors Affecting Fire Disaster Occurrence and Severity

Fires may accompany natural disasters such as earthquakes or volcanic eruptions. Sources of ignition for fire disasters include lightning, human carelessness, arson, and malfunctioning equipment. Fire disasters have occurred above the ground (in tall buildings and on planes), on the ground, and below the ground (in mines and caves). Sometimes they occur in circumstances that are unexpected or unpredictable. Seven descriptive categories of fire disasters along with selected examples, are shown in Table 18-2 *(5, 6)*.

Natural Factors

The first category listed in Table 18-2 is disasters resulting from forest fires. The three examples provided occurred either before or during the early 1900s and involved three states. During that period, information dissemination, warning systems, firefighting equipment, and control capabilities were not as sophisticated as those available today. Forest fires now have far greater impact on the environment than on the health of the surrounding communities. Each year such fires destroy thousands of acres of valuable grass and timberland, but their impact on human morbidity and mortality is small. For example, the 1947 Maine fire resulted in 16 deaths, 1,200 structures damaged, and 206, 000 acres of timber and scenic forest destroyed; the 1964 Cayote, California, fire resulted in 1 death, 188 structures damaged, and 175, 000 acres of watershed land destroyed; and the 1977 Santa Barbara, California, fire left no deaths, 250 structures damaged, and 800 acres of watershed land destroyed.

Tangentially related but basically different are firestorms—both naturally occurring and human-generated. Natural storms develop from forest fires. Firestorms result in a convection plume consisting of hot gases that causes air to be drawn inward at the base of the plume. This plume of wind then begins to rotate and form a fire-induced cyclone that, like a tornado, has counterclockwise winds in the Northern Hemisphere. The worst known natural firestorm occurred in Pehtigo, Wisconsin, in 1871. It burned more than 2,000 square miles of forest and killed approximately 2,300 people. Near Sundance, Ohio, in 1967, a firestorm had surface winds of 50 mph and peak winds of 120 mph; it lasted for 9 hours. This fire storm destroyed 70 square miles of land. Nowadays, the incidence of natural firestorms has been so reduced through building and fire-control practices that any adverse public health impact is small.

Table 18-2 Selected Fire Disaster, by Category, Date and Associated Mortality, United States (1871–1980)

Category	Location	Date	Number of Fatalities
Forests			
	Michigan and Wisconsin	1871	1,000
	Minnesota	1894	894
	Minnesota and Wisconsin	1918	1,000
Cities			
	Chicago	1871	766
	Peshtigo, Wisconsin	1871	800
	San Francisco	1906	1,188
	Chelsea, Massachusetts	1908	18
Ships			
	New York Harbor	1904	1,000
	Rhode Island coast	1954	103
Hotels			
	Winecoff (Atlanta)	1946	119
	LaSalle (Chicago)	1946	61
	MGM Grand (Las Vegas)	1980	84
Places of entertainment			
	Theater (Chicago)	1903	602
	Dance Hall (Mississippi)	1940	207
	Nightclub (Massachusetts)	1942	492
	Circus (Connecticut)	1944	163
	Supper Club (Kentucky)	1977	164
Health Care Facilities			
	Hospital (Oklahoma)	1918	38
	Nursing Home (Missouri)	1957	72
	Hospital (Connecticut)	1961	16
	Nursing Home (Ohio)	1963	63
	Nursing Home (Ohio)	1970	31
Schools			
	Collinwood, Ohio	1908	161
	Chicago, Illinois	1958	93

Sources: Lyons JW. *Fire*. New York: Scientific American Library, 1985 (5); Eckert WG. The medico-legal and forensic aspects of fires. *Am J Forensic Med Pathol* 1981;2(4):347–356 (6).

Human-Generated Factors

Human-generated firestorms resulted from incendiary bombing during World War II. In Hamburg, Germany, on February 27, 1943, the Allied Forces dropped bombs that caused a firestorm with winds up to 100 mph; the fire storm destroyed 3.2 square miles of the city and killed 21, 000 residents. In Dresden, Germany, on February 13 and 14,

1945, bombs induced a firestorm that had surface winds up to 80 mph, burned 4.6 square miles of the city, and killed 135, 000 people. On March 20, 1945, an incendiary attack on Tokyo resulted in a firestorm that killed 84, 000 persons.

As with forest-fire disasters, citywide conflagrations in the United States were most devastating before or during the early 1900s. Sources of ignition for these fire disasters were both human (Chicago fire) and natural (San Francisco earthquake fire). The source of combustion was frequently wooden structures crowded onto small areas. The contemporary risk of this category of fire disaster has been minimized by developing and enforcing building codes, setting standards to ensure that all fire equipment is compatible with sources of water (e.g., fire hydrants), and regulating combustible materials in buildings. However, buildings are still susceptible to massive fires that are deliberately caused; a recent example is the fire that resulted from the bomb explosion at the World Trade Center in New York City.

On Friday, February 26, 1993, a bomb exploded beneath the twin towers of the World Trade Center, a seven-building complex where 40, 000 people work and another 80, 000 people visit each day (7). The intense fire caused by the bomb blast sent smoke up the elevator shafts, onto the tower's floors, and then into the stairwells. Of the 548 people treated for disaster-related morbidity, 485 (88.8%) were treated for smoke inhalation, 38 (7.0%) for minor trauma, 9 (1.6%) for major trauma, 3 (0.5%) for cardiac conditions, 1 (0.2%) for psychological conditions, and 10 (1.8%) for other conditions. Risk factors for hospitalization included older age, having a preexisting cardiopulmonary condition, being trapped in an elevator, and not evacuating the premises quickly.

The third category of historical fire disasters consists of fires in places where groups of generally healthy persons reside on a temporary basis (e.g., ships or in hotels). In recent times, building codes have increased the safety of such places by establishing criteria for interior passages, stairwells, and exits. These criteria are designed to prevent passageways and stairwells from becoming chimneys or corridors for fires and to ensure that people have ample means of escape. Public health problems can result when existing building codes are not followed. In the United States from 1934 to 1961, 130 hotel fires killed 1,204 people (5). In November 1980, the Las Vegas MGM Grand Hotel fire killed 84 people. Investigation of this disaster showed that three of the four stairwells and their access panels did not comply with all fire codes (5). The fire and products of combustion that killed people spread through these stairwells. A fire in the Dupont Plaza Hotel in San Juan, Puerto Rico, on December 31, 1986, killed 97 people and injured more than 140 others (8). This fire was of incendiary origin and was started in a stack of new furniture still in boxes. Autopsy results indicated that burns rather than smoke inhalation caused the majority of deaths.

Places of entertainment present special problems for the enforcement of fire codes. In such locations, large numbers of people are crowded into unfamiliar and enclosed spaces. The exits may malfunction or be too few or the furnishings and decorations may be made of flammable materials. Perhaps the most famous fire disaster in this category was the Coconut Grove nightclub fire in Boston in November 1942. In this incident, most exits were either locked or they malfunctioned. A total of 492 persons died, and many others sustained serious burns.

Locations such as health care facilities and schools, in which many people depend upon others for safety and well-being, are associated with even higher risks than are hotels and places of entertainment. These risks are reduced when (1) the buildings are designed with the understanding that some occupants will require assistance in the event of a fire, (2) evacuation plans are developed and practiced, and (3) modern safety features (e.g., fire doors and sprinklers) are installed.

Public Health Impacts of Fire Disasters: Historical Perspective

For children and adults combined, burn injuries are the second most frequent cause of death in the home, preceded only by falls (9). For adults, burn injuries result in more catastrophic fatalities than any other cause (1). In the United States the annual number of burn injuries among adults is estimated at 1 million (10). Estimates of adult rates of burn injuries requiring hospitalization range from 26 to 37 burn injuries per 100, 000 adults (11–15). With respect to number of years of life lost by death from specific causes (16), the prevention of one death from burns results in more years of life saved than the prevention of one death from cancer or cardiovascular disease (17).

An analysis of annual mortality data of the National Center of Health Statistics (NCHS) shows that from 1978 through 1984, an average of 4,897 persons died each year in residential fires (18). Groups with the highest death rates due to fires included blacks, adults 65 years of age or older, and children 5 years of age or younger. Most of these deaths occurred when a structure caught fire (conflagration), rather than when clothes caught fire. A similar analysis of data from 1979 through 1985 indicates that smoke inhalation accounted for two-thirds of the deaths and burns accounted for one-third (19).

The most current data available from the NFPA are shown in Table 18-3. In the United States during 1992, there were almost 2 million fires, only 35 of which were

Table 18-3 Fires in the United States, 1992

	All Fires	Catastrophic Fires*
Number of Fires	1,964,500	35
Number of Civilian Deaths	4,730	176
Number of Civilian Injuries	28,700	Not reported

*As defined by the NFPA—residential fires, resulting in 5 or more deaths or nonresidential fires resulting in 3 or more deaths.

Sources: Trembley KJ. Catastrophic fires and deaths drop in 1992. NFPA Journal 1993;(Sept./Oct.):56–69 (20); Karter MJ. Fire loss in the United States in 1992. NFPA Journal 1993;(Sept./Oct.):78–87. (21)

Table 18-4 Fires, Deaths, and Injuries by Type of Fire, United States, 1992

Type of Fire	Fires		Deaths*		Injuries*	
	No.	%	No.	%	No.	%
Residential						
One or Two Family	358,000	18.22	3,160	66.81	15,275	53.22
Apartments	101,000	5.14	545	11.52	5,825	20.38
Hotels and Motels	6,000	.31	30	.63	250	.87
Other	7,000	.36	30	.63	250	.87
Nonresidential	165,500	8.42	175	3.70	2,725	9.49
Highway Vehicles	385,500	19.62	665	14.06	2,750	9.58
Other Vehicles	19,500	.99	65	1.37	250	.87
All Others[†]	922,000	46.93	60	1.27	1,375	4.79
Total	1,964,500	100.00	4,730	100.00	28,700	100.00

*Civilian mortality and morbidity.

[†]Includes 743,000 fires in rubbish, bush, grass, or wildland with no dollar value or financial loss involved.

Source: Trembley KJ. Catastrophic fires and deaths drop in 1992. *NFPA Journal* 1993;(Sept./Oct.):56–69. *(20)*

catastrophic. The vast majority of all fire-related mortality and morbidity resulted from noncatastrophic fires. Relevant characteristics of noncatastrophic fires are shown in Table 18-4. Although fires in one- and two-family residences accounted for only 18% of all fires, this category of fire accounted for 67% of all mortality and 53% of all morbidity. Therefore, the key to public health prevention of fire-related mortality and morbidity is to focus on risk factors associated with one- and two- family residential fires.

Factors Influencing Morbidity and Mortality Due to Fire Disasters

Natural Factors

Perhaps the most important natural factor in fire disasters—certainly the one that receives the most media attention—is forests or grasslands, which serve as sources of combustion. Although the greatest impact of this type of fire is certainly on the ecology, these fires do have some effect on public health, and that effect is different from the public health effects of residential fires.

For 5 days beginning on August 30, 1987, dry lightning strikes ignited more than 1,500 fires that destroyed more than 600, 000 acres of California forests *(22)*. Selected medical information obtained from hospital emergency departments in the six counties most severely affected by smoke or fire showed that, during the period of major forest-fire activity, the number of people seeking treatment for asthma, chronic obstructive pulmonary disease, sinusitis, upper-respiratory infections, and laryngitis increased over the number normally expected. These increases in respiratory morbidity show that people with preexisting respiratory disease are a sensitive subpopulation who should be targeted for public health intervention when they are likely to be exposed to forest-fire smoke.

A grass wildfire swept through parts of Alameda County, California, on October 20–21, 1991. Lasting nearly 3 days, the fire covered 1,600 acres of mixed urban and wildland terrain and destroyed more than 3,800 housing units *(23)*. Overall, this fire resulted in 26 deaths and more than 225 injuries *(23)*. Emergency department records showed that more than twice as many people sought treatment for smoke-related disorders than did so for burns and other traumatic injuries *(24)*. Of the persons with smoke-related disorders, 61% had documented bronchospasm. Researchers concluded that health advisories should be targeted toward persons with asthma or chronic lung disease, warning them either to stay indoors or to vacate areas affected by smoke.

Many forest and grassland fires may eventually reach residential areas where they can cause mortality and morbidity. However, with sufficient warning, evacuation of residents at risk can minimize any public health impact. Consequently, one- or two-family residence fires ignited by means other than forest fires are a far greater public health concern.

Human-Generated Factors

The greatest impact on public health is from fires that occur in one- and two-family residences. Three-quarters of all people in the United States live in one- or two-family residences. Data from the United States Fire Administration are collected as part of the National Fire Incident Reporting System (NFIRS). Included are data from more than 13, 500 fire departments across the United States *(25)*. The most recent data are for

Table 18-5 Annual Mortality and Morbidity Due to Fire in One- and Two-Family Homes, United States, 1983–1990

	No. of Deaths	No. of Injuries
1983	3825	16,450
1984	3290	15,100
1985	4020	15,250
1986	4005	14,650
1987	3780	15,200
1988	4125	17,125
1989	3545	15,255
1990	3370	15,250

Source: National Fire Data Center, United States Fire Administration. *Fire in the United States 1983–1990.* Washington, D.C.: Federal Emergency Management Agency, 1993. *(25)*

Table 18-6 Fire Mortality and Fire Morbidity in One- and Two-Family Dwellings by Time of Occurrence, United States, 1990

Time	Fires (%)	Mortality (%)	Morbidity (%)
12:00– 2:59 A.M.	8.7	19.9	12.2
3:00– 5:59 A.M.	6.7	20.4	11.1
6:00– 8:59 A.M.	8.6	10.7	8.8
9:00–11:59 A.M.	12.9	12.3	12.6
12:00– 2:59 P.M.	14.9	7.4	13.8
3:00– 5:59 P.M.	17.4	5.7	14.8
6:00– 8:59 P.M.	18.0	9.0	14.6
9:00–11:59 P.M.	12.8	14.6	12.1
Total	**100.0**	**100.0**	**100.0**

Source: National Fire Data Center, United States Fire Administration. *Fire in the United States 1983–1990.* Washington, D.C.: Federal Emergency Management Agency, 1993. *(25)*

1990 and provide characteristics of fires and associated mortality and morbidity that occur in one- and two-family residences.

Annual incidences of deaths and injuries resulting from fires in one- and two-family residences are shown in Table 18-5. The trends for deaths and injuries went down slightly from 1983 to 1990 but retained the same relative magnitude of public health importance.

The incidences of fires, deaths, and injuries in one- and two-family residences during 1990 are shown by time of occurrence in Table 18-6. Most fires and injuries due to fires occur between 5:00 and 7:00 P.M., when people are most frequently preparing meals. In contrast, deaths due to fires tend to peak late at night and early in the morning, when dropped smoking materials may serve as sources of ignition.

The 1990 distribution of fires and deaths by month are shown in Table 18-7. Both fires and deaths in one- and two-family residences generally peak in the midwinter, perhaps because of increased use of heating sources.

The causes of fires, deaths, and injuries in one- and two-family residences in 1990 are shown in Table 18-8. With respect to numbers of fires, heating is a leading cause of residential fires at 24%, followed by cooking at 20%, and arson at 13%. Fire deaths are most frequently caused by careless smoking (24% of all deaths). Many careless smoking deaths result from cigarettes being dropped on upholstered furniture or bedding. Fires related to heating are a second-leading cause of deaths at 19%, and fires caused by arson are third at 17%. For injuries, fires from cooking are first and account for 22% of all injuries. These injuries often result from unattended cooking, from oil or grease catching on fire, and from ignition of loose clothing. Heating is the second-leading cause of injuries at 16%, and careless smoking is third at 12%.

The rooms where fires began in the residences where fires, deaths, and injuries occurred in 1990 are shown in Table 18-9. More than twice as many fires occurred in the

Table 18-7 Percentages of Fires and Fire
Mortality in One- and Two-Family Dwellings
by Month of Year, United States, 1990

	Fires (%)	Mortality (%)
January	10.4	15.4
February	9.6	10.4
March	9.4	7.3
April	7.8	8.2
May	7.0	5.1
June	6.9	6.0
July	7.3	4.5
August	6.7	6.3
September	6.5	5.1
October	7.6	7.9
November	8.9	10.4
December	12.0	13.6

Source: National Fire Data Center, United States Fire Administration. *Fire in the United States 1983–1990.* Washington, D.C.: Federal Emergency Management Agency, 1993. *(25)*

kitchen than in any other area. Most of these fires, of course, were associated with cooking. The second most common location is the bedroom, and chimney fires are close behind in third place. Chimneys often have creosote buildup that may serve as a source of combustion. For deaths, the leading area is the lounge area, where people may fall asleep on upholstered furniture while smoking. For injuries, the kitchen is the most common location because of the large number of burns associated with cooking.

Table 18-8 Percentages of Fires, Fire Mortality, and Fire Morbidity in One- and Two-Family Dwellings by Known Causes, United States, 1990

Cause	Fire (%)	Mortality (%)	Morbidity (%)
Incendiary	13.3	17.3	9.4
Children playing	4.8	6.8	10.0
Careless smoking	5.0	24.1	12.0
Heating	23.8	18.7	16.0
Cooking	19.5	9.3	22.0
Electrical distribution	10.2	9.1	7.5
Appliances	8.0	3.5	4.9
Open flame	6.5	6.1	7.1
Open heat	1.4	2.6	1.6
Other equipment	1.2	1.1	8.1
Natural	2.3	.4	.7
Exposure	4.0	.9	.8

Source: National Fire Data Center, United States Fire Administration. *Fire in the United States 1983–1990.* Washington, D.C.: Federal Emergency Management Agency, 1993 (25).

Table 18-9 Percentages of Fires, Fire Mortality, and Fire Morbidity in One- and Two-Family Dwellings by Rooms of Origin, United States, 1990

Rooms	Fires (%)	Mortality (%)	Morbidity (%)
Lounge area	9.0	31.9	14.9
Bedroom	11.5	23.8	23.4
Dining room	—	2.3	—
Kitchen	23.6	14.6	30.1
Laundry room	4.0	2.0	—
Heating equipment room	—	2.0	3.1
Garage, carport	—	—	3.6
Chimney	11.2	—	—
Other/unknown	6.0	9.4	2.8

Source: National Fire Data Center, United States Fire Administration. *Fire in the United States 1983–1990.* Washington, D.C.: Federal Emergency Management Agency, 1993. *(25)*

Data pertaining to smoke-detector performance during fires and deaths occurring in one- and two-family residences in 1990 are shown in Table 18-10. It is important to note that there was no operating detector in 76% of the fires and in 87% of the deaths (excluding those fires and deaths where the presence of a detector was unknown).

Inhalation injury is even more important in the context of fire-related mortality. Inhalation injury is an important co-morbid factor in burn injury and increases the number of deaths substantially *(26)*. Most victims succumb to the asphyxiating effect of carbon monoxide long before the flames or heat affect them directly *(27, 28)*. Also, carbon dioxide poisoning or oxygen deficiency may play be fatal *(29)*. During fire disasters within buildings, the confines of the structure assist in retaining and concentrating the toxic combustion products and smoke from the fire *(30, 31)*. Contents of the building also can contribute to deaths. A smoldering mattress or sofa in a standard-size room can produce lethal levels of carbon monoxide in as little as 30 seconds *(32)*.

It is also important to realize that some fire-associated mortality may not result directly from the fire or it products. First, a fire may start after a death *(32)*; e.g., a person

Table 18-10 Percentages of Fires, Fire Mortality, and Fire Morbidity in One- and Two-Family Dwellings by Smoke-Detector Performance, United States, 1990

Smoke-Detector Status	Fires (%)	Mortality (%)
Present/operational	15.2	8.2
Present/not operational	16.9	8.3
No detector	35.8	47.2
Unknown	37.1	35.8

Source: National Fire Data Center, United States Fire Administration. *Fire in the United States 1983–1990.* Washington, D.C.: Federal Emergency Management Agency, 1993. *(25)*

could have a fatal cardiac collapse while smoking, while using matches or a lighter, or while being near an open flame (candle or stove). Although firefighters are one of the occupational groups at greatest risk of dying on the job, the direct effects of fires are not the greatest killers of firefighters *(33)*. Most firefighters who die while responding to fires die from heart attacks or vehicular accidents *(33)*.

Of the host characteristics that have been assessed, age appears to be an important risk factor. In 1984, 53% of all persons killed in residential fire disasters were younger than 15 years of age, compared with only 22.2% of the general population at risk *(4)*. Persons in this age group either may be too young to react on their own or may react improperly because of insufficient knowledge of safe behavior. Interestingly, elderly persons (those older than 65 years of age) accounted for only 5.8% of deaths in all residential fire disasters and did not represent a high-risk group. However, this may merely be a consequence of a greater chance of living in multiple-family dwellings such as apartment buildings, retirement communities, or nursing homes.

Although not specific to catastrophic fires alone, an important host characteristic for sustaining burn injuries is any predisposing medical condition or factor. In one study of 500 hospitalized adult burn patients, "poor judgment" was implicated as a contributing factor in persons sustaining burn injuries *(34)*. Elderly adults are more prone to severe burn injuries than are younger adults, possibly because of more limited defensive and reactive capabilities *(35)*. Three studies that examined the contributory influence of predisposing medical factors to burn injuries in adults showed that approximately one-fourth of all adults who sustained burn injuries had some type of predisposing medical condition *(35, 36)*. These studies show that the two most important factors are alcoholism and epilepsy. Other studies have shown that 5%–10% of all adult burn injuries are sustained by individuals subject to epileptic seizures *(37–42)* and that alcoholism also plays a prominent role in the occurrence of adult burn injuries *(43, 44)*.

A retrospective study of 277 adults consecutively hospitalized for burns showed predisposing factors to include living alone, alcohol and drug abuse, physical or mental illness, and advanced age *(45)*. A study of residential fires in Maryland showed that 47% of the fires and 45% of the fire-related deaths were associated with cigarettes *(46)*. A study of 55 people who died during house fires showed that more than half of the deaths resulted from cigarette-ignited fires and that 39% of the people who died in such fires were not the cigarette smokers themselves *(19)*. A published review of ten studies showed that nearly half of those who die in fires are legally intoxicated, having a blood alcohol concentration greater than 0.10% *(47)*. Since it appears unlikely that 50% of the general population is intoxicated at any given time, alcohol intoxication may be a risk factor for fire death.

Because smoking and alcohol consumption are correlated behaviors, studies that evaluate only alcohol consumption do not necessarily indicate a causal role. An analysis of 116 deaths and injuries from residential fires reported to the Washington State Fire Incident Reporting System from 1984 and 1985 showed that smoking, rather than alcohol consumption, was the more important risk factor *(48)*.

Public Health Implications and Prevention Strategies for Fires

Historically, in the United States there has been a tremendous public health problem associated with fires. The problem is still of major concern, although its complexity and nature have changed over time. Fires should be viewed as preventable problems that certainly deserve greater attention from and efforts of public health professionals.

In terms of public health implications, a burn injury is one of the most serious insults the human body can experience. Burn injuries that require hospitalization are both serious and costly *(49)*. They require more bed-days per patient than any other type of injury *(12, 50)*. Furthermore, severe burn injuries are one of the most difficult medical problems to treat *(17)*. Approximately 5% of all burn patients sustain concomitant traumatic injuries that affect their medical care *(51)*. Patients with burns may need multiple surgical procedures and may be left with lifelong disfigurement and deformity. Severe burn injuries subject both the patient and the patient's family to profound psychological and financial stress *(52)*.

Burn injuries can result in loss of bodily function (sensory or motor or both) and serious disfigurement, even though the extent of the injuries may be small. Persons with preexisting renal, cardiovascular, or pulmonary disease cannot tolerate burn injuries as well as those without such disease. For persons with occlusive vascular disease, burn injuries to the lower extremities (especially the feet) are particularly serious. Gangrene requiring amputation is not uncommon after burn injuries to the feet or legs of adults with peripheral arteriosclerosis.

Burn injuries may lead to new cardiovascular or pulmonary disease. The most common types of pathologic pulmonary conditions include pneumonia and atelectasis. Ophthalmic *(53)*, renal *(54)*, and neurologic *(55)* disease may develop after some types of burn injuries.

Two major types of concomitant injuries, inhalation injuries and fractures, may result from catastrophic fire events that cause burn injuries. An inhalation injury, caused by breathing in noxious gases, is the most serious concomitant injury *(56)*. Smoke from some fires contains nitrogen dioxide and sulfur dioxide, which may cause bronchiolitis *(57)*, alveolitis *(58)*, and bronchospasms *(59)*. Clinical features of inhalation injury include nasal-membrane irritation, pharyngeal edema, hoarseness, and bronchorrhea. Fractures may also compound the burn injury in accordance with their severity. The presence of fractures along with burns complicates treatment and prognosis for both the burn injury and fracture *(60, 61)*.

Prevention and Control Measures

Epidemiology: Surveillance and Research

Epidemiology can play an important role in preventing or mitigating the public health impact of fires. At present, few descriptive or analytic data on the public health impact of fire disasters are available. Data are basically limited to surveillance statistics maintained and published by a few agencies and gathered from case reports of fire disasters. Limitations in these data include the lack of denominator data needed to draw more valid conclusions about risk factors, insufficient description of .ssociated morbidity, and insufficient information about the circumstances of the fire and associated human behavior.

A full spectrum of epidemiologic activities encompassing both surveillance and research would almost certainly assist in the further prevention or mitigation of fire-associated mortality and morbidity.

Engineering and Legal Controls

Public acceptance of skyscrapers and high-rise buildings in the United States has resulted in part from the establishment and enforcement of building codes. The first U.S. building codes were implemented by municipalities in the late nineteenth century. These early codes addressed the prevention of conflagration and were designed to minimize the risk that fires would spread to neighboring buildings. These codes provided specifications for roofing, exterior materials, and characteristics (such as thickness and fire resistance) of common walls.

At the initiation of insurance companies, the National Fire Protection Agency (NFPA) was established in 1896. This organization has played a vital role in establishing or augmenting building codes and regulations. For example, NFPA codes have been developed for fire-wall performance, separation between freestanding structures, and storage of combustible materials.

The evolution of codes is in some ways associated with the evolution of fire disasters in this country. The early threats of fire focused around urban conflagration. Today, however, this type of fire represents little public health threat. The chief concerns today deal with fire inside—rather than among—buildings. For the threat of fires within commercial buildings, codes provide for public safety by detailing stipulations for interior passages, stairwells, and doors. These codes provide for protective strategies involving both containment of fire and evacuation of people.

Although the greatest contemporary risk of fire involves single-family residences and duplexes, building codes for these structures are different from those for commercial buildings in several ways. First, these codes tend to involve less expensive strategies, since individuals rather than businesses must bear the cost. Second, the containment of fire within certain areas of the structure is not a viable approach, because of the size of residences. Third, because of the lack of access for inspection and the number of residential buildings, codes that require routine inspection of the inside of buildings are not practical. Consequently, residential building codes have focused on aspects of structures not seen or difficult to correct once construction of the residential building is complete (e.g., the design of chimneys and the placement of electrical circuits and wiring). These codes are enforced when the building is being constructed or remodeled.

A recent engineering control is the smoke detector. These inexpensive devices increase the length of warning time. The data presented, though limited, support the need for this control to be utilized within residential homes. A recent survey of several hundred primary-care physicians (internists) showed that 85% seldom or never talked to their patients about using smoke detectors even though they were aware the risks of burn injury and the efficacy of detectors (62). On the other hand, smoke detectors can have limited efficacy, since they are not an entirely passive prevention measure; they must be purchased, properly installed, and maintained with fresh batteries. Also, residents must be able to respond properly to the alarm, an action that may be difficult for the young, the aged, the disabled, and the intoxicated (63).

A study of residential fires in which 57 New Mexico children died concluded that strategies to prevent such fatalities should address housing conditions (substandard homes) along with adult safety practices (64), since enhanced prehospital emergency or burn-unit care is unlikely to greatly affect childhood fire-mortality rates (64).

Because the cigarette-initiated fire is the major cause of residential fire deaths, the most effective potential solution for the cigarette-initiated fire lies with the cigarette itself (63). Public education of the "careless" smoker may never be efficacious, since it has been estimated that 99.99% of the 600 billion cigarettes smoked each year are disposed of safely (65). A legal control involving the development of cigarettes that would fail to ignite the majority of furnishings currently in homes would greatly reduce the occurrence of residential fires in the United States.

Response to and Suppression of Fires

In the United States, the training of firefighters and the fighting of fires are old and established practices. The earliest response to fires consisted of ad hoc bucket brigades. The first firefighting company of trained individuals was founded in the 1730s by Benjamin Franklin (5).

The ability of fire departments to reach any portion of their catchment area within minutes of receiving a fire alarm has minimized the risk of injury to persons and damage to property once residential fires have been discovered. Each year in the United States, fire departments respond to approximately 1 million residential fires (5). Given the resources committed to and the realized accomplishments of fire response and suppression over the years, additional substantial improvements in firefighting strategy that would further impact on the public health implications of fire disasters are not very likely.

An important but often unrecognized function of fire departments is to inspect buildings to enforce compliance with codes that govern construction, maintenance, and occupancy. The development of firefighting techniques for control and prevention of fires has augmented such codes that minimize the risk of fire for whole sections of cities and communities. If a fire does break out, it is more likely to be dealt with in a timely and productive matter. However, the focus of most building inspections by fire departments is nonresidential structures. Also, some of the firefighting strategies for large buildings are not suited for single-family dwellings and duplexes. For example, a house fire cannot purposely be allowed to burn beyond the room in which it started (a technique sometimes used in fighting nonresidential fires) since there is no realistic way to contain it before it envelops the entire structure.

Medical Treatment and Rehabilitation

Extensive clinical and epidemiologic work has focused on the triage, management, and rehabilitation of victims of fire disasters *(66–70)*. For example, a fire at a football match in Bradford City, United Kingdom, resulted in 56 deaths and over 200 injuries *(71)*. Key components of an efficacious medical response to this fire disaster included warning time and content of the warning's language, efficient triage by a physician skilled with burn-injury diagnosis and treatment, adequate resources made available by prior planning, capability to address inpatient and family needs, and utilization of coordinated outside help. On November 18, 1987, a fire broke out at the end of the evening rush hour at King's Cross Underground Station, London *(72)*. Thirteen people were killed, and 45 others sustained burn injuries in the fire flashover in the main ticket concourse. Local emergency medical services were quickly saturated. This disaster showed that hospitals responding to disasters need both a disaster contingency plan and the key medical and administrative staff to implement and operate it, and that all major trauma units should have medical and plastic surgery capability to deal with burn patients. An example of a situation where emergency medical care components of a disaster plan were successfully implemented occurred when 1,700 fire victims from the MGM Grand Hotel fire in Las Vegas were effectively triaged and cared for by the local EMS system *(73)*.

Published studies about the medical implications and severity of burn injuries are only slightly indicative of the tremendous amount of available scientific knowledge concerning the medical consequences and treatment of burn injuries. Burn units in hospitals or entire hospitals devoted to burns operate throughout the United States. Surgical and medical treatment have maximized not only the likelihood of survival but also the aesthetic and functional potential for victims of serious burns. Current medical practice acknowledges that children are not miniature adults and require different types of burn management *(74)*.

As a means of tertiary prevention, medical treatment and rehabilitation have reached a plateau in ensuring survivorship and reducing morbidity associated with fire disasters. As a result, further significant reduction in fire-disaster morbidity and mortality will depend heavily on primary prevention activities during the pre-event phase of the disaster to prevent fires, reduce human exposure to the thermal energy of fire, or decrease the susceptibility of humans to injury. Primary prevention approaches may not only minimize public health impacts but may also improve adverse economic (e.g., lost jobs) and social conditions (e.g., homeless families) associated with fires. To realize future reductions in the public health impacts of fire disasters, any additional resources should be expended on primary prevention strategies, such as public education and awareness.

Public Awareness and Education

For any public health problem, once risk factors and prevention strategies have been identified by research and accepted by public health professionals, any reduction in the magnitude of the problem depends on the awareness and education of the public at risk. Certainly, fires are no exception. In fact, the need for public awareness and education may be more important for fires than for other public health problems if one considers the size of the population at risk and the incidence of fires. Most of the U.S. population lives in single-family homes or duplexes, and 1 million fires occur in such residencies each year.

People need to understand the risk of fire associated with their residences. Since 1980, national attention to major fires in hotels has sensitized the portion of the public who regularly use hotels to the need to be knowledgeable about appropriate means of egress and reaction during fires. However, the entire adult public should be able to apply the same basic knowledge to fires in their homes. Parents and teachers should train children who are old enough about what to do if there is a fire, and plans should be made at home and at school to take care of young children in the event of a fire. Families should hold rehearsals to help instill knowledge about appropriate safety actions. Adults should recognize the risks that auxiliary heaters and cigarettes pose as sources of ignition for residential fires. Smoke detectors should be installed and maintained on each level of the home.

Over 75% of the hospitals that belong to the American Hospital Association deliver specialized care to patients in their residences, including intravenous alimentation, home dialysis, and ventilatory support (75). One hospital-based home care staff directed a burn care prevention program at homebound patients (76). This program combined fire-prevention activities (fire-safety education and smoke-detector installation) with home health care for this high-risk population.

If an educational program to prevent fire injuries is to be successful, it must not only educate the persons at risk but also modify their behavior (77). Overall burn prevention campaigns aimed at public education have failed to provide the expected decrease in burn injuries (78). Education may increase knowledge but does not necessarily lead to behavioral and/or lifestyle change. More effort is needed in evaluating the efficacy of educational programs aimed toward behavior modification and ensuring that such behavior is effective.

On November 14, 1987, the blanket factory at Kibbutz Urim in Israel was completely destroyed by fire (79). The factory was a high-roofed building with multiple openings

and contained smoke detectors that were tested every month. An evacuation plan had
been rehearsed every six months. At the time of the fire, 62 workers were in the factory.
Although 45 of the workers received mild injuries from the smoke, no serious injuries
or skin burns occurred. This disaster showed that the fire evacuation plan had been
successfully implemented and prevented any serious injuries or deaths.

Critical Knowledge Gaps

Public health professionals may lack knowledge concerning the characteristics and public health impact of fire disasters in the United States. Their concept of a fire disaster
should be adjusted to reflect the fact that a large number of fire disasters involve only
a few deaths and usually occur in the home. Although quite different from what is
usually perceived to be a disaster, this kind of incident represents the contemporary
fire-disaster problem.

Available data for fires and their health impacts are often inadequate in terms of
completeness, accuracy, and comparability between data sets *(80)*. Sources of data
include the National Center for Health Statistics, the National Fire Protection Agency,
various members of the insurance industry, the National Fire Protection and Control
Administration, the National Household Fire Survey, and State Fire Marshals. Statistics
published by various sources may differ because of different objectives, assumptions,
and methods of collection and analysis. Much of the data in this chapter, for instance,
represents statistics published by the National Fire Protection Agency and appear to be
the most comprehensive and detailed information available, but may vary from data
compiled from other sources.

Very little information is available on morbidity associated with fire disasters. Currently laws for mandatory reporting of all burn injuries exist in only 12 states *(81)*.
Most available information does not cover nonfatal injuries. As with other injury scenarios, numerous serious burn injuries and even more minor burn injuries occur for
every fatality associated with a fire disaster. Given the potential for the tremendous
burden hospitalization for burn injuries places on medical, economic, and social systems, sufficient public health knowledge about these injuries is essential.

Detailed information for risk assessment is lacking. Available data for fire disasters
are limited mainly to surveillance data based on the aggregation of individual case
reports. With the lack of denominator data and detailed characteristics, only crude
conclusions about risk can be drawn. Furthermore, limitations in existing data make it
extremely difficult to determine the efficacy of various types of prevention strategies.

Current literature does not directly address differences and similarities between fire
disasters and all fire incidents. It is helpful to understand which characteristics of fire
disasters are unique and which are similar for all types of fires. This understanding
would assist in setting priorities for research needs and detailed preventive strategies.

A review of the literature does not provide a complete appreciation for the operating assumptions adopted by groups addressing either the prevention or suppression of fires. With public health implications, there appear to be two different assumptions: the goal may be to prevent fire, or the goal may be to control the fire or evacuate the people. Such knowledge would be helpful in developing a thorough understanding of progress to date and in anticipating future needs and advances of these groups.

Most deaths from fire disasters result from the inhalation of combustion materials produced by the fire. Fundamental knowledge needed for prevention of these deaths includes how gases are produced by and distributed during a fire and how best to detect and warn potential victims about the presence of such gases. We need to understand general gas processes involved in ignition, smoldering combustion, and the spread of flaming combustion, and we need to understand distribution dynamics in rooms and corridors during a fire disaster.

Most building codes in the United States focus on nonresidential buildings, although existing data show that the contemporary problem of fire is with residential structures. More information is needed concerning the appropriateness and effectiveness of augmenting existing residential building codes.

The threat of urban conflagration in peacetime is no longer a major public health problem in the United States; however, there is a critical knowledge gap concerning the potential new threat of suburban conflagration in some states. For example, to minimize the potential of erosion in some desert states, the chaparral has been allowed to remain close to walls or yards in hillside residential and commercial developments (residential-wildland interface). This practice may increase the risk of conflagration from brushfires.

As with most public health problems in this country, state and federal efforts to prevent fire disasters augment those activities at the local level. Currently, there is a lack of detailed knowledge about strength, success, and needs of local efforts.

A key prevention strategy appears to be public awareness and education, yet the extent of the general public's basic understanding of fire disasters is unclear. More data on baseline levels of public knowledge about fires is needed, especially for high-risk parts of the country, and the ways behavior is actually affected by education should be determined.

Methodologic Problems of Epidemiologic Studies of Fire Disasters

Although fire disasters may often result from just a single causal factor, it is usually necessary to consider several factors jointly in order to better understand the disaster scenario and the relative contributions of these individual factors. Epidemiologists have used stratified analyses but have encountered problems because of the necessity of using small numbers. In some instances in the literature, even the most frequent pattern of factors is relatively insignificant because only a small percentage of fires is represented in the relevant study. An increased knowledge of the comparability of databases is essential in order to facilitate data aggregation so that larger numbers may be obtained for multivariate statistical analyses.

There are very few studies focusing on the epidemiology of fire disasters. Most investigations have been cross-sectional studies or hospital-based case series. Consequently, they focus on the more severe burn injuries. Investigations of this kind are limited in types of variables that can be examined. Most available descriptive information about fire disasters is limited to surveillance statistics maintained by agencies such as the National Center for Health Statistics, the United States Fire Administration, and the National Fire Protection Agency.

Research Recommendations

The following activities are recommended to improve the identification and efficacy of prevention strategies designed to prevent or mitigate public health impacts of fires:

- Both public and health professionals should become better educated about the true, insidious nature of public health impacts of contemporary fires.
- Appropriate agencies and public health professionals should develop greater concern for and focus more efforts on morbidity from fires.
- Efforts should be undertaken to maximize uniformity and comparability of data sources.
- Existing data systems should be modified or new systems developed as appropriate to provide descriptive data with more detailed characteristics of human and environmental factors and applicable denominator data.
- Since most information about characteristics of fires and the public health impact of fires derives from surveillance, epidemiologic studies that provide analytical data about risk factors should be designed and conducted.
- Through consultation with appropriate fire-prevention agencies, the need for specific epidemiologic studies should be determined and supported. For example, population surveys of level of education about fire disasters or safety practices are appropriate. Also, most available information focuses on the environmental characteristics of fires. More emphasis on the epidemiologic characteristics of the host is needed so that the importance of such factors as behavior, knowledge, awareness, planning, perception, and predisposing medical factors can be determined more accurately.
- Prevention strategies need to encompass specific actions to address and minimize the risk of young children who are dependent on the knowledge and behavior of others.

- Groups such as health departments, fire departments, and civic associations should conduct more studies to determine the extent of and provision for smoke detectors in residential dwellings.
- Public health and fire-protection professionals should increase emphasis on public education and awareness of the proper selection, installation, usage, and maintenance of smoke detectors.
- Public health and fire-protection professionals should stress that cigarette smoking is potentially dangerous, not only in terms of personal health, but also as a cause of fire disasters that destroy lives and property.

Summary

Contemporary fires should be viewed as an unnecessary and preventable problem that deserves the attention and efforts of public health professionals.

The literature contains limited statistics about the characteristics and adverse public health impact of fires with the greatest public health concern—fires that occur in one- and two-family residences. However, these data still allow for identifying important contributing factors to fire disasters, such as the role of residential fires, sources of ignition that include cigarettes, and the need for widespread use of smoke detectors.

Appropriate prevention strategies can be divided into five broad categories of activities in order to reduce the public health impact of fire disasters: (1) epidemiologic surveillance and research, (2) engineering and legal controls, (3) mitigation response and suppression, (4) medical treatment and rehabilitation, and (5) public awareness and education.

References

1. Metropolitan Life Insurance Company. Catastrophic accidents, a 35-year review. *Stat Bull Metrop Insur Co* 1977;58:1–4.
2. Reig A, Tejerina C, Baena P, Mirabet V. Massive burns: a study of epidemiology and mortality. *Burns* (England) 1994;20(1):51–54.
3. Baker SP, O'Neil B, Kerpf R. *Injury fact book.* Lexington, MA: DC Health and Company, 1992.
4. Curtis MH, Hall JR, LeBlan PR. Analysis of multiple-death fires in the United States during 1984. *Fire J* 1985;18–30, 74–81.
5. Lyons JW. *Fire.* New York: Scientific American Library, 1985.
6. Eckert WG. The medico-legal and forensic aspects of fires. *Am J Forensic Med Pathal* 1981; 2(4):347–357.
7. Quenemoen LE, Davis YM, Malilay J, *et al. The World Trade Center bombing: injury prevention strategies for high-rise building fires.* Unpublished report. Atlanta, GA: Centers for Disease Control and Prevention, National Center for Environmental Health, 1994.

8. Levin BC, Rechani PR, Gurman JL, *et al.* Analysis of carboxyhemoglobin and cyanide in blood from victims of the Dupont Plaza Hotel Fire in Puerto Rico. *J Forensic Sci* 1990; 35(1):151–168.

9. National Safety Council. *Accident facts.* Chicago: National Safety Council, 1983.

10. Sanderson LM. *An epidemiologic description and analysis of lost workday occupational burn injuries* [dissertation]. Houston: Univ. of Texas School of Public Health, 1981.

11. Feck G, Baptiste M, Greenwald P. The incidence of hospitalized burn injury in upstate New York. *Am J Public Health* 1977;67:966–967.

12. National Center for Health Statistics. *Inpatient utilization of short-stay hospitals by diagnoses: United States, 1971.* Vital and Health Statistics series 13, no. 16. Washington, D.C.: U.S. Government Printing Office, 1974.

13. Clark WR, Lerner D. Regional burn survey: two years of hospitalized burn patients in central New York. *J Trauma* 1978;18:524–532.

14. Linn BS, Stevenson SE, Feller I. Evaluation of burn care in Florida. *N Engl J Med* 1977; 296:311–315.

15. Greenwald P, Crane KH, Feller I. Need for burn care facilities in New York State. *N Y State J Med* 1972;72:2677–2680.

16. Dickinson FG, Welker EL. What is the leading cause of death? *JAMA* 1948;138:528–529.

17. Feck G, Baptiste MS, Tate CL. *An epidemiologic study of burn injuries and strategies for prevention.* DHEW Environmental Health Sciences Division. Washington, D.C.: U.S. Government Printing Office, 1978.

18. Gulaid JA, Sattin RW, Waxweiler RJ. Deaths from residential fires, 1978–1984. *MMWR* 1988;37(ss-1):39–45.

19. Mierley MC, Baker SP. Fatal house fires in an urban population. *JAMA* 1983;249(11):1466–1468.

20. Trembley KJ. Catastrophic fires and deaths drop in 1992. *NFPA Journal* 1993;(Sept./Oct.):56–69.

21. Karter MJ. Fire loss in the United States in 1992. *NFPA Journal* 1993;(Sept/Oct):78–87.

22. Duclos P, Sanderson LM, Lipsett M. The 1987 forest fire disaster in California: assessment of emergency room visits. *Arch Environ Health* 1990;45(1):53–58.

23. Bedian K, Arcus A, Frankel-Cone C, *et al. Emergency medical response to the Oakland/ Berkeley Hills fire of October 1991.* Sacramento, CA: California Department of Health Services, 1994.

24. Shusterman D, Kaplan JZ, Canabarro C. Immediate health effects of an urban wildfire. *West J Med* 1993;158:133–138.

25. National Fire Data Center, United States Fire Administration. *Fire in the United States 1983– 1990.* Washington, D.C.: Federal Emergency Management Agency, 1993.

26. Tredeget EE, Shankowsky HA, Taerum TV, *et al.* The role of inhalation injury in burn trauma. *Ann Surg* 1990;212(6):720–727.

27. Zikria BA, Weston GC, Chodoff M. Smoke and carbon monoxide poisoning in fire victims. *J Trauma* 1972;12:641–645

28. Zikria BA, Stormer WO. Respiratory tract damage in burns: pathophysiology and therapy. *Ann N Y Acad Sci* 1968;150:618–626.

29. Gormsen H, Jeppersen N, Lund A. The causes of death in fire victims. *Forensic Sci Int* 1984; 24:107–111.

30. Federal Emergency Management Agency and the United States Fire Administration. *Highlights of fire in the United States*, 2nd ed. Washington, D.C.: U.S. Government Printing Office, 1980.

31. Karter MJ. Fire loss in the United States during 1979. *Fire J* 1980;75:52–56.

32. Sopher IM. Death caused by fire. *Clin Lab Med* 1983;3(2):295–307.
33. Clark WE. Sudden death: How fire fighters get killed. *Fire Chief Magazine* 1984;Oct:38–40.
34. Bowers LF. Accidental burns. *Int Surg* 1966;46:338–339.
35. Beverly EV. Reducing fire and burn hazards among the elderly. *Geriatrics* 1976;31:106–110.
36. MacLeod A. Adult burns in Melbourne: a five-year survey. *Med J Aust* 1970;2:772–777.
37. Colebrook L, Colebrook V. The prevention of burns and scalds: a review of 1000 cases. *Lancet* 1949;2:181–188.
38. Nasilowski W, Zielkiewicz W. Evaluation of a thousand cases of burns: circumstances of the accidents and prevention measures. *Pol Med J* 1968;7:1410–1414.
39. Maisels DO, Gosh J. Predisposing causes of burns in adults. *Practitioner* 1968;201:767–773.
40. Jackson DM. The treatment of burns: an exercise in emergency surgery. *Ann R Coll Surg Engl* 1953;13:236–257.
41. Maissels DO, Koups BM. Burned epileptics. *Lancet* 1964;1:1298–1301.
42. Richards EH. Aspects of epilepsy and burns. *Epilepsia* 1968;43:646–648.
43. Crikelair CF, Symonds FC, Ollstein RN, Kirsner AI. Burn causation: its many sides. *J Trauma* 1968;8:572–581.
44. Juillerat EE. Survey of fatal clothing fires. *Bull N Y Acad Med* 1967;43:646–648.
45. Brodzka W, Thornhill HL, Howard S. Burns: causes and risk factors. *Arch Phys Med Rehabil* 1985;66(11):746–752.
46. Birky MM, Clarke FB. Inhalation of toxic products from fires. *Bull N Y Acad Med* 1981; 57:997–1013.
47. Howland J, Hingson R. Alcohol as a risk factor for injuries or death due to fires or burns: a review of the literature. *Public Health Rep* 1987;102:475–483.
48. Ballard JE, Koepsell TD, Rivara F. Association of smoking and alcohol drinking with residential fire injuries. *Am J Epidemiol* 1992;136(1):26–34.
49. Moore FD. The burn-prone society. *JAMA* 1975;231:281–282.
50. Jamieson KG, Wigglesworth EC. The dimension of the accident problem in Australia. *Aust N Z J Surg* 1977;47:135–138.
51. Purdue GF, Hunt JL. Multiple trauma and the burn patient. *Am J Surg* 1989;158:536–539.
52. Pegg SP, Gregory JJ, Hogan PG, *et al.* Epidemiology pattern of adult burn injuries. *Burns* 1979;5:326–334.
53. Long JC. A clinical and experimental study of electric cataract. *Am J Ophthalmol* 1963; 56:108–133.
54. Artz CP. Electrical injury stimulates renal injury. *Surg Gynecol Obstet* 1967;125:1316–1317.
55. Levine NS, Atkins A, McKell DW, Peck SD, Pruitt BA. Spinal cord injury following electrical accidents [case reports]. *J Trauma* 1975;15:459–463.
56. Aschaver BM, Allyn PA, Furnas AW, Bartlett RH. Pulmonary complications of burns. *Ann Surg* 1973;177:311–319.
57. Zikrin BA, Ferrer JM, Floch NF. Chemical factors contributing to pulmonary damage in smoke poisoning. *Surgery* 1972;71:704–709.
58. Aub JC, Puttman H, Brues AM. The pulmonary complication: a clinical symptom. *Ann Surg* 1943;117:834–840.
59. Perez-Guerra F. Walsh RE, Sagel SS. Bronchiectasis obliterans and tracheal stenosis. *JAMA* 1970;218:1568–1570.
60. Japlan JZ, Pruitt BA. Orthopedic management of the burn patient. In: Heppenstill RB, editor. *Fracture healing and treatment.* Philadelphia: W. B. Saunders, 1979.

61. Pruitt BA. Complications of thermal injury. *Clin Plast Surg* 1974;1:667–691.
62. Johnson KC, Ford DE, Smith GS. The current practices of internists in prevention of residential fire injury. *Am J Prev Med* 1993;9(1):39–44.
63. Botkin JR. The fire-safe cigarette. *JAMA* 1988;260(2):226–229.
64. McLoughlin E, Vince CJ, Lee AM *et al.* Project burn prevention: outcome and implications. *Am J Public Health* 1982;72:241–247.
65. Parker DJ, Sklar DP, Tanberg D *et al.* Fire fatalities among New Mexico Children. *Ann Emerg Med* 1993;22(3):517–522.
66. Kutsumi A, Kuroiwa Y, Taketa R. Medical report on casualties in the Hokuriku Tunnel train fire in Japan with special reference to smoke-gas poisoning. *Mt Sinai J Med* 1979;46:469–472.
67. Duignan JP, McEnee GP, Scully B, Corrigan TP. Report of a fire disaster: management of burns and complications. *Ir Med J* 1984;77(1):8–10.
68. Cope O. The management of the Coconut Grove burns at the Massachusetts General Hospital: treatment of surface burns. *Ann Surg* 1982;117:885–897.
69. Das RAP. 1981 Circus fire disaster in Bangalore, India: causes, management of burn patients and possible presentation. *Burns* 1983;10:17–29.
70. Pegg SP. Burn management in a disaster. *Aust Fam Physician* 1983;12(12):848–852.
71. Sharpe DT, Foo ITH. Management of burns in major disasters. *Injury* 1990;21:41–44.
72. Sturgeon D, Rosser R, Shoenberg P. The King's Cross fire, Part 1: the physical injuries. *Burns* (England) 1991;17(1):10–13.
73. Buerk CA, Bartdorf JW, Cammack KU, Ravenholt HO. The MGM Grand Hotel fire: lessons learned from a major disaster. *Arch Surg* 1982;117:641–644.
74. Ngim, RCK. Epidemiology of burns in Singapore children: an 11-year study of 2288 patients. *Ann Acad Med Singapore* 1992;21(5):667–671.
75. Nassif JZ. There is still no place like home. *Generations* 1986;Winter 1986–87:5.
76. Schmeer S, Stern N, Monafo W. An outreach burn prevention program for home care patients. *J Burn Care Rehabil* 1988;9(6):645–647.
77. Wade J, Purdue GF, Hunt JL, Childers L. Crawl on your belly like GI Joe. *J Burn Care Rehabil* 1990;11(3):261–263.
78. Linares AZ, Linares HA. Burn prevention: the need for a comprehensive approach. *Burns* (England) 1990;16(4):281–285.
79. Benmeir P, Sagi A, Rosenberg L. An example of burn prevention: The ''Urim'' factory fire. *Burns* (England) 1989;15(4):252–253.
80. National Fire Data Center, U.S. Fire Administration, U.S. Department of Commerce. *Fire in the United States*. Washington, D.C.: U.S. Government Printing Office, 1978.
81. Hammond J. The status of statewide burn prevention legislation. *J Burn Care Rehabil* 1993; 14(4):473–475.

19

Nuclear Reactor Incidents

ROBERT C. WHITCOMB, JR.
MICHAEL SAGE

Background and Nature of Problem

Electrical power demand has steadily increased in the United States. The generation of electricity by nuclear power has also steadily increased since the mid-1950s. By September 1994, the United States had 109 operating nuclear reactors producing about 21% of its electrical energy, compared with 56 nuclear reactors producing about 77% of the electrical energy in France (1).

As the use of nuclear power expanded, the potential for incidents at nuclear reactors increased. Three nuclear reactor incidents have caused measurable exposures of the public: Windscale in 1957, Three Mile Island (TMI) in 1979, and Chernobyl in 1986.

Scope and Relative Importance of the Problem

Nuclear power production is only one step in the nuclear fuel cycle. The cycle includes mining and milling uranium ores, converting uranium to a chemical form suitable for enrichment, enriching the isotopic content of uranium-235, fabricating fuel elements, producing energy in reactors, reprocessing irradiated fuel (a process that has ceased indefinitely in the United States), transporting materials throughout the fuel cycle, decommissioning facilities and equipment, and, finally, disposing of radioactive wastes. During each step in the nuclear fuel cycle, there is the potential for incidents (2).

397

A radiological incident can result in both short-term (acute) and long-term (chronic) exposure. The actual or potential doses to exposed persons vary from facility to facility and from one location to another. Generally, the doses decrease rapidly with distance from the source. In most cases, the primary health concern is the long-term increased risk of cancer. Protecting the public from nuclear incidents begins with designing and locating nuclear facilities and includes emergency response planning and preparedness.

Factors Affecting Problem Occurrence and Severity

Characteristics of Nuclear Reactors

In any complex industrial process, incidents should be anticipated. Those planning for or responding to potential incidents at nuclear reactors need thorough understanding of the design and operational characteristics of those reactors. It should be emphasized that each reactor design must be evaluated individually. For example, the Chernobyl reactor should be evaluated differently from reactors in the United States because it does not have the concrete containment building as do U.S. commercial reactors. This chapter's discussion focuses on typical U.S.-designed reactors.

A nuclear reactor has unique characteristics that pose special problems for emergency planners and responders. In a typical reactor vessel or core, uranium nuclei are split by neutrons, and thermal energy is released. Two or more smaller atoms are created from the fission of each large uranium nucleus. Many of these new atoms are radioactive. These "fission products" and the radionuclides produced as they decay make up the core inventory. The fission process and the decaying of fission products generate heat, which is removed by a coolant system (usually water) for conversion into steam and finally into electricity.

There are three main barriers to prevent the release of fission products. The first barrier is the fuel cladding. Uranium fuel pellets are placed inside this fuel cladding and arranged in specific patterns within the core. During normal operation, fission products are trapped inside the fuel rods, but if excessive heat builds up inside the core, the fuel cladding can rupture or melt and release fission products such as radioactive noble gases, iodine, and cesium. The second fission product barrier is the reactor coolant system. This barrier includes the pipes, pumps, and valves that supply cool water to the core and remove the heat generated in the core. Breaks or leaks in this system can result in liquid and gaseous releases. The third fission product barrier is the containment building. This concrete structure surrounds the core to provide physical containment of fission products and house mechanical safety features, including emergency cooling and filtration systems. It is designed to withstand postulated incidents within the plant and natural disasters such as earthquakes, storms, and collisions from aircraft. Breach of this barrier is indicative of a major incident.

In addition to these barriers are other safety systems that are also designed to prevent a release of radioactive material into the environment. For example, filters and other absorption media can trap most large particulates and reactive compounds before they reach the environment, and containment sprays can reduce the escape of fission products. However, a release to the environment can occur if safety systems or the containment building is damaged by mechanical failure, human error, or a natural disaster such as an earthquake.

The Nuclear Fuel Cycle

Incidents can happen at any stage within the nuclear fuel cycle, not just during the operation of the nuclear reactor. Uranium must first be mined and milled to produce yellow cake, a combination of all uranium isotopes. Since only certain isotopes of uranium can be fissioned in a conventional power reactor, the yellow cake is chemically processed and converted into a gaseous compound for enrichment. The fissionable isotopes are then separated and concentrated into a solid uranium oxide. Uranium oxide is shaped into pellets at a fuel-fabrication facility and loaded into fuel rods. A typical reactor must be refueled about every 18 months. Because the questions of how to permanently dispose of high-level waste has not been resolved, spent fuel rods are stored on site in spent fuel pools, with coolant systems to prevent the buildup of heat from the decay of fission products. Movement of the fuel rods into or out of the core (or within the storage facility) also poses the risk of an incident that could cause a release of fission products.

The processing of uranium involves a variety of hazardous chemicals, which could be released during an incident. For example, the incident in December 1985 at a uranium-conversion facility in Gore, Oklahoma, produced a cloud of hydrogen fluoride. One worker was killed and others were hospitalized from the acute effects of this vapor (*3*). Chemicals such as these could be released into water supplies or into the atmosphere during a fire or other incident. A partial list of the chemicals used at nuclear reactors and their potential health effects are shown in Table 19-1.

Public Health Impacts: Historical Perspective

Many nuclear reactor incidents in the United States have involved test or experimental reactors. Four of these incidents did not cause a release of radiological material to the environment despite damage to the core. These incidents involved the Chalk River Reactor, the Idaho Experimental Breeder, the Westinghouse Test Reactor, and Detroit Edison's Fermi Reactor (breeder). Significant quantities of radioiodine were released during reactor incidents at two facilities, one in the United States and one in England. Of these, the Windscale reactor in England and the SL-1 reactor in the United States

Table 19-1 Chemicals Used at Nuclear Power Plants

Chemical	Health Effects
Sulfuric acid	Irritating to eyes, nose, throat, respiratory tract, and skin; may cause pulmonary edema, bronchitis, emphysema, conjunctivitis, stomatitis, dental erosion, tracheobronchitis, skin and eye burns, and dermatitis.
Chlorine	Irritating to eyes, skin, nose, and mouth; may cause lacrimation, rhinorrhea, cough, choking, substernal pain, nausea, vomiting, headache, dizziness, syncope, pulmonary edema, pneumonia, hypoxemia, dermatitis, and eye and skin burns.
Ammonia	Irritating to eyes, nose, and throat; may cause dyspnea, bronchospasm, chest pain, pulmonary edema, pink frothy sputum, skin burns, and vesiculation.
Sodium hydroxide	Irritating to nose; may cause pneumonitis, burns to the eyes and skin, and temporary loss of hair.
Hydrazine	Irritating to eyes, nose, and throat; may cause temporary blindness, dizziness, nausea, dermatitis, and skin and eye burns. Also an animal carcinogen.

Sources: U.S. Department of Transportation. *1990 emergency response guidebook. Guidebook for first response to hazardous materials incidents.* Washington, D.C.: U.S. Department of Transportation, 1990; U.S. Department of Health and Human Services, National Institutes of Occupational Safety and Health (NIOSH). *Pocket guide to chemical hazards.* Washington, D.C.: Department of Health and Human Services, 1990.

did not have containment buildings and were not for commercial use or power production.

Two significant incidents have occurred at commercial power reactors. The incident at Three Mile Island, Pennsylvania, resulted in substantial damage to the core and the release of radioactive noble gases and radioiodine. The more recent incident at Chernobyl in the Ukraine (former Soviet Union) was the most serious incident recorded at any nuclear power facility. It produced massive damage to the core and allowed millions of curies of fission products to escape into the environment. Table 19-2 presents a summary of these incidents.

Chernobyl, Ukraine

The incident at the Chernobyl nuclear reactor, located in the Ukraine, occurred on April 26, 1986. It caused extensive contamination in the local area and also caused radioactive material to be widely dispersed and deposited throughout Europe and the northern hemisphere. An estimated 50 million curies of radioactive material were released into the environment. Twelve million curies (nearly 25% of the total) were released during the first day of the incident. Over the next 9 days, another 38 million curies escaped from the burning graphite core (*4*).

The reactor was one of many graphite-moderated, light-water-cooled reactors that produced electrical power in the former Soviet Union (*5*). Though construction features

Table 19-2 Incidents Involving Core Damage to Nuclear Reactors

Description of Incident	Site	Date	Collective Effective Dose (person Sv)*
Minor core damage (no release of radiological material)	Chalk River	1952	NA†
	Breeder Reactor, Idaho	1955	NA
	Westinghouse Test Reactor	1960	NA
	Detroit Edison Fermi	1966	NA
Major core damage (radioiodine released)			
Noncommercial	Windscale, England	1957	2000
Commercial	Three Mile Island, Pennsylvania	1979	40
	Chernobyl, Ukraine	1986	600,000
Other incidents (fission product release)	Kyshtym, Chelyabinsk, Russia	1957	2500

*Source: United Nations Scientific Committee on the Effects of Atomic Radiation (UNSCEAR). *Sources and effects of ionizing radiation*. Report to the General Assembly. New York: United Nations, 1993. (5)

†Not applicable; no release to the environment.

of this reactor are unique to Russian graphite-moderated reactors, the basic cause of the incident was human error. During a low-power test procedure, operators switched off critical safety systems. Instabilities within the reactor caused explosions and fire, damaging the reactor and releasing the core contents. The fire and release were terminated 10 days after the incident.

Fallout from the release spread over large parts of Europe and the Northern Hemisphere. Rain caused large variations in the deposition of radionuclides, which resulted in localized hot spots. Long-term exposures will continue as a result of the consumption of food grown on contaminated soil and direct irradiation from deposited radionuclides.

Evacuation of the general population was begun the morning of April 27, 1986. The evacuation of the entire 30-kilometer exclusion zone was completed by May 6, 1986. About 115,000 people were eventually evacuated from the affected areas (5). The zone remains evacuated today, although some people have been allowed to return to their homes in the less contaminated areas and others have returned to their homes in areas of the exclusion zone despite government efforts to deter them.

Other protective actions were taken after the incident. To reduce the amount of radioactive iodine accumulating in the thyroid gland, health officials distributed potassium iodide to the population on April 26 and several days after. Potassium iodide prophylaxis was given to 5.4 million people in the former Soviet Union, including 1.7

million children. Thousands of cattle and other livestock were removed from the contaminated areas. Officials also took actions to prevent or reduce contamination to surface water and groundwater, property, food, and land.

Thirty deaths occurred within 3 months of the incident. The initial explosion killed 2 workers. About 145 firefighters and emergency workers suffered acute radiation sickness, and 28 died within the 3 months following the event (4).

The estimated collective effective dose (the estimated effective dose to a reference individual of the population multiplied by the number of potentially exposed people in that population) from the Chernobyl event was approximately 600, 000 person sieverts (Sv). (The sievert is a special unit used to express the quantity of dose, discussed in further detail later in this chapter.) Of this amount, 40% was received in the former Soviet Union, 57% in the remainder of Europe, and 3% in other countries in the Northern Hemisphere (5).

Three Mile Island, Pennsylvania

On March 28, 1978, at the Three Mile Island power plant near Middletown, Pennsylvania, a series of mechanical failures and human errors led to a loss of coolant in the Unit 2 reactor, which allowed the core to overheat. During the incident, large amounts of radioactive materials were released into containment, but environmental releases were relatively small. Volatile radionuclides did escape through the ventilation system, but only after passing through a filtration system that removed the chemically active compounds, including most of the radioiodine. The principal radionuclides released were xenon and small quantities of iodine.

The estimated collective effective dose from Three Mile Island was approximately 40 person Sv. Individual doses averaged 15 μSv within 80 km of the plant. The maximum effective dose that any member of the public may have received from external gamma exposure is estimated to have been 850 μSv.

Windscale, England

When the United Kingdom began production of nuclear weapons, plutonium-producing reactors were constructed at a site on the northwest coast of England called Windscale. In 1957, a fire in one reactor released a substantial amount of fission products. Because radioiodine was released during the incident, protective actions for milk were implemented. Other food products and water did not require protective action. Ingestion of radioiodine in milk was considered the most likely pathway of exposure.

The estimated collective effective dose received in the United Kingdom and in Europe from all radionuclides and pathways was approximately 2,000 person Sv. Of this amount, 900 person Sv was due to inhalation, 800 was due to ingestion of milk and other foods, and 300 was due to external exposure to radionuclides deposited on the ground (5).

Kyshtym, Chelyabinsk, Russia

On September 29, 1957, a major incident occurred at a reprocessing facility in the former Soviet Union. Although this incident did not occur at a nuclear power plant, the results are typical of what might be expected from a catastrophic incident. The event occurred as a result of the failure of process-monitoring equipment, which led to a loss of cooling in a waste storage tank. The explosion and fire released about 1 EBq of radioactive materials, 90% of which was deposited locally and the remainder of which (about 100 PBq) was dispersed away from the site of the explosion. (A becquerel [Bq] is the unit of activity expressed in disintegrations per second. The prefix E is a multiplier of 10^{18}, and the prefix P is a multiplier of 10^{15}.). The radioactive plume reached a height of about 1 km, and fallout from this release extended to a distance of about 300 km from the site.

The estimated collective effective dose received by the evacuated populations was approximately 1,300 person Sv. The collective effective dose received by the nonevacuated populations was estimated to be approximately 1,200 person Sv (5).

Factors Influencing Morbidity and Mortality

Routes of Exposure

An atmospheric plume of airborne radioactive material from the plant is the principal source of public exposure during the initial stages of nuclear reactor incidents. Exposure can include an external dose received while immersed in the plume and an internal dose from inhaling gases or particulates. The plume is composed of varying mixtures of noble gases (e.g., krypton, xenon), iodines, and particulate material. The period of release may be short (a few hours) or last for several days.

If the original release contains primarily inert radioactive gases, surface contamination and the resultant potential for long-term exposure are small. However, if large quantities of particulates are released from the plant, surface contamination will be substantial and a long-term source of exposure. Long after the initial release from the plant, public exposure from radionuclides deposited on the ground, cars, homes, machinery, food crops, or water can continue both by direct external radiation and through several ingestion pathways. Radionuclides can be ingested directly by consuming water or by eating fruits and vegetables contaminated by radioactive materials. Food crops will also absorb and assimilate radionuclides from the soil so that long-term contamination of locally grown fruits and vegetables or animal feed can be a health concern. In addition, indirect pathways can develop through the food chain, such as through milk or meat from cows that ingested pasture grass, feed, or drinking water contaminated with radionuclides. The most common radionuclides in this pathway are iodine, strontium, and cesium.

Potential Health Effects

Adverse health effects associated with a nuclear reactor incident can be caused by direct injury (e.g., transportation accidents that can occur during an evacuation), by the stress of the situation (e.g., myocardial infarction, psychological distress), or by exposure to radioactive material or chemicals released during the incident. Only radiation exposures that have adverse health effects are considered here, because they are unique to radiological incidents.

A radiological incident can result in both short-term (acute) and long-term (chronic) exposure. The actual or potential doses to exposed persons vary from facility to facility and from one location to another. Generally, the doses decrease rapidly with distance from the source. The primary health concern is the long-term increased risk for cancer.

The biological effects of radiation exposure depend on the absorbed dose, the type of radiation, the rate of exposure, how much of the body is exposed, and the specific organs exposed (e.g., thyroid gland). Because genetic material is particularly sensitive to radiation, tissues that divide rapidly (e.g., blood-forming tissues, intestinal-lining cells) are more sensitive to damage than those that divide more slowly (e.g., muscle, nervous system tissue).

The exposure of only a part of the body, such as an arm or leg or a single organ, is less damaging than the exposure of the whole body to the same dose. Dose rate also has a significant influence on the recipients biological response. Because of the body's repair mechanisms, the effects from a dose of 5 Sv delivered instantaneously is quite different from those caused by the same dose given over a month or more. Adverse health effects increase with the combination of the total dose, the proportion of the body exposed, and the dose rate.

Dose Quantities

Radiation is energy emitted from radioactive materials as waves or particles. Three types of radiation are alpha, beta, and gamma. Alpha and beta radiation are particles released from the nucleus of an atom. Gamma rays are electromagnetic waves with energy similar to that of X rays.

The absorbed dose is the amount of energy deposited in the body during radiation exposure. Absorbed dose is measured in joules per kilogram (J/kg). The special unit used to express this quantity is the gray (Gy). One gray is equal to 1 J/kg (6).

Because different types of radiation (e.g., gamma rays, beta particles, alpha particles) produce different tissue damage at the same absorbed dose, the absorbed dose is often multiplied by a radiation-weighting factor to give what is called an equivalent dose. The special unit used to express this quantity is the sievert (Sv) (7).

Another measure of dose, the effective dose, is used to account for the fact that a particular radiation dose to one part of the body does not produce the same potential health impact as the same dose to another part. For example, when radioiodine is taken internally, it is selectively concentrated in the thyroid gland. When the radioiodine decays, most of its energy is deposited in the thyroid. To calculate the effect that the dose received by the thyroid has on the whole body (i.e., the effective dose), one must multiply the thyroid dose by the tissue-weighting factor.

When large populations or population groups are exposed, a unit of collective effective dose (person Sv) is employed. It represents the estimated effective dose to a reference individual of the population multiplied by the number of potentially exposed people in that population.

Acute Effects

Acute doses result from an instantaneous or short-term exposure (of less than a few days) to radiation or radioactive materials. After an acute, whole-body dose of <1 Sv, an individual may have no outward symptoms but may show increased chromosomal aberrations in blood lymphocytes and lower blood count. A higher dose may produce acute radiation syndrome, a condition with dose-dependent symptoms. Acute, whole-body doses of >1 Sv may cause vomiting, hemorrhage, and an increased risk for infection due to reduced white-blood-cell counts. Treatment may include antibiotic therapy, blood transfusions, and possibly bone-marrow transplantation. Acute, whole-body doses of >10 Sv will damage the gastrointestinal tract, causing diarrhea and electrolyte imbalance, and may affect the central nervous system, causing seizures, gait disturbances, and coma. Ninety percent of people exposed to such doses will die. Fortunately, such acute, whole-body radiation doses in peacetime are very rare.

Chronic Effects

Chronic doses result from long-term exposure (over several days, many years, or a lifetime) to radiation or radioactive materials deposited in the environment or internally in the body. The most pressing health concerns associated with nuclear-reactor incidents are the delayed effects from long-term exposure to low levels of radiation (8). Data on the biological effects of radiation have been collected from animal studies and studies of humans exposed to diagnostic, therapeutic, occupational, and wartime irradiation. Exposed people include children exposed prenatally during abdominal X rays received by their mothers during pregnancy, people who underwent treatment for ankylosing spondylitis, radium-dial painters, uranium miners, and survivors of the atomic bombing of Hiroshima and Nagasaki in World War II. These studies provide evidence for three types of delayed effects: somatic effects on the exposed person, teratogenic effects on the developing fetus exposed in utero, and genetic effects on the offspring of the exposed person.

Risk Factors and Health Effects

Risk factors for exposure during a radiological release are numerous. Obviously, both living adjacent to and downwind from a nuclear power plant increase an individual's chance of exposure if an incident occurs. People such as farmers or construction workers who work outdoors are also at additional risk because they probably take longer to return home for sheltering or evacuation. To alert these people in case of an incident, emergency officials should use sirens to supplement radio or television warnings. In addition, systems should be developed for alerting the hard of hearing. People who have difficulty evacuating are also at risk. For example, the physically challenged, nursing-home and hospital patients, and prisoners require special aid and additional time to evacuate. In areas surrounding nuclear facilities, individuals who will need assistance should be clearly identified in the local community emergency-response plan. Plans should also be developed to alert local schools, hospitals, and prisons of any unintentional release. Some population groups more sensitive to radiation exposure, such as children and fetuses, require extra consideration when protective actions are implemented. For example, children and pregnant women may be evacuated before the rest of the population or at lower expected dose levels. By developing county and state emergency response plans, additional risk to these special groups can be reduced.

Many risk factors for long-term environmental exposure after the plume has passed are identical to factors that can increase exposure during a radioactive release. Children and fetuses are more sensitive to radiation than adults. Children are more vulnerable to exposure from radionuclides in milk because they generally drink more milk than adults. People who live in rural areas and people of low socioeconomic status may eat more locally grown fruits and vegetables and are at greater risk of ingesting contaminants from these sources. A population that uses surface water (from reservoirs or rivers) may receive additional exposure from drinking water contaminated by surface runoff or by direct deposition from the plume.

The main somatic effect of radiation exposures is cancer, especially leukemia, thyroid cancer, breast cancer, and lung cancer. According to current estimates of the risk to members of the public from low-level radiation exposure, a whole-body dose of 1 Sv increases an individual's lifetime risk for fatal cancer by about 5%, the risk for nonfatal cancer by 1%, and the risk for severe genetic effects by 1.3%. For someone exposed to 1 Sv, the total increased risk is thus 7.3% (7, 9).

The principal teratogenic effects described in studies of survivors of the atomic bombings of Nagasaki and Hiroshima have been mental retardation and reduced head size, especially among people who were exposed as fetuses 8–15 weeks after conception. After 12 weeks of gestation, maternal exposure to significant quantities of radioactive iodine can destroy the fetal thyroid gland.

Genetic effects among offspring of the exposed population may include mutations and chromosomal aberrations. These changes may be transmitted and become manifest as disorders in the offspring of the exposed individual. Radiation has not been shown to cause such effects in humans, but experimental studies on plants and animals suggest that such effects are possible.

None of these risk estimates for low-level exposures are precise, because they are extrapolated from risks associated with relatively high radiation exposure. The exact risk at low levels of exposure is not known. Nevertheless, because the interaction of radiation with human tissue is believed to be harmful even at low levels, radiation exposures beyond natural background radiation should be reduced.

Public Health Implications and Prevention Strategies in Radiation Disasters

Acute Exposures

If, despite precautions to prevent exposure, some people are exposed to external or internal sources of radiation following a nuclear plant incident, much of the morbidity and mortality from these exposures can still be prevented. For acute exposures, emergency lifesaving assistance to prevent shock from trauma or to maintain respiration has highest priority. People exposed externally or internally may require symptomatic treatment at a specialized hospital if their whole-body dose is >50 rem (the United States continues to use traditional dose units, although it is moving toward using the International System of units and measurements: 100 rem = 1 Sv). However, people whose skin or clothing has been contaminated by radioactive material may also pose a hazard to the hospital staff and other patients. Therefore, these people must go through decontamination procedures both to prevent adverse health effects to them and to protect other people from being exposed.

Treatment for radiation injuries depends on the degree of exposure and on whether the exposure is internal or external. It is extremely unlikely that a live patient will be so contaminated as to pose an acute radiation risk to rescue or medical personnel. Therefore, for any acutely exposed radiation victims, the usual priorities of emergency care (the saving of life and the prevention of further injury) take precedence over decontaminating the patient or minimizing the exposure of attending personnel.

Clinical assessment of a person's level of exposure is generally more accurate than the assessment of the general populations exposure. Personal dosimeter readings, direct measurements of radioactivity in and on the body, and clinical assessments of symptoms, signs, and white blood cell counts may provide evidence of the level of exposure. For the general population, exposures can be estimated from levels of radiation measured by detectors around the plant and by factors such as peoples distance and direction from the plant and the time they spent at different exposed locations. Analysis of biological samples and whole-body radiation counters can be used to detect internal levels of radionuclides. Although studies of chromosomal aberrations in blood lymphocytes may detect exposures as low as 10 rem within a few hours after an incident, medical examinations and treatment should be confined to people who are highly exposed or contaminated or who have ingested or inhaled significant quantities of radioactive material.

Chronic Exposures

For low-level chronic exposures, both internal and external, it is unclear whether long-term follow-up and monitoring can reduce subsequent morbidity and mortality. However, clinical assessment should be continued, especially for people who have ingested or inhaled radioactive materials. This follow-up is essential in order to assess the material's assimilation in and elimination from the body and ultimately to provide an improved estimate of the total dose to that individual. Epidemiologic studies based on registries of exposed people may provide further information on the effects of low-level radiation, although their low statistical power may make interpretation difficult (8).

Prevention and Control Measures

Design and Placement Factors

The prevention of a nuclear reactor incident should be a priority during the initial stages of designing a nuclear plant. One of the most important safety factors is the choice of plant location, which involves geographic and meteorologic considerations. A site should not be selected in an area with high seismic activity, although it may not be possible to choose a site with no history of seismic vibrations. The probability of earthquakes can be estimated for a general area on the basis of past seismic activity and the location of faults. The site should not be located in areas such as floodplains or in tornado- or hurricane-prone areas. The potential health effects from a release can also be limited by locating the plant in an area with a low population density and by establishing an uninhabited area around the plant to act as a barrier between the reactor and the population.

After the site is selected, the plant should be designed in accordance with the conditions at that particular site. Special construction features can increase the safety of the plant. For instance, in areas in which tornadoes or earthquakes may occur, plants should be built to withstand high winds and impact from blowing debris; and in areas in which earthquakes may occur, plants should be built to withstand vibrations from minor earthquakes.

Factors Relating to Plant Operation

Though many of a nuclear reactor's safety systems are computer-controlled, operators are essential to the safe operation of the plant. To lower the probability of human error, plant personnel are trained to respond to unusual conditions within the plant and are assigned specific responsibilities during an incident. However, fatigue from rotating shifts, boredom, and inadequate training or supervision can lead to serious human error. In fact, all radiological incidents can be partially attributed to human error. To deter deliberate sabotage of the reactor, plant personnel can use security systems to prevent unauthorized personnel from being on site and to limit access to sensitive areas of the plant.

Off site, elected officials and emergency workers such as firefighters and police officers should also learn to help in activities such as evacuation and to protect themselves and others from radiation hazards. State and federal emergency response plans provide a blueprint for agencies to use in responding to emergencies and to help them reduce possible errors in human judgment during an incident.

Surveillance for Incidents

The Nuclear Regulatory Commission (NRC) and the Federal Emergency Management Agency (FEMA) have established a system to identify unusual occurrences at nuclear facilities. The operator of a nuclear power facility must notify the NRC of changes in the plant's normal status so that officials can prepare to respond immediately to any release that occurs. A tiered classification system based on four emergency action levels defines the severity of the status of a reactor incident and the potential for a release. Investigation of reports of unusual occurrences can clarify the types of incidents that occur at a nuclear facility. Other nuclear power plant operators are notified of the results from these investigations so that they can evaluate the safety of their own procedures and avoid similar incidents. The emergency action levels defined by NRC are described in Table 19-3.

Emergency-Response Planning

Since the Three Mile Island incident in 1979, FEMA has developed a national contingency plan, the Federal Radiological Emergency Response Plan (FRERP), to coordinate federal response to peacetime radiological emergencies (*10*). (FEMA issued draft revisions in 1994.) The FRERP describes the federal government's concept of operations for responding to radiological emergencies, outlines federal policies and planning assumptions that underlie this concept of operations and on which federal agency response

Table 19-3 Emergency Action Levels Defined by the Nuclear Regulatory Commission

Emergency Action Level	Plant Status
Notification of unusual event	Potential degradation of the normal level of plant safety with no release of radioactivity requiring offsite response.
Alert	Actual or potential degradation of plant safety at a substantial level; any potential release expected to be well below established emergency action levels.
Site-area emergency	Actual or probable failure of safety systems that normally provide protection for the public; potential releases not expected to exceed established action levels except in areas near the plant boundary.
General emergency	Actual or imminent core degradation or melting with a potential for loss of containment integrity; potential releases expected to exceed established action levels.

Source: U.S. Nuclear Regulatory Commission. *Response technical manual*. RTM-92, vol. 1, rev. 2. Washington, D.C.: U.S. Nuclear Regulatory Commission, Division of Operational Assessment, Office for Analysis and Evaluation of Operational Data, 1992. (*17*)

plans (other than agency-specific policies) are based, and specifies the authorities and responsibilities of each federal agency that has a substantial role in dealing with such emergencies.

Individual federal agencies (e.g., the Centers for Disease Control and Prevention) have developed more specific plans applicable to their unique capabilities and responsibilities (*11, 12*). All operating nuclear power plant sites have state and local off-site emergency-preparedness plans, but they have not all been approved by FEMA. The General Accounting Office has reported to the U.S. Congress on "further actions needed to improve emergency preparedness around nuclear power plants," especially the need for better centralized federal agency control and coordination (*13*).

Neighboring countries have begun developing plans that establish cooperative efforts and response to potential incidents that have potential transboundary effects. One such plan is in development between the United States and Canada (*14*).

"Tabletop" and field exercises are regularly conducted by FEMA to test federal plans for radiological emergency response. All agencies with primary responsibility participate in these exercises to test their own readiness and to refine the federal response plan. State and local officials also participate in these FEMA-sponsored exercises so that methods for local, state, and federal interactions can be developed. However, no exercise can fully test an emergency-response plan or can fully anticipate political, economic, or social issues that influence public health recommendations during an emergency.

Reducing Off-Site Exposures from a Nuclear Reactor Incident

The U.S. Environmental Protection Agency (EPA) has set *protective action guides (PAGs)*, which are levels at which action should be taken to lower the potential radiation dose to the public. These are not actual doses but are projected or estimated doses that would be received if no action is taken.

Actions to reduce or eliminate exposure of the public following a nuclear power plant incident should be based on the realization that a potentially serious problem is developing and may continue many years after the actual release of radioactive material. Federal emergency-response plans contain specific requirements regarding the notification of local, state, and federal officials. The degree of response by state and federal agencies depends on the severity of the incident and the size of the potentially exposed population. Decisions to initiate a particular protective action are based on factors such as local weather conditions and the conditions at the plant, which influence the probability of a release and the probability of which isotopes will be released. To be effective, protective actions should meet the following criteria (15):

- The action must be effective in reducing or preventing exposure to the public and must not carry health risks greater than those of the incident itself (i.e., if a release has already begun, the benefits of evacuation must be weighed against the expected dose people would receive during the evacuation).
- The implementation of the protective action must be feasible both logistically and financially.
- The agency or agencies responsible for implementing the protective action must be clearly identified and must have the authority to implement the action.
- The protective action's economic impact on the public, business, industry, or government must not exceed the health and economic impacts of the incident itself.

Early-Phase Protective Action

The early phase of a nuclear reactor incident is also known as the plume phase. This phase begins with the notification of an event and ends with the termination of the release or plume passage in the affected area.

For the general population, EPA recommends that protective action be taken if the projected thyroid dose is at least 25 rem or if the projected whole-body dose is from 1 to 5 rem (16). However, more stringent limits may be applied by state health authorities, particularly for pregnant women and children. Protective actions may include evacuating, sheltering, or administering potassium iodide (KI) to the potentially exposed population. The current early phase PAGs recommended by the EPA are presented in Table 19-4.

One of the first decisions to be made is whether to advise people to evacuate or remain in their homes with their windows and doors shut and ventilation turned off while the radioactive plume passes. By remaining in their homes and using respiratory protection such as wet handkerchiefs or towels, people can lower their inhalation of particulates but not of noble gases. Sheltering can also reduce gamma exposure from the plume by a factor of 2–10, but it is an alternative only for short periods of time

Table 19-4 Protective Action Guides (PAGs) for the Early Phase of a Nuclear Incident

Protective Action	PAG Projected Dose	Comments
Evacuation (or sheltering)	1–5 rem*	Evacuation (or for some situations, sheltering) should normally be initiated at one rem.
Administer stable iodine	25 rem†	Requires approval of state medical officials.

*The sum of the effective dose equivalent resulting from external exposure and the committed effective dose equivalent incurred from all significant inhalation pathways during the early phase.

†Committed dose equivalent to the thyroid from radioiodine.

Source: U.S. Nuclear Regulatory Commission. *Response technical manual.* RTM-92, vol. 1, rev. 2. Washington, D.C.: U.S. Nuclear Regulatory Commission, Division of Operational Assessment, Office for Analysis and Evaluation of Operational Data, 1992. (*17*)

because of the infiltration of gases and vapors into the dwelling by normal air exchange with outside air. The decision to have people seek shelter in the area rather than evacuate is questionable if the release period is unpredictable or likely to be longer than several hours. Evacuation is a more costly but generally more effective method for reducing public exposure before a release has occurred. Officials who must decide whether to order an evacuation must consider such factors as adverse weather conditions (which may make evacuation an unsuitable alternative), the likelihood of a release, the availability of shelters for the evacuees, and the quality of the evacuation routes. If a release has already begun, the benefits of evacuation must be weighed against the expected dose received during the evacuation.

If radioiodine is released from the plant, the administration of stable iodide in potassium iodide (KI) tablets can lower or block the uptake of radioiodine by the thyroid. However, KI tablets will not protect against external radiation exposure or exposure to other inhaled radionuclides. To be effective, KI should be administered about 3 hours before exposure to radioiodine (*17*). Although some people may also suffer side effects after taking KI, a risk assessment by the Food and Drug Administration (FDA) suggests that the risk from a projected thyroid dose of 25 rem outweighs the risk from short-term use of KI (*18*). During an actual release, the potential dose of radioiodine to the thyroid is estimated by using dispersion modeling based on the actual or imminent conditions at the plant. The decision to use or not use KI and the determination of how it should be distributed are left to the individual states. However, the rapid distribution of KI tablets required during an emergency is difficult, stockpiling for an unlikely release is costly, and the KI tablets have a limited shelf life.

Intermediate-Phase Protective Actions

The intermediate phase is also known as the relocation or reentry phase of the incident and extends through the first year following the release. The PAG for this phase is 2

Table 19-5 Protective Action Guides (PAGs) for Exposure to Deposited Radioactivity During the Intermediate Phase of a Nuclear Incident

Protective Action	PAG Projected Dose	Comments
Relocate the general population.	≥2 rem	Beta dose to skin may be up to 50 times higher.
Apply simple dose reduction techniques.	<2 rem	These protective actions should be taken to reduce doses to as low as practicable levels.

Source: U.S. Nuclear Regulatory Commission. *Response technical manual*. RTM-92, vol. 1, rev. 2. Washington, D.C.: U.S. Nuclear Regulatory Commission, Division of Operational Assessment, Office for Analysis and Evaluation of Operational Data, 1992. (*17*)

rem. This projected dose includes the sum of the effective dose equivalent from external gamma radiation and the committed effective dose equivalent from inhalation of resuspended materials received in the first year. If projected doses in the first year are equal to or greater than 2 rem, residents should be evacuated or, if already evacuated, permanently relocated outside the contaminated area. The current intermediate-phase PAGs recommended by the EPA are presented in Table 19-5.

Additionally, access to highly contaminated areas can be restricted to prevent the public from entering. In less severe situations, dilution and removal of contamination can be attempted by washing surfaces, soaking or plowing soil, or removing soil from highly concentrated areas. Weathering from rain or snow also decreases the concentration of radionuclides on structures and on the ground surface, although surface runoff may recontaminate local lakes and streams after each heavy rain.

Ingestion Pathway Protective Actions

Protective actions for the ingestion pathway can take place anytime during the intermediate phase and continue many years after the release. These actions are concerned with limiting the intake of radioactive materials contained in foods. There are two types of protective actions that can be taken during this period—preventive and emergency. Preventive actions, such as placing dairy cows on stored feed, have a minimal impact on radioactive contamination of human food or animal feed. Emergency actions, which have a larger impact, include isolating food containing radioactivity to prevent its introduction into commerce, or condemning and disposing of contaminated foods. The FDA preventative PAGs are a projected dose of 0.5 rem to the whole body, bone marrow, or any other organ, or 1.5 rem to the thyroid. The emergency PAGs are a projected dose of 5 rem to the whole body, bone marrow, or any other organ, or 15 rem to the thyroid. The current ingestion PAGs recommended by the FDA are presented in Table 19-6 (*19*). (The FDA issued draft revisions to its guidance in 1994.)

Table 19-6 FDA Protective Action Guides (PAGs) for Ingestion of Contaminated Foods

PAG	Organ of Interest	Projected Dose Commitment
Preventive (lower impact)	Whole body, bone marrow, or any other organ	0.5 rem
	Thyroid	1.5 rem
Emergency (high impact)	Whole body, bone marrow, or any other organ	5 rem
	Thyroid	15 rem

Source: U.S. Nuclear Regulatory Commission. *Response technical manual.* RTM-92, vol. 1, rev. 2. Washington, D.C.: U.S. Nuclear Regulatory Commission, Division of Operational Assessment, Office for Analysis and Evaluation of Operational Data, 1992. (*17*)

The ingestion of contaminated food or water can be prevented by supplying fresh food and drinking water to residents if necessary. Normal food preparation such as peeling or washing can remove the contamination on some fruits and vegetables. Food that cannot be appropriately decontaminated may need to be destroyed. Significant contamination of milk can be avoided by providing uncontaminated feed and water to cattle. The success of this action depends on the availability of stored feed and fresh water and the ability of farmers to remove cows from pastures in a short time.

Late-Phase Protective Actions

The late phase is also known as the recovery phase of an incident. During this phase, the main concern is reducing radiation in the environment to levels that will allow the general population to have unrestricted access to the once contaminated area. This phase may last many years.

Research Recommendations

- Collect information on the optimal ways to educate the public about the potential risks from nuclear reactors, the effects of any radiological release, and protective actions that can be taken in the event of a release. Such education may alleviate the public's anxiety about possible incidents and minimize their exposure if one does occur.
- Conduct further research on ways to control human error associated with radiological incidents. For example, examine whether safety systems should be designed so that plant operators cannot turn them off, whether rotating shifts should be eliminated, whether current training programs need improvement, and how quality work can be maintained during off-shifts such as weekends or nights.

- Because incidents can occur throughout the nuclear fuel cycle, ensure that federal emergency-response planning places more emphasis on planning for incidents at all parts of the cycle rather than concentrating efforts solely on preparation for a catastrophic event at a nuclear power reactor.
- Conduct additional research to determine which isotopes will most likely be the greatest source of exposure during a variety of release scenarios. Until the Three Mile Island incident, emergency plans for reactors centered on a large release of radioiodine. However, during the Three Mile Island incident, significantly less radioiodine was released than expected. At Chernobyl, long-lived isotopes continue to pose a more significant hazard than would have been estimated previously.
- Examine ways of providing state and federal agencies with additional expertise in emergency response and radiological safety.
- Provide states with more-concrete guidance on the value of stockpiling potassium iodide or distributing it during an incident.
- Reevaluate traditional methods for treating victims of a major radiological incident in view of the experience gained in the treatment of trauma and severe radiation exposure during and following the disaster at Chernobyl.

Summary and Conclusions

The reactor core is the central component of a nuclear power plant. Complex mechanical systems cool and protect the reactor, convert the thermal energy to electricity, and filter effluents. Natural disasters, mechanical failures, and human errors can all contribute to an incident by damaging the safety systems or the core itself. A release of radioactive material such as noble gases and radioiodine is most likely to be caused by a series of malfunctions or errors rather than by a single event. To prevent exposures, engineers must design nuclear power plants so that the possibility of an incident is reduced. Plant personnel can also be trained to maintain safety systems within the plant and to respond appropriately if an incident does occur.

Health effects from a radiological release can be acute or chronic. Relatively high doses of radiation can damage the bone marrow, intestinal lining, and nervous system. Cancer or genetic defects induced by radiation exposure may not appear until many years after exposure and may be induced by low levels of exposure. Chemicals stored on-site at nuclear facilities can also pose a health hazard during an incident. The publics exposure can be avoided or reduced with proper planning and response to possible incidents at a nuclear facility. The public around a nuclear plant can be evacuated or sheltered before or during an unintentional release to prevent external exposure and inhalation of radionuclides. After the release has ended, food and water pathways and surface contamination can be important sources of exposure. Supplying fresh food and water can reduce the direct ingestion of radionuclides. However, radionuclides can also build up in foods (e.g., the cow–milk–human pathway) and may require different strategies to prevent exposure. If exposure occurs despite protective actions, morbidity and mortality can be reduced through appropriate medical care for acute effects and possibly through long-term screening for cancer.

Populations and individuals that are more sensitive to radiation may be at higher risk from an incident. Children and fetuses are more sensitive to radiation effects than adults and are more likely to be exposed through the cow–milk–human pathway. People living closest to a reactor are at a higher risk for exposure during an incident, as are those who work outdoors. People who eat vegetables and fruit from local gardens are more likely to ingest radionuclides through food pathways. People who are elderly, physically challenged, or hospitalized require special assistance during an emergency. Protective actions to reduce the risks that a radiological release poses for such people should be addressed in radiological emergency-response plans.

Planning for nuclear power plant incidents has expanded, and continues to expand, after the incidents at Three Mile Island and Chernobyl. State emergency plans and exercises to test those plans are required around nuclear facilities. Federal plans have also been developed and tested through exercises. Multinational plans are being developed to address facilities located near national borders. In all plans, however, exercises are not likely to fully explore the political, economic, social, and technical problems that will develop during an actual emergency. Therefore, emergency response plans must be flexible, and state and federal agencies must maintain the technical and managerial expertise to cope with emergency-response issues.

References

1. American Nuclear Society. World list of nuclear power plants. *Nuclear News* 1994;37:57–76.
2. Organization for Economic Co-Operation and Development, Nuclear Energy Agency. *The safety of the nuclear fuel cycle*. Washington, D.C.: Organization for Economic Co-Operation and Development, Nuclear Energy Agency. 1992.
3. U.S. Nuclear Regulatory Commission. *Assessment of the public health impact from the accidental release of UF6 at the Sequoyah Fuels Corporation facility at Gore, Oklahoma*. U.S. Nuclear Regulator Commission NUREG 1189. Washington, D.C.: U.S. Government Printing Office, 1986.
4. The International Chernobyl Project. *Assessment of radiological consequences and evaluation of protective measures. Technical report by the International Advisory Committee*. Vienna: International Atomic Energy Agency, 1992.
5. United Nations Scientific Committee on the Effects of Atomic Radiation (UNSCEAR). *Sources and effects of ionizing radiation*. Report to the General Assembly. New York: United Nations, 1993.
6. International Commission on Radiation Units and Measurements. *Quantities and units in radiation protection dosimetry*. ICRU Report 51. Bethesda, MD: International Commission on Radiation Units and Measurements, 1993.

7. International Commission on Radiological Protection. *1990 recommendations of the International Commission on Radiological Protection.* ICRP Publication 60. New York: Pergamon Press, 1991.

8. National Research Council, Committee on the Biological Effects of Ionizing Radiations (BEIR). *Health effects of exposure to low levels of ionizing radiation.* BEIR V. Washington, D.C.: National Academy Press, 1990.

9. National Council on Radiation Protection and Measurements. *Limitation of exposure to ionizing radiation.* NCRP Report No. 116. Bethesda, MD: National Council on Radiation Protection and Measurements, 1991.

10. Federal Emergency Management Agency. Federal radiological emergency response plan. *Federal Register* 1984;49(178):35896–35925.

11. U.S. Department of Health and Human Services (HHS). *HHS radiological emergency response plan.* Washington, D.C.: Department of Health and Human Services, 1985.

12. U.S. Department of Health and Human Services. *Centers for Disease Control emergency response plan.* Washington, D.C.: Department of Health and Human Services, 1990.

13. U.S. General Accounting Office. *Further actions needed to improve emergency preparedness around nuclear power plants.* Gaithersburg, MD: U.S. General Accounting Office, 1984.

14. Governments of Canada and the United States of America. *Joint radiological emergency response plan.* Draft October 11, 1994.

15. International Commission on Radiological Protection. *Protection of the public in the event of a major radiation accident.* ICRP Publication 40. New York: Pergamon Press, 1984.

16. U.S. Environmental Protection Agency. *Manual of protective action guides and protective actions for nuclear incidents.* Washington, D.C.: Environmental Protection Agency, 1992.

17. U.S. Nuclear Regulatory Commission. *Response technical manual.* RTM-92, vol. 1, rev 2. Washington, D.C.: U.S. Nuclear Regulatory Commission, Division of Operational Assessment, Office for Analysis and Evaluation of Operational Data, 1992.

18. Food and Drug Administration. *Potassium iodide as a thyroid-blocking agent in a radiation emergency: recommendations on use.* Washington, D.C.: Department of Health and Human Services, 1982.

19. Food and Drug Administration. *Accidental radioactive contamination of human food and animal feed: recommendations for state and local agencies.* Washington, D.C.: Department of Health and Human Services, 1982.

Recommended Readings

American Medical Association. *A guide to the hospital management of injuries arising from exposure to or involving ionizing radiation.* Chicago: American Medical Association, 1984.

Arnold L. Windscale 1957: anatomy of a nuclear accident. London, U.K.: MacMillan Academic and Professional Ltd., 1992.

Dohrenwend BP. Psychological implications of nuclear accidents: the case of Three Mile Island. *Bull N Y Acad Med* 1983;59:1060–1076.

Eichholz G. *Environmental aspects of nuclear power.* Ann Arbor, MI: Ann Arbor Science, 1982.

Fabrikant J. The effects of the accident at Three Mile Island on the mental health and behavioral responses of the general population and nuclear workers. *Health Phys* 1983:45:579–586.

Gardner MJ, Winter PD. Mortality in Cumberland during 1959–78 with reference to cancer in young people around Windscale. *Lancet* 1984:1:216–217.

Goldhaber MK, Tokuhata GK, Digon E, *et al*: The Three Mile Island population registry. *Public Health Rep* 1983;98:603–609.

Goldhaber MK, Staub SL, Tokuhata GK. Spontaneous abortions after the Three Mile Island nuclear accident: a life table analysis. *Am J Public Health* 1983;73:752–759.

Health Physics Society. *Guide for hospital emergency departments on handling radiation accident patients*. McLean, VA: Health Physics Society, 1985.

Hubner KF. Decontamination procedures and risks to health care personnel. *Bull N Y Acad Med* 1983;59:1119–1128.

Lester MS. Public information during a nuclear power plant accident: lessons learned from Three Mile Island. *Bull N Y Acad Med* 1983;59:1080–1086.

National Council on Radiation Protection and Measurements. *Protection of the thyroid gland in the event of releases of radioiodine No. 55*. Bethesda, MD: National Council on Radiation Protection and Measurements, 1977.

Nuclear Regulatory Commission. *Reactor safety study: an assessment of accident risks in U.S. commercial nuclear power plants*. Springfield, VA: U.S. Nuclear Regulatory Commission, 1975.

Nuclear Regulatory Commission. *Population dose and health impact of the accident at the Three Mile Island nuclear station*. Washington, D.C.: U.S. Nuclear Regulatory Commission, 1979.

Nuclear Regulatory Commission. *Report on the accident at the Chernobyl nuclear power station*. Washington, D.C.: U.S. Government Printing Office, 1987.

Shleien B. *Preparedness and response in radiation accidents*. Washington, D.C.: Food and Drug Administration, 1983.

Shleien B, Schmidt GD, Chiaechierini RP. *Background for protective action recommendations: accidental radioactive contamination of food and animal feeds*. Washington, D.C.: Food and Drug Administration, 1984.

Sutherland RM, Mulcahy RT. Basic principles of radiation biology. In: Rubin P, Bakermeier RF, Krackov SK, editors. *Clinical oncology for medical students and physicians*, 6th ed. Rochester, NY: American Cancer Society, 1983:40–57.

Urguhart J, Palmer M, Cutler J. Cancer in Cumbria: the Windscale connection. *Lancet* 1984; 1:217–218.

Wald N. Diagnosis and therapy of radiation injuries. *Bull N Y Acad Med* 1983;59:1129–1138.

20

Complex Emergencies: Refugee and Other Populations

MICHAEL J. TOOLE

Background and Nature of Complex Emergencies

Since the end of the cold war in 1991, the frequency of violent civil conflicts has increased worldwide. Recent examples that have attracted widespread media attention include the Kurdish exodus from northern Iraq in 1991, Somalia in 1992–93, Bosnia and Herzegovina in 1992–93, and Rwanda in 1994. Moreover, equally severe though less visible conflicts during the past several years have affected millions of people in Angola, Burundi, Mozambique, southern Sudan, Liberia, Afghanistan, Tajikistan, Azerbaijan, and Georgia. Wars have increasingly targeted civilian populations, resulting in high civilian casualty rates, widespread human rights abuses, forced removal of communities from their homes or "ethnic cleansing," and, in some countries, the total collapse of governance. The deliberate use of food as a weapon of war in some instances has led to severe famine. A new term—*complex emergency*—has been coined to describe these relatively acute situations that affect large civilian populations and usually involve a combination of war or civil strife, food shortages, and population displacement that results in significant excess mortality.

Violent civil wars are not unique to the post–cold war era; conflicts in Ethiopia, Cambodia, Vietnam, East Timor, and Afghanistan caused millions of civilian deaths during the 1970s and 1980s. However, since 1991, several developments have heightened both the real risk and the perceived frequency of conflicts worldwide. First, the two former superpowers no longer have the ability to influence their former client-states to facilitate the resolution of internal conflicts. Second, since the end of the cold war, civil conflicts have tended to be of an ethnic or religious nature, unleashing intense historical forces for independence and nationhood. Third, since the fall of the "Iron Curtain," international media organizations have been able to gain access to zones of conflict more readily and new satellite technology has enabled scenes from the battle-front to be beamed directly into living rooms the world over. While this "CNN effect" has sometimes promptly mobilized public concern for emergency victims, it has also led to short memories. The transient coverage of disasters in foreign lands has inhibited international efforts to learn from past mistakes and to incorporate those lessons into emergency-preparedness planning.

Scope and Relative Importance of Complex Emergencies

Since 1980, approximately 130 armed conflicts have occurred worldwide; 32 have each caused more than 1,000 battlefield deaths (*1*). Between 1975 and 1989, civil conflicts were estimated to have caused approximately 750,000 deaths in Africa, 150,000 in Latin America, 3,400,000 in Asia, and 800, 000 in the Middle East (*2*). Since 1990, the carnage has increased as new wars have ignited in Somalia, Burundi, Rwanda, Angola, and Sri Lanka. In addition, since 1990, three European conflicts—in the former Yugoslavia, Azerbaijan, and Georgia—have caused at least 300,000 deaths. UNICEF estimates that 1.5 million children have been killed in wars since 1980 (*3*).

Factors Affecting Problem Occurrence and Severity

There is a fairly predictable sequence of events in the evolution of complex humanitarian emergencies. Political instability, the persecution of certain minorities, and human rights abuses lead to civil unrest and violence. Governments and ruling elites respond with greater repression, causing widespread armed conflict. The direct destruction of infrastructure, the diversion of resources away from community services, and general economic collapse lead to a deterioration in medical services, especially prevention programs such as child immunization and antenatal care. Medical treatment facilities are overwhelmed by the needs of war casualties; the routine management of medical problems suffers from lack of staff and shortages in essential medical supplies.

Deliberate diversion of food supplies by various armed factions, disruption of transport and marketing, and economic hardship often cause severe food deficits. Local farmers may not plant crops as extensively as usual, the supply of seeds and fertilizer may be disrupted, irrigation systems may be damaged by the fighting, and crops may be intentionally destroyed or looted by armed soldiers. In countries that do not normally produce agricultural surpluses or that have large pastoral or nomadic communities, the impact of food deficits on the nutritional status of civilians may be severe, particularly in sub-Saharan Africa. If adverse climatic factors intervene, as often happens in drought-prone countries such as Sudan, Somalia, Mozambique, and Ethiopia, the outcome may be catastrophic.

In some countries, such as Liberia and Somalia, governance has completely collapsed and the normal functions of a modern nation-state have ceased. When this degree of anarchy develops, the provision of effective humanitarian assistance becomes logistically difficult and extremely dangerous for relief personnel. Relief convoys are prey to bandits and local warlords, massive diversion of relief supplies occurs, and the implementation of sustainable, community-supported programs becomes virtually impossible. The proliferation and loose control of weapons in many countries have compounded the problem. In many developing nations, growth in military spending has far exceeded domestic economic growth rates. One study found that 29 of 134 surveyed countries spent a greater proportion of their national budget on the military than on health and education combined (2).

Mass migration and food shortages have been responsible for most deaths following civil conflicts in Africa and Asia. The most visible form of migration occurs when refugees cross international borders. *Refugees* are defined under several international conventions as persons who flee their country of origin through a well-founded fear of persecution for reasons of race, religion, social class, or political beliefs (4). The number of dependent refugees under the protection and care of the United Nations High Commissioner for Refugees (UNHCR) has steadily increased, from approximately 5 million in 1980 to almost 23 million in late 1994, and shows no sign of stabilizing (Table 20-1) (5). For example, more than 600,000 refugees fled Burur di for Rwanda, Tanzania, and Zaire during a two-week period in late October and early November 1993. During three days in mid-July 1994, an estimated 1 million Rwandan refugees fled into eastern Zaire, provoking the most serious refugee crisis in 20 years. In addition to those persons who meet the international definition of refugees, an estimated 25 million people have fled their homes for the same reasons as refugees but remain *internally displaced* in their countries of origin (Table 20-2). The reasons for the flight of refugees and internally displaced persons are generally the same: war, civil strife, and persecution. Food shortages and hunger are usually complicating factors rather than primary causes of population migration. For example, a severe drought in Somalia during 1992 exacerbated rather than initiated the flow of refugees fleeing the civil war across the border into Kenya.

Public Health Impacts: Historical Perspective

Focus on Somalia

Somalia provides a graphic example of a recent complex emergency. The country has a homogeneous ethnic population that shares a common language but is characterized

Table 20-1 Estimated Number of Refugees Arriving in Countries of Asylum, 1990–1994

Country of Origin	Country of Asylum	Year of Arrival	Estimated Population
Liberia	Guinea	1990	300,000
Liberia	Côte d'Ivoire	1990	200,000
Somalia	Djibouti	1990	30,000
Somalia	Ethiopia	1990–91	200,000
Sudan	Ethiopia	1990	40,000
Kuwait, Iraq	Jordan	1990	750,000
Mozambique	Malawi	1990–92	250,000
Azerbaijan	Armenia	1990–92	290,000
Armenia	Azerbaijan	1990–92	200,000
Iraq	Iran	1991	1,100,000
Iraq	Turkey	1991	450,000
Sierra Leone	Guinea	1991	185,000
Ethiopia	Sudan	1991	51,000
Somalia	Kenya	1991–92	320,000
Croatia, Bosnia-Herzegovina	Former Yugoslav republics	1991–93	750,000
Croatia, Bosnia	Western Europe	1991–93	512,000
Georgia	Russia	1991–93	140,000
Somalia	Yemen	1992	50,000
Ethiopia	Kenya	1992	80,000
Sudan	Kenya	1992	20,000
Mali, Niger	Algeria	1992	40,000
Myanmar	Bangladesh	1992	250,000
Bhutan	Nepal	1992	75,000
Mozambique	Zimbabwe	1992	60,000
Tajikstan	Afghanistan	1993	60,000
Togo	Ghana	1993	120,000
Togo	Benin	1993	120,000
Burundi	Tanzania	1993	350,000
Burundi	Rwanda	1993	370,000
Rwanda	Tanzania	1994	400,000
Rwanda	Burundi	1994	100,000
Rwanda	Zaire	1994	1,000,000

Source: US Committee for Refugees and United Nations High Commissioner for Refugees.

by distinct tribes or clans with long histories of rivalries and hostilities dating back centuries. After independence in the 1960s, Somalia had a brief experiment with democracy that ended with a military coup, followed by 24 years of rule by a military dictator. In January 1991, various clans and factions banded together to overthrow the government; the civil war took an estimated 14,000 combatant and civilian lives in Mogadishu alone (6). Ten months later, a second civil war erupted between the crumbling alliances of numerous rival clans and subclans. The country was plunged into chaos and fragmented into at least five ''mini-states.''

In the process, the country's economy, social and political institutions, and infrastructure were destroyed. By 1992, there were no electricity, running water, or sanitation

Table 20-2 Estimated Numbers of Internally
Displaced Persons, by Country, July 1994

Sudan	4,000,000
South Africa	4,000,000
Mozambique	2,000,000
Rwanda	2,000,000
Afghanistan	2,000,000
Angola	2,000,000
Bosnia and Herzegovina	1,300,000
Iraq	1,000,000
Liberia	1,000,000
Lebanon	700,000
Somalia	700,000
Zaire	700,000
Peru	600,000
Sri Lanka	600,000
Azerbaijan	600,000
Burundi	500,000
Ethiopia	500,000
Philippines	500,000
Russian Federation*	300,000
Cyprus	250,000
El Salvador	200,000
Myanmar	200,000
Sierra Leone	400,000
Croatia	350,000
Colombia	300,000
Kenya	300,000
Haiti	300,000
Cyprus	265,000
Iran	260,000
India	250,000
Georgia	250,000
Guatemala	200,000
Eritrea	200,000
Togo	150,000
Cambodia	95,000

*Displaced from Chechnya into neighboring regions of Russia.

Source: US Committee for Refugees and UNHCR.

facilities in most areas. Transportation systems and schools had been decimated; fuel
and spare parts were scarce. Agriculture and trade were disrupted as tens of thousands
of farmers fled the countryside to avoid the warfare. Irrigation systems and water wells
had been blown up. Many hospitals and clinics had been leveled or completely looted.
Medical personnel had been killed or exiled. There were no police, no jails, no courts,
and no law. Looting and banditry had become a way of life and a means of survival.
Superimposed on the warfare and chaos was a severe and prolonged drought, which
began when the rainy season failed in early 1991. Crops planted by the few remaining

farmers were devastated; the combination of drought and social disintegration resulted in catastrophic famine. There were massive population migrations of up to 900, 000 people out of war-torn rural and urban areas to refugee camps in Kenya, Ethiopia, Djibouti, and Yemen. Many of the refugees traveled on foot over hundreds of kilometers to cross the borders of Somalia seeking safety and food; many reportedly died of hunger.

The Land Mine Epidemic

In civil conflicts, antipersonnel land mines have been consistently used as a means of disrupting normal activities of farming and herding, accelerating the ex-migration of local populations, and preventing the use of land by opposing combatants and their civilian supporters. The health and economic impact of mines is great and unfortunately long-lasting. First, land mines can result in death, serious injury, and lifelong disability. Second, the disruption of agricultural activities creates conditions for famine and economic hardship. Third, since the potency of land mines remains even after the onset of peace, strategic areas and agricultural lands can remain unsettled and unused for many years, creating long-term economic losses and population disruption.

The United Nations estimates that at least 100 million antipersonnel mines currently lie in more than 60 countries worldwide (7). At least 1 million uncleared mines are thought to exist in each of the following countries: Afghanistan, Angola, Iraq, Kuwait, Cambodia, Mozambique, Bosnia, Somalia, Croatia, Sudan, and Ethiopia/Eritrea. The vast number of uncleared land mines in border areas of war-afflicted countries has been a major constraint to refugee repatriation programs planned by UNHCR. In addition, the presence of land mines has forced relief agencies in some areas to deliver food aid by air, adding significantly to the cost of humanitarian assistance programs. Aid workers themselves have been killed or injured by land mines in Somalia, Cambodia, Afghanistan, and Angola.

Public Health Consequences

Direct Impact

Injuries
Deaths, injuries, and disabilities caused by war-related violence are the most immediate public health consequences of complex emergencies on civilian populations. Fewer than 20% of casualties in World War I were civilians; the proportion rose to almost 50% by World War II and was estimated to be 80% during the 1980s (3, 8). A recent example of this trend can be seen in the vicious war in the former Yugoslavia. The goal of this war has been to create ''ethnically cleansed'' zones by intentionally killing, injuring, disabling, intimidating, and removing civilians from their homes. The exact death toll

may never be known; estimates in late 1994 ranged between 150,000 and 250,000. In the Bosnian capital Sarajevo alone, for example, there were 4,600 war-related deaths and 16,000 injuries during the first year of the war, and by the end of 1994 more than 10,000 Sarajevans had died (9). UNICEF estimates that 15,000 children have been killed and 35,000 injured throughout the former Yugoslavia since the onset of the war (10). In the central Bosnian province of Zenica, the proportion of all hospital admissions due to war-related trauma rose from 22% in April 1992 to a peak of 71% in December of the same year (9).

Land Mines

The public health impact of antipersonnel land mines on combatants and civilians has been well documented in a number of published reports, including the most comprehensive summary by the International Committee of the Red Cross (ICRC) (11). The number of deaths and injuries caused by land mines globally is not known; few population-based epidemiologic studies of the problem have been conducted. Nevertheless, the ICRC has estimated the following ratios of mine-related amputees to population in three countries: Cambodia, 1:236; Angola, 1:470; and northern Somalia, 1:1,000.

ICRC estimates that land mines have killed between 100,000 and 200,000 people in Afghanistan during the past ten years. The case-fatality rate (CFR) among civilians with land mine injuries is probably very high, because most incidents occur in remote areas with poor access to hospitals that have appropriate surgical and resuscitative facilities. A 1991 study by Physicians for Human Rights found that the average Cambodian land mine victim arrived at a hospital 12 hours after the initial injury (12). A 1994 study in Mozambique found that the cumulative incidence of land mine injuries and deaths in Sofala Province since 1980 was 20.2 per 1,000 residents (13). Since the beginning of the war in the early 1980s, an estimated 10, 000 Mozambicans have died because of land mine injuries (13).

Torture and Sexual Assault

In civil conflicts in Central and South America during the 1980s, the systematic torture of civilians was particularly common (2). Widespread rape of civilian women by military forces has been documented in recent conflicts in Bangladesh, Uganda, Myanmar, Somalia, and the former Yugoslavia (2, 14). The number of women raped by men on various sides of the conflict in Bosnia-Herzegovina is not known; however, investigations by Amnesty International and the European Commission concluded that tens of thousands of Muslim girls and women have been raped as part of a systematic campaign of terror (14, 15).

Indirect Impact

The indirect public health consequences of complex emergencies have resulted from food shortages and hunger, mass migration, and the destruction of public utilities and medical facilities. They have been most severe in developing countries where food reserves are already insufficient, hygienic conditions poor, and basic medical services inadequate. The most common outcome, especially in Africa, has been a high rate of severe undernutrition and death. While studies have demonstrated that undernourished individuals—particularly children—are at higher risk of mortality, the immediate cause of death is usually a communicable disease. Malnutrition causes an increased CFR in the most common childhood communicable diseases, such as measles, diarrheal diseases, and acute respiratory infections. Those at highest risk of premature mortality during complex emergencies are young children, women, and the elderly. The crowded and unsanitary conditions of refugee camps, the violence of forced migrations, and the adverse psychological effects of uncertainty and dependency contribute to the health problems experienced by affected communities.

Mortality

Mortality rates are the most specific indicators of the health status of emergency-affected populations. Mortality rates have been estimated from hospital and burial records, community-based surveys, and 24-hour burial-site surveillance. Among the many problems in estimating mortality under emergency conditions are recall bias in surveys, families' failure to report perinatal deaths, inaccurate denominators (overall population size, births, age-specific populations), and lack of standard reporting procedures. In general, however, bias tends to underestimate mortality rates, since deaths are usually under-reported or undercounted, and population size is often exaggerated (16). Most reports of emergency-related mortality have come from displaced populations. It is possible that mortality rates are lower in those communities in which people remain in their original villages and homes; however, comparison of mortality in displaced vs. non-displaced populations is problematic because displacement itself may reflect a more serious baseline situation. Nonetheless, comparisons between displaced and nondisplaced populations during complex emergencies show that in nearly all cases the displaced experience a significantly higher crude mortality rate (CMR) (16).

Since 1990, death rates among Sudanese refugees in Ethiopia (July 1990), newly arrived Somali refugees in Ethiopia (June 1991), Somali refugees in Kenya (January 1992), Bhutanese refugees in Nepal (May 1992), and newly arriving Mozambican refugees in Zimbabwe and Malawi (July 1992) have been elevated between 5 to 12 times the CMR in the country of origin (Table 20-3) (17). Death rates among Bhutanese and Mozambican refugees returned to normal levels within three months; however, improvement was more gradual among Sudanese and Somali refugees, who were housed in large camps in remote areas of Ethiopia and Kenya, where water supply was often inadequate and the logistics of food delivery were problematic. Between March and May 1991, the CMR among 400,000 Kurdish refugees on the Turkey-Iraq border was 18 times higher than the normal rate reported in Iraq (18).

Table 20-3 Estimated Crude Mortality Rates* (CMR) in Selected Refugee Populations, 1990–1994

Date	Host Country	Country of Origin	Baseline CMR	Refugee CMR
July 1990	Ethiopia	Sudan	1.7	6.9
June 1991	Ethiopia	Somalia	1.8	14.0
March–May 1991	Turkey/Iraq	Iraq	0.7	12.6
March 1992	Kenya	Somalia	1.8	22.2
March 1992	Nepal	Bhutan	1.3	9.0
June 1992	Bangladesh	Myanmar	0.8	4.8
June 1992	Malawi	Mozambique	1.5	3.5
August 1992	Zimbabwe	Mozambique	1.5	10.5
Dec 1993	Rwanda	Burundi	1.8	9.0
May 1994	Tanzania	Rwanda	1.8	1.8
June 1994	Burundi	Rwanda	1.8	15.0
July 1994	Zaire	Rwanda	1.8	102.0

*Deaths per 1,000 per month.

During the month following the massive influx of Rwandan refugees into the North Kivu region of eastern Zaire in July 1994, the CMR was estimated on the basis of surveillance data to have been between 60 and 100 per 1,000, depending on the population denominator used (*19*). Population surveys conducted in the same refugee camps estimated that between 7% and 9% of the refugees died during this period. The massacres in Rwanda in early 1994 and the high death rate among Rwandan refugees in eastern Zaire led to an unprecedented number of unaccompanied children among the refugee population. By mid-August, more than 12,000 such children, most of whom were probably orphans, had been registered in north Kivu, and death rates in the sites where they were placed reached as high as 100 per 10,000 per day.

The risk of death is usually highest during the period immediately after refugees arrive in the country of asylum, a phenomenon that reflects long periods of inadequate food and medical care. For example, during 1992, more than 150,000 Mozambicans fled to refugee camps in neighboring Zimbabwe and Malawi. During July and August 1992, the CMR among Mozambican refugees who had been in Chambuta camp for less than one month was 4 times the death rate of refugees who had been in the camp between 1 and 3 months, and 16 times the death rate normally reported for nondisplaced populations in Mozambique (Fig. 20-1) (*20*).

Political and security factors may obstruct the accurate documentation of death rates among internally displaced populations; however, a few situations have been well documented. In Mozambique (1983), Ethiopia (1984–85), and Sudan (1988), CMRs estimated by surveillance or population-based surveys of internally displaced persons ranged between 4 and 70 times the death rates in nondisplaced populations in the same country (Table 20-4) (*17*). Population surveys conducted in various parts of central and southern Somalia during the civil war found that the average CMRs among internally

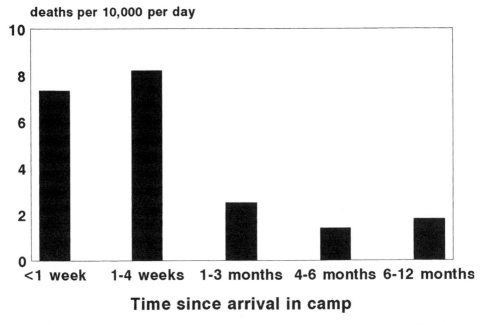

deaths per 10,000 per day

Time since arrival in camp

Figure 20-1. Crude death rate by time of stay in refugee camp. Mozambican refugees, Chambuta, Zimbabwe, July–August 1992.

displaced populations between April 1991 and January 1993 ranged from 7 to 25 times the baseline rate of 2 per 1,000 per month (*21*). Since 1990, increased fighting and food shortages in southern Sudan have led to displacement of large numbers of persons. Population surveys conducted in March 1993 at three sites found average monthly CMRs for each site during the previous year that were 6 to 12 times baseline rates (*22*).

Table 20-4 Mean Crude Monthly Mortality Rates* (CMR) for Internally Displaced Persons, 1990–1994

Country	Date	Baseline CMR	Internally Displaced Persons CMR
Liberia	Jan–Dec 1990	1.2	7.1
Iraq	March–May 1991	0.7	12.6
Somalia (Merca)	Apr 1991–March 1992	2.0	13.8
Somalia (Baidoa)	Apr– Nov 1992	2.0	50.7
Somalia (Afgoi)	Apr–Dec 1992	2.0	16.5
Sudan (Ayod)	Apr 1992–March 1993	1.6	23.0
Sudan (Akon)	Apr 1992–March 1993	1.6	13.7
Bosnia (Zepa)	Apr 1992–March 1993	0.8	3.0
Bosnia (Sarajevo)	Apr 1993	0.8	2.9

*Deaths per 1,000 per month

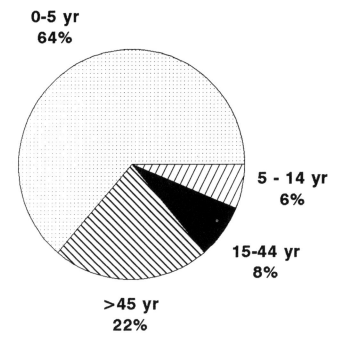

Figure 20-2. Deaths by age, Kurdish refugees, March 29–May 24, 1991, Turkey-Iraq border.

Most deaths in refugee populations have occurred among children less than 5 years of age; for example, 64% of deaths among Kurdish refugees on the Turkish border occurred in the 17% of the population less than 5 years of age (Fig. 20-2) (*22*). Although absolute death rates are highest in infants, the *relative* increase in mortality during emergencies may be highest in children 1–12 years of age (*23*). In the Rwandan refugee camps of eastern Zaire, however, under-5 death rates were no higher than other age-specific rates during the first month after the influx, because most deaths in this population were caused by cholera, which equally affects all age groups (*19*). Sex-specific mortality analyses are not often performed; however, among Burmese refugees in Bangladesh, the death rate among girls was 2–4 times the rate for boys (*17*). Since sex-specific mortality data is among the easiest to collect, it should be collected by more agencies in the future.

Factors Influencing Morbidity and Mortality

Cause-Specific Mortality
The major reported causes of death among refugees and displaced populations have been malnutrition, diarrheal diseases, measles, acute respiratory infections, and malaria (*16*). These diseases consistently account for 60%–95% of all reported causes of death in these populations. Measles epidemics caused high death rates among refugees during

the 1980s. During a 3-month period of 1985, for example, more than 2,000 measles-associated deaths were documented in one refugee camp in eastern Sudan. This represented a case fatality rate (CFR) based on reported cases of 30% (*24*). Since 1990, measles outbreaks have been reported among new refugees in camps in Nepal, Zimbabwe, and Malawi, contributing to high death rates in those camps. However, refugee camps in Ethiopia, Turkey, Tanzania, and Zaire have been spared measles epidemics because high measles vaccination coverage rates were achieved.

Epidemics of severe diarrheal disease have been increasingly common; cholera epidemics have occurred in refugee camps in Malawi, Zimbabwe, Swaziland, Nepal, Bangladesh, Turkey, Afghanistan, Burundi, and Zaire (*17*). Cholera CFRs in refugee camps have ranged between 3% and 30%. In addition, outbreaks of dysentery caused by *Shigella dysenteriae* type I have been reported since 1991 in Malawi, Nepal, Kenya, Bangladesh, Burundi, Angola, Rwanda, Tanzania, and Zaire (*17, 19, 25*). Dysentery CFRs have been as high as 10% among young children and the elderly. In eastern Zaire, between 40,000 and 45,000 Rwandan refugees may have died from cholera or dysentery (80% to 90% of all deaths) in July–August 1994 (*19*).

Malnutrition

Acute protein-energy malnutrition has often been a major contributing factor to high death rates from communicable diseases among refugees and internally displaced persons. The close correlation between malnutrition prevalence and crude mortality during a relief operation for Somali refugees in eastern Ethiopia in 1988–89 is clearly demonstrated in Figure 20-3. Malnutrition prevalence was estimated by serial cross-sectional cluster sample surveys of children less than 5 years of age, and monthly CMRs were estimated retrospectively by a population-based survey in August 1989 (*26*). During the period of high malnutrition prevalence and high mortality (March through May 1989), food rations provided an average of approximately 1,400 kilocalories per person per day instead of the recommended minimum of 1,900 kilocalories per person per day (*27*).

In stable developing countries not affected by emergencies, the prevalence of acute malnutrition among children less than 5 years of age in stable, non-emergency-affected developing countries is normally less than 5% (*16*). In Rwandan refugee camps in eastern Zaire, one month after the influx, the prevalence of acute malnutrition was between 18% and 23%. Surveys found that children living in households headed by single women and children with a history of recent dysentery were at significantly higher risk of malnutrition than other refugee children (*19*). The highest malnutrition rates have been reported among internally displaced populations in Somalia and southern Sudan. In Somalia, acute malnutrition prevalence rates in displaced children ranged between 47% and 75% during 1992 (*21*). In March 1993, population surveys of internally displaced communities in southern Sudan found prevalences as high as 81% (*22*). High acute malnutrition prevalence has not always been associated with food shortages.

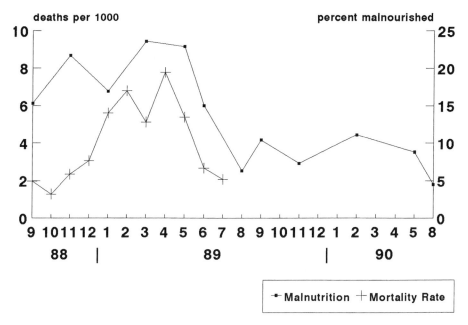

Figure 20-3. Acute malnutrition prevalence (percent weight/height <80% median) in children less than 5 years of age and crude mortality rates (deaths per 1,000 per month), in the Hartisheik A Camp, eastern Ethiopia, 1988–1990.

For example, in 1991, the malnutrition prevalence among Kurdish refugee children 12–23 months of age was 13.5% (*28*). This elevated rate was associated with the high incidence of diarrhea in this age group while the children were in mountain camps where water and sanitation were inadequate.

In addition, a high incidence of micronutrient-deficiency diseases has been reported in many refugee camps, especially in Africa (*29*). The typical rations provided in large-scale relief operations lack vitamin A, putting these populations at high risk. In addition, those communicable diseases that are highly incident in refugee camps, measles and diarrhea, are known to deplete vitamin A stores rapidly. Consequently, young refugee and displaced children are at high risk of developing vitamin A deficiency. In 1990, more than 18,000 cases of pellagra, caused by food rations deficient in niacin, were reported among Mozambican refugees in Malawi (*30*). Numerous outbreaks of scurvy (vitamin C deficiency) were documented in refugee camps in Somalia, Ethiopia, and Sudan between 1982 and 1991 (*31*). The prevalence of scurvy was highly associated with the period of residence in camps, a reflection of the time exposed to rations lacking in vitamin C; higher prevalence rates have been identified among women and the elderly. Iron-deficiency anemia has been reported in many refugee populations, affecting mainly women of childbearing age and young children.

Psychological Trauma

Increases in morbidity, mortality, and malnutrition are the most obvious consequences of population displacement; however, there have been symptoms of severe psychological trauma among refugees, expressed as anxiety, fear, and aggression in the early phase of flight from their homes and progressing to apathy, dependency, and depression as their displaced status becomes chronic (*32, 33*). The psychological impact of complex emergencies on children may be especially severe. UNICEF surveys in Sarajevo have found that 30% of children have lost a family member, 40% have been shot at by snipers, 19% have witnessed a massacre, and 72% have seen their homes shelled or attacked (*10*). The outcome of this childhood stress on the future mental health of Bosnians may not be known for many years.

Impact of Damaged Public Utilities

Recent violent conflicts in urban settings have caused extensive damage to water, electricity, sewage, and heating systems, with potentially important public health implications. In Sarajevo, the capital, and other large cities in Bosnia-Herzegovina, municipal water supplies were destroyed by shelling; similar breakdowns in sewage systems and cross-contamination of piped water supplies led to widespread contamination of drinking water. These problems were compounded by the lack of electricity and diesel fuel needed to run generators. In the summer of 1993, Sarajevans had on average only 5 liters of water per person per day, compared with the minimum of 15–20 liters recommended by WHO. Although widespread epidemics of diarrheal disease were avoided, local health department data showed that the incidence of communicable diseases had increased significantly since the beginning of the war. For example, the incidence of hepatitis A increased 6-fold in Sarajevo, 12-fold in Zenica, and 4-fold in Tuzla between 1991 and 1993. The incidence of dysentery caused by *Shigella sp* increased 12-fold and 17-fold in Sarajevo and Zenica, respectively, during the same period (*9*).

Impact of Disrupted Health Services

The breakdown of routine health services may contribute heavily to the public health impact of complex emergencies. In Bosnia-Herzegovina, where changes in morbidity and mortality due to communicable diseases and malnutrition have been relatively moderate, the impact of disruption of medical services has been well documented. Many essential prevention programs have collapsed because health services have been diverted toward treating the war injured. In addition, the conflict has prevented much of the population from reaching health facilities; furthermore, many of those facilities have been destroyed or heavily damaged. There have been numerous reports of intentionally destroyed medical facilities, including the heavily damaged Kosevo General Hospital in Sarajevo. Consequently, antenatal care and child immunization programs have been severely curtailed. Only between 22% and 34% of children in Sarajevo, Zenica, Bihac, and Tuzla have been immunized against measles; an average of only 49% against polio; and 55% against diphtheria and whooping cough (9). Outbreaks of these diseases have not yet been reported; they are inevitable, however, if vaccination rates remain low. The incidence of new cases of tuberculosis has reportedly been rising due to the shortage of appropriate drugs and the difficulty of access by patients to treatment facilities. Shortages of drugs such as insulin, laboratory reagents to test blood for the human immunodeficiency virus, and kidney-dialysis filters have severely affected the quality of medical care.

Public health surveillance data indicate serious deterioration in child health status; for example, perinatal mortality increased in Sarajevo from 16 deaths per 1,000 live births in 1991 to 27 per 1,000 during the first four months of 1993. The rate of premature births increased from 5.3% to 12.9%, the stillbirth rate increased from 7.5 per 1,000 to 12.3 per 1,000, and the average birth weight decreased from 3,700 gm to 3,000 gm during the same period (9). There has also been a dramatic increase in spontaneous and therapeutic abortions, which by mid-1993 were twice as numerous as births at the Kosevo Hospital in Sarajevo. These problems can be directly linked to the deterioration in quality of antenatal and perinatal care in the city.

Prevention, Preparedness, and Response

The frequency and degree of complexity of humanitarian emergencies has been increasing in the past five years; armed conflict is the common risk factor in each situation. Genocide in Rwanda and its sequelae in neighboring countries dominated the news during 1994, and violent conflicts continue almost unabated in Angola, Bosnia-Herzegovina, Afghanistan, Kashmir, Sri Lanka, Azerbaijan, Georgia, Tajikistan, and the breakaway Russian republic of Chechnya. Meanwhile, several African countries are well on the path to total collapse; these include Zaire, Togo, Burundi, Algeria, and—perhaps less far down the path—Nigeria and Kenya. Unless decisive steps are taken by the international community in three areas—prevention, preparedness, and response—complex emergencies will continue to take a heavy toll on civilian populations.

Prevention

The most urgent need is to develop more effective diplomatic and political mechanisms that might resolve conflicts early in their evolution—prior to the stage when food shortages occur, health services collapse, populations migrate, and significant adverse public health outcomes emerge. One of the major obstacles is the almost sacred notion of national sovereignty embodied in the United Nations Charter. The prohibition against the ''threat or use of force'' on the territory of independent sovereign member states of the United Nations has forced the international community to stand by and watch extreme examples of human rights abuses until, in certain cases, a threshold of tolerance has been crossed and public indignation has demanded action, as in the case of Somalia. By the time such action is taken, the conflict has often advanced to a stage where any involvement by outside forces is perceived by belligerents as taking sides. This perception may result in the entanglement of the international community in the conflict itself, as occurred in Somalia. Cautious, neutral, but determined diplomacy of the kind the Atlanta-based Carter Center practiced in Ethiopia, Sudan, Haiti, and Bosnia-Herzegovina might serve as a model for future conflict-resolution efforts. Epidemiologists and behavioral scientists might play a role in this process by systematically studying the dynamics and characteristic behaviors that sustain conflict situations and by seeking to identify measures that might reduce the level of tension between opposing sides.

Preparedness

Early Detection
Emergency-detection activities in the form of early-warning systems and risk mapping have existed for some time; however, these systems have tended to focus on monitoring natural rather than man-made hazards. For example, the Famine Early Warning System (FEWS) funded by the U.S. Agency for International Development routinely monitors crop yields, food availability, staple cereal prices, rainfall, and household income in a number of African countries, and also conducts periodic "vulnerability assessments." FEWS data is published and disseminated widely in timely bulletins and has proven useful in predicting natural disasters, such as the drought throughout southern Africa in 1992. Nevertheless, systems like FEWS have not developed early indicators related to human rights abuses, ethnic conflict, political instability, and migration. Other groups, such as Africa Watch, Physicians for Human Rights, Amnesty International, and African Rights have conducted assessments of vulnerability in countries such as Burundi relatively early in the evolution of civil conflict. The problem with such assessments is that the results are often ignored by the governments of wealthy donor nations if the situations are perceived not to be in their security interests. For example, early in 1992, several excellent reports on the deteriorating situation in Somalia were largely ignored by the international community (6, 34). In addition to the work they do with population surveys that measure the effects of complex emergencies (i.e., late indicators such as mortality rates and malnutrition prevalence), epidemiologists may be able to play an important role in developing and field-testing the sensitivity and specificity of a broad range of early-warning indicators that will predict emerging unstable situations.

Contingency Planning
The inability of the world to promptly address the explosive epidemic of cholera among Rwandan refugees in eastern Zaire, in July 1994 underscored the lack of emergency preparedness planning at a global level. This epidemic highlighted the inadequate reserves of essential medical supplies and equipment for establishing and distributing safe

water, and revealed a lack of technical consensus on the most appropriate interventions. Agencies that did have the appropriate skills and experience, such as Oxfam and MSF, lacked the needed resources, and those agencies with the resources and logistics, such as the U.S. military, lacked technical experience in emergency relief. Preparedness planning for complex emergencies needs to take place both at a coordinated international level and at the individual country level. The creation of a single, global "superagency" to respond to all emergencies worldwide is unlikely at this time and, many would say, undesirable; however, donor nations would be wise to invest funds in strengthening the existing network of experienced relief organizations. These agencies need resources to implement early-warning systems, maintain technical expertise, train personnel, build reserves of relief supplies, and develop their logistic capacity. At the country level, all health-development programs should have an emergency-preparedness component that should include the establishment of standard public health policies (e.g., immunization and management of epidemics), treatment protocols, staff training, and the maintenance of reserves of essential drugs and vaccines for use in disasters.

Personnel Training

It has been clear from observations during recent emergency relief programs that there is considerable variation in the expertise and effectiveness of relief workers, both expatriate and local, particularly in the health sector. The frontline relief workers in complex emergencies are often volunteers recruited by nongovernmental organizations (NGOs) who sometimes lack specific training and experience in emergency relief. They require knowledge and practical experience in a broad range of subjects, including food and nutrition, water and sanitation, disease surveillance, immunization, communicable-disease control, epidemic management, and maternal and child health care. They should be able to conduct rapid public health needs assessments, establish priorities, work closely with affected communities, train local workers, coordinate with a complex array of relief organizations, monitor and evaluate the impact of their activities, and efficiently manage scarce resources. In addition, they need to function effectively in an often hostile and dangerous environment; such skills are specific to emergencies and are not necessarily present in the average graduate of a Western medical or nursing school. Therefore, relief agencies need to allocate more resources to relevant training and orientation of their staff, as well as provide adequate support in the field. Indigenous health workers in emergency-prone countries, while often familiar with the management of common endemic diseases, also need training in the particular skills required to work effectively under emergency conditions.

Emergency Response

Overview

In the complicated, dangerous, and unpredictable environment of a complex emergency, there can be no single, perfect formula for mounting an effective and appropriate response. Every situation is unique in terms of the political, environmental, cultural, economic, and public health context; what works in Angola may not work in Rwanda or Bosnia. Nevertheless, there are principles and practices that are relevant to every emergency; the paramount priority is to ensure the protection and safety of the affected population. These principles and practices include the following: (1) intervene early; (2) support, not undermine, community coping strategies; (3) try to prevent communities from migrating; (4) avoid establishing large and crowded camps; (5) collect, analyze, and disseminate useful, accurate, and timely information; (6) ensure that the allocation of resources does not further divide communities; (7) focus on disease prevention; (8) work through existing structures and institutions, rather than constructing new and poorly sustainable facilities; (9) insist that women control the distribution of relief supplies (this will ensure more equitable apportionment); (10) ensure open communication and coordination among agencies.

Framework

The United Nations has created the Department of Humanitarian Affairs (DHA) to mobilize and coordinate international disaster preparedness and response. However, in the event of a complex emergency, other U.N. agencies with more operational resources are usually designated lead relief agencies. For example, when refugees cross international borders, the U.N. High Commission for Refugees (UNHCR) is automatically this lead agency. In the case of an emergency involving internally displaced persons or conflict-affected communities that have not migrated, other agencies may be designated—for example, UNICEF in Somalia and the World Food Programme in Angola. In the former Yugoslavia, UNHCR has been designated the lead relief agency in all republics. Normally, the government of the emergency-affected country would have the authority to coordinate and implement emergency relief programs; however, in recent situations, such as Somalia, Rwanda, and Liberia, where governments have totally collapsed, the U.N. has taken on this role. In other settings, such as southern Sudan and Bosnia-Herzegovina, where governments have been major parties to the conflict and have obstructed international relief efforts, the U.N. has often acted unilaterally to ensure the effective delivery of relief aid.

The International Committee of the Red Cross (ICRC) has a unique role in responding to conflict situations. Under its mandate, as described by the Geneva Conventions, the ICRC negotiates with all sides of a conflict in order to gain access to civilian populations where it provides protection and assistance. The ICRC maintains strict neutrality and will rarely make public criticisms of warring parties; ICRC delegates are usually Swiss citizens, although the agency's technicians may be recruited among other nationalities. While the ICRC relies on the cooperation of all sides, there have been a number of recent instances where access to conflict zones has been denied, even by governments of countries that are signatories of the Geneva Conventions. In addition to ICRC, the International Federation of Red Cross and Red Crescent Societies coordinates the activities of its member national societies, which often play a key role in emergency relief.

There exists a vast array of nongovernmental organizations (NGOs), both indigenous and expatriate. Certain international NGOs, with branches in many countries, have developed considerable technical and management expertise in the delivery of emergency assistance. Some of the more experienced NGOs include Médecins sans Frontières (Doctors without Borders), OXFAM, Save the Children, the International Rescue Committee, CARE, World Vision, and Caritas (or Catholic Relief Services in the U.S.). There are many thousands of NGOs worldwide, some of them small but highly effective, while others are large and wealthy, but less predictable in their level of technical expertise. An encouraging trend has been the emergence of highly motivated and competent NGOs based in developing countries, including Bangladesh, India, Thailand, and the Philippines. Their role in providing emergency-relief assistance may grow in the coming years.

Military Forces
Since the end of the cold war, military forces of various nations have played an increasingly visible role in providing emergency humanitarian assistance. The first such major relief effort took place in Turkey and northern Iraq at the end of the Gulf War in 1991 when the allied military forces led the relief effort for Kurdish refugees. In addition to establishing a secure zone for Kurds in northern Iraq, military units from the United States, France, the United Kingdom, the Netherlands, and other nations participated in the actual transport and distribution of relief supplies to refugees in mountain camps. Their role during this operation was facilitated by the ready availability of military transport and resources left over from the military operation in Iraq and Kuwait and by the presence of large U.S. military Civil Affairs units whose expertise in various technical and management areas was highly relevant to the needs of refugees (*35*). Since that time, military forces have played a prominent role in relief operations in Somalia, the former Yugoslavia, Rwanda, and Haiti.

The role of the military in the humanitarian assistance program in northern Iraq stands out as a relative success; however, inherent in any involvement by the military in humanitarian relief is the danger of being drawn into the conflict. This problem was graphically illustrated in Somalia, where military relief efforts ended in failure when various armed factions perceived the military forces under U.N. command to have taken sides. The resulting attacks on the U.N. forces and armed reprisals eventually led to the withdrawal of the U.N. from the country (*36*). The involvement of the military is often ambiguous, confusing the various tasks of peacekeeping, peace-enforcing, and providing relief. No one would doubt the logistical advantage of the military; however, this advantage is not always matched with appropriate experience in the technical aspects of a relief operation. Furthermore, military assistance is expensive; for example, in the Rwandan camps of eastern Zaire, each U.S. soldier involved in providing clean water to the refugees was accompanied by a squad of armed soldiers for his protection. Finally, because military deployment depends on political decisions by national governments, it cannot always be integrated into disaster-preparedness planning.

Elements of Emergency Response

Prompt resolution of the conflict that has led to an emergency situation is the first response priority; at the very least, civilian populations should be protected from the violence and deprivation caused by war. The international community has so far achieved few successes in this area. In the absence of conflict resolution, those communities that are totally dependent on external aid for their survival, because they have either been displaced from their homes or are living under a state of siege, must be provided the basic minimum resources necessary to maintain health and well-being. The provision of adequate food, clean water, shelter, sanitation, and warmth will prevent the most severe public health consequences of complex emergencies. The following measures represent the basic elements of emergency response:

- Provide food rations containing adequate calories, protein, and essential micronutrients. General food rations should contain at least 1,900 kilocalories of energy per person per day (more in cold climates), as well as the minimum daily allowances of protein and micronutrients recommended by the United Nations (*27*). Food should be distributed regularly to family units, taking care that socially vulnerable groups such as female-headed households, unaccompanied minors, and the elderly receive their fair share. In addition, adequate cooking fuel, utensils, and facilities to grind whole-grain cereals need to be distributed. The evidence that vitamin A deficiency is associated with increased childhood mortality and disabling blindness is now so convincing that supplements of Vitamin A should be provided routinely to all refugee children under 5 years of age at first contact and every 3–6 months thereafter (*37*).

  Although *supplementary feeding* programs are often popular with relief agencies, their effectiveness in refugee camps in the absence of adequate general rations has been questioned (*38*). When the family ration is insufficient to provide adequate energy to all family members, then the supplementary ration (usually 400–600 kilocalories per day) may be the only food source for young children. This is not enough to maintain nutrition. If adequate general rations are provided, children who are clinically undernourished may benefit from daily food supplements, but only if efforts are made to identify them in the community and to ensure their attendance at feeding centers. Therapeutic feeding programs should be established to provide total nutritional rehabilitation of severely malnourished children (*39*).

- Provide clean water in sufficient quantity and adequate sanitation facilities. UNHCR recommends that a minimum of 15 liters of clean water be provided per person per day for domestic needs— cooking, drinking, and bathing (*40*). In general, ensuring access to adequate quantities of relatively clean water is probably more effective in preventing diarrheal disease, especially bacterial dysentery, than providing small quantities of pure microbe-free water. When refugee camps are unavoidable, the proximity to safe water sources needs to be recognized as the most important criterion for site selection. Adequate sanitation is an essential component of diarrheal disease prevention. While the eventual goal of sanitation programs should be the construction of one latrine per family, interim measures may include the designation of separate defecation areas. For maximal impact, these measures should be complemented by community hygiene education and regular distribution of soap.

- Implement appropriate interventions for the prevention of specific communicable diseases. Immunization of children against measles is probably the single most important (and cost-effective) preventive measure in emergency-affected populations, particularly those housed in camps. Since infants as young as 6 months of age frequently contract measles in refugee-camp outbreaks and are at greater risk of dying due to impaired nutrition, it is recommended that measles-immunization programs in emergency settings target all children between the ages of 6 months and 12 years (41). When undernutrition affects the entire population, and when previous exposure to measles is unknown, it may be prudent to extend the coverage to children 6–14 years of age. Immunization programs should eventually include all antigens recommended by WHO's Expanded Programme on Immunization. Malaria control in refugee camps is more difficult. Under the transient circumstances that characterize most refugee camps, vector-control techniques have generally been impractical and expensive. Prompt identification and treatment of symptomatic individuals is a more effective measure to reduce malaria mortality, although the spread of chloroquine resistance means that effective case management will become more expensive and technically more challenging in the future.
- Institute appropriate curative programs with adequate population coverage. An essential drug list and standardized treatment protocols are necessary elements of a curative program. It is not necessary to develop totally new guidelines in each refugee situation: several excellent manuals already exist, from which guidelines can be adapted to suit local conditions (42, 43). WHO has also developed guidelines for the clinical management of dehydration from diarrhea and for acute respiratory infections; these can be used by trained community health workers (CHWs) (44, 45). Some relief programs, such as those in Somalia, Sudan, and Malawi, have successfully trained large numbers of refugees as CHWs to detect cases of diarrhea and acute respiratory infections, provide primary treatment, and refer severely ill patients to a clinic, thereby increasing coverage by health services and diminishing reliance on expatriate workers.
- Establish a health information system. A surveillance system is an essential part of the relief program and should be established immediately (16). Only information of public health importance should be collected. Mortality surveillance is critical and may require creative methods such as 24-hour graveyard surveillance. In addition, surveillance of nutritional status and important epidemic diseases such as measles, cholera, and dysentery should be instituted. Information on program cov-

erage and effectiveness should also be systematically collected; such data should include the average quantity of food rations distributed, per capita clean water available, ratio of families to latrines, immunization coverage, and supplementary feeding program attendance. Information collected by the surveillance system needs to be analyzed and widely disseminated in timely bulletins.

Summary

Epidemiologic data have identified those health problems that recurrently cause most deaths and severe morbidity in emergency settings and have shown that young children and women are most at risk of these adverse outcomes. Relief programs need to focus more clearly on these public health problems—measles, diarrheal diseases, malnutrition, malaria, and acute respiratory infections—especially among women and young children. In addition, new solutions to recurring problems need to be explored. Emergencies will continue to occur, and refugees will continue to seek refuge, in remote regions of the world where the provision of basic needs requires innovative approaches. There is a need for systematic operational and evaluation research in certain areas of nutrition, water supply, and disease control.

Relief-management decisions need to be based on sound technical information, and assistance programs need to be systematically evaluated, not merely for their quantity and content, but for their impact and effectiveness. Responsibilities for technical coordination and implementation of relief programs should increasingly be shared with proven, competent, and experienced NGOs. Greater resources need to be allocated to personnel training, emergency-preparedness planning, and the maintenance of regional reserves of essential relief supplies. These activities need to include government and nongovernment agencies in developing countries where emergencies are likely to occur. The increasingly favored option of military intervention often reflects the lack of attention given to conflicts in the early stages of their evolution. Determined diplomacy applied early in a conflict might preclude the need for later military toughness with all its associated problems, such as those observed recently in Somalia. Ironically, well-intentioned humanitarian programs in Bosnia (e.g., involvement of UN peacekeepers) have inadvertently created more obstacles to more effective initiatives to stop the violence and may actually prolong the conflict. This is due to the fear by those responsible for relief programs that if UN personnel intervene forcefully to stop or prevent human rights abuses witnessed by them, armed retaliation might result, causing the complete disruption of the humanitarian relief program. The public health community has an important role in developing sensitive and accurate early-warning systems, carefully documenting the public health consequences of emergencies, and designing effective, focused relief programs. Finally, public health professionals may act as credible advocates for prompt humanitarian responses at the highest levels of political decision-making.

References

1. Cobey J, Flanigin A, Foege W. Effective humanitarian Aid: our only hope for intervention in civil war. *JAMA* 1993;270:632–634.
2. Zwi A, Ugalde A. Political violence in the third world: a public health issue. *Health Policy and Planning* 1991;6:203–217.
3. United Nations Children's Fund. *The state of the world's children, 1994*. New York: United Nations Children's Fund, 1994.
4. United Nations High Commissioner for Refugees. *Convention and protocol relating to the status of refugees*. HCR/INF/29/Rev 3. Geneva, Switzerland: United Nations High Commissioner for Refugees, 1992.
5. U.S. Committee for Refugees. *World refugee survey, 1994*. Washington, D.C.: U.S. Committee for Refugees.
6. Physicians for Human Rights and Africa Watch. *No mercy in Mogadishu*. New York: Africa Watch, 1992.
7. Human Rights Watch and Physicians for Human Rights. *Landmines: a deadly legacy*. New York: Africa Watch, 1993.
8. Garfield R, Neugut A. Epidemiologic analysis of warfare: an historical review. *JAMA* 1991; 266:688–692.
9. Centers for Disease Control and Prevention. Status of public health—Bosnia and Herzegovina, August–September 1993. *MMWR* 1993;42:973, 979–982.
10. United Nations Childrens Fund. *A Programme of hope for Sarajevo*. New York: United Nations Childrens Fund, 1993.
11. Coupland RM, Korver A. Injuries from antipersonnel mines: the experience of the International Committee of the Red Cross. *Br Med J* 1991;304:1509–1512.
12. Stover E, McGrath R. *Land mines in Cambodia—The coward's war*. Boston: Physicians for Human Rights, 1991.
13. Physicians for Human Rights & Africa Watch. *Landmines in Mozambique*. New York: Africa Watch, 1994.
14. Swiss S, Giller J. Rape as a Crime of War. *JAMA* 1993:270:612–615.
15. Toole M, Galson S, Brady W. Are war and public health compatible? *Lancet* 1993;341:935–938.
16. Centers for Disease Control and Prevention. Famine-affected, refugee, and displaced populations: recommendations for public health issues. *MMWR* 1992;41(RR-13):1–76.
17. Toole M, Waldman R. Refugees and displaced persons: war, hunger, and public health. *JAMA* 1993;270:600–605.
18. Centers for Disease Control. Public health consequences of acute displacement of Iraqi citizens: March–May 1991. *MMWR* 1991;40:443–446.
19. Goma Epidemiology Group. Public health impact of Rwandan refugee crisis. What happened in Goma, Zaire, in July 1994? *Lancet* 1995;345:339–343.
20. Centers for Disease Control and Prevention. Mortality among newly arrived Mozambican refugees, Zimbabwe and Malawi, 1992. *MMWR* 1993;42:468–469,475–477.
21. Boss LP, Toole MJ, Yip R. Assessments of mortality, morbidity, and nutritional status in Somalia during the 1991–1992 famine. *JAMA* 1994;272:371–376.
22. Centers for Disease Control and Prevention. Nutrition and mortality assessment—southern Sudan, March 1993. *MMWR* 1993;42:304–308.
23. de Waal A. Famine mortality: a case study of Darfur, Sudan, 1984–85. *Population Studies* 1989;43:5–24.
24. Shears P, Berry AM, Murphy R, Nabil MA. Epidemiologic assessment of the health and

nutrition of Ethiopian refugees in emergency camps in Sudan. *Br Med J* 1987;295:314–318.

25. Centers for Disease Control and Prevention. Health status of displaced persons following civil war— Burundi, December 1993–January 1994. *MMWR* 1994;43:701–703.

26. Toole MJ, Bhatia R. A case study of Somali refugees in Hartisheik A camp, eastern Ethiopia: health and nutrition profile, July 1988–June 1989. *Journal of Refugee Studies* 1992;5:313–326.

27. United Nations Administrative Committee for Coordination, Sub-Committee for Coordination, Sub-Committee on Nutrition (ACC/SCN). *Improving nutrition in refugees and displaced persons in Africa. Report of a workshop in Machakos, Kenya, December 1994.* Geneva: ACC/SCN, 1995.

28. Yip R, Sharp TW. Acute malnutrition and high childhood mortality related to diarrhea. *JAMA* 1993;270:587–590.

29. Toole MJ. Micronutrient deficiency diseases in refugee populations. *Lancet* 1992;333;1214–1216.

30. Centers for Disease Control and Prevention. Outbreak of pellagra among Mozambican refugees— Malawi, 1990. *MMWR* 1991;40:209–213.

31. Desenclos JC, Berry AM, Padt R, Farah B, Segala C, Nabil AM. Epidemiologic patterns of scurvy among Ethiopian refugees. *Bull World Health Organ* 1989;67:309–316.

32. Kunz EF. The refugee in flight: kinetic models and forms of displacement. *International Migration Review* 1973;7(3).

33. Hansen A. Once the running stops: assimilation of Angolan refugees into Zambian border villages. *Disasters* 1979;3:369–374.

34. Manoncourt S, Doppler B, Enten F, *et al.* Public health consequences of civil war in Somalia, April 1992. *Lancet* 1992;340:176–177.

35. Sharp TW, Yip R, Malone JD. US military forces and emergency international humanitarian assistance. *JAMA* 1994;272:386–390.

36. Toole MJ. Military role in humanitarian relief in Somalia. *Lancet* 1993;342:190–191.

37. Nieburg P, Waldman RJ, Leavell R, *et al.* Vitamin A supplementation for refugees and famine victims. *Bull World Health Organ* 1988;66:689–697.

38. Gibb C. A review of feeding programmes in refugee reception centres in Eastern Sudan, October 1985. *Disasters* 1986;10:17–24.

39. Dick B. Supplementary feeding for refugees and other displaced communities—questioning current orthodoxy. *Disasters* 1986;10:53–64.

40. United Nations High Commissioner for Refugees. *Water manual for refugee situations.* Geneva: United Nations High Commissioner for Refugees, 1992.

41. Toole MJ, Steketee RW, Waldman RJ, Nieburg P. Measles prevention and control in emergency settings. *Bull World Health Organ* 1989;67(4):381–388.

42. Desenclos JC, editor. *Clinical guidelines. Diagnostic and treatment manual*, 2nd ed. Paris (France): Médecins Sans Frontières, 1992.

43. Mears C, Chowdhury S, editors. *Health care for refugees and displaced people.* Oxford, U.K.: Oxfam, 1994.

44. World Health Organization. *The treatment of acute diarrhea.* WHO/CDD/SER/80.2. Rev. 1. Geneva, Switzerland: World Health Organization, 1984.

45. World Health Organization and UNICEF. *Basic principles for control of acute respiratory infections in children in developing countries.* Geneva, Switzerland: World Health Organization, 1986.

Index